Clinical Dec

A Case Study Approach

• • • • • • • • • • • •

Clinical Decision Making

A Case Study Approach

SECOND EDITION

• • • • • • • • • • • • • • •

Denise L. Robinson, PhD, RN, FNP

Professor
Director, MSN Program
Northern Kentucky University
Highland Heights, Kentucky

Family Nurse Practitioner
Northern Kentucky Family Health Centers, Inc.
Covington, Kentucky

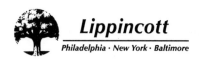
Lippincott
Philadelphia · New York · Baltimore

Acquisitions Editor: Lisa Stead
Managing Editor/Development: Karin McAndrews
Project Editor: Nicole Walz
Senior Production Manager: Helen Ewan
Managing Editor/Production: Barbara Ryalls
Art Director: Carolyn O'Brien
Cover Design: BJ Crim
Manufacturing Manager: William Alberti
Indexer: Gaye Taralla
Compositor: Peirce Graphic Services, Inc.
Printer: R. R. Donnelley & Sons—Crawfordsville

2nd Edition

9 8 7 6 5 4 3 2 1

Library of Congress Cataloging-in-Publication Data
Robinson, Denise L.
  Clinical decision making : a case study approach/Denise L. Robinson.—2nd ed.
    p. ; cm.
  Rev. ed. of: Clinical decision making for nurse practitioners. c1998.
  Includes bibliographical references and index.
  ISBN 0-7817-2994-7 (alk. paper)
  1. Nursing—Case studies. 2. Nursing—Decision making. 3. Clinical competence.
4. Nursing—Problems, exercises, etc. I. Robinson, Denise L. Clinical decision making for nurse practitioners. II. Title.
  [DNLM: 1. Nursing Diagnosis—Case Report. 2. Nursing Diagnosis—Examination Questions. 3. Clinical Medicine—Case Report. 4. Clinical Medicine—Examination Questions. 7. Diagnosis, Differential—Case Report. 8. Diagnosis, Differential—Examination Questions. 9. Nurse Practitioners—Case Report. 10. Nurse Practitioners—Examination Questions. 11. Patient Care Planning—Case Report. 12. Patient Care Planning—Examination Questions. WY 18.2 R659c2002]
  RT 42.R63 2002
  610.73—dc21

2001037686

Care has been taken to confirm the accuracy of the information presented and to describe generally accepted practices. However, the authors, editors, and publisher are not responsible for errors or omissions or for any consequences from application of the information in this book and make no warranty, express or implied, with respect to the content of the publication.

The authors, editors, and publisher have exerted every effort to ensure that drug selection and dosage set forth in this text are in accordance with the current recommendations and practice at the time of publication. However, in view of ongoing research, changes in government regulations, and the constant flow of information relating to drug therapy and drug reactions, the reader is urged to check the package insert for each drug for any change in indications and dosage and for added warnings and precautions. This is particularly important when the recommended agent is a new or infrequently employed drug.

Some drugs and medical devices presented in this publication have Food and Drug Administration (FDA) clearance for limited use in restricted settings. It is the responsibility of the health care provider to ascertain the FDA status of each drug or device planned for use in his or her clinical practice.

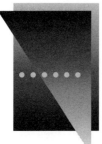

Contributors

Janet Andrews, PhD, RN-C, WHNP
Associate Professor
International Liaison
Family Nursing Department
Georgia College and State University
Milledgeville, Georgia
Cases 9, 31

Carol Abbott, MSN, FNP
Bernstein Allergy Group
Cincinnati, Ohio
Case 28

Ellen Benton, MSN, RN, FNP
Asthma and Allergy Affiliates
Cincinnati, Ohio

Kim Hudson Benton, RN, MSN, WHCNP
Family Nursing Department
Georgia College and State University
Milledgeville, Georgia
Case 14

Patricia Birchfield, DSN, ARNP
Associate Professor
College of Nursing
University of Kentucky
Lexington, Kentucky
Cases 5, 37

Ginger Conway
Case 36

Leslie Cooper, MSN, RN, CS, FNP
School Health Coordinator
Boone County Schools
Florence, Kentucky

Family Nurse Practitioner
Warsaw Family Medicine
Warsaw, Kentucky
Case 33

Christine Colella, MSN, CS, C-ANP
Assistant Professor of Clinical Nursing
University of Cincinnati School of Nursing
Cincinnati, Ohio
Case 3

Jean DeMartinis
Case 25

Ann Dollins, PhD, CNM
Assistant Dean
College of Professional Studies
Northern Kentucky University
Highland Heights, Kentucky
Case 24

Anita Kay Emery, ARNP-C, MSN
Tri-State Gastroenterology Associates
Edgewood, Kentucky
Case 12

Laura Flesch
Case 7

Jason Gregg, RN, BSN, MSN, FNP-C
Family nurse practitioner
Falmouth, Kentucky
Case 32

Cheryl P. Kish, EdD, RNC, WHNP
Professor and Coordinator
Graduate Programs in Health Sciences
Georgia College and State University
Milledgeville, Georgia
Cases 19, 26

Alice B. Loper RN, MN, FNP
Assistant Professor of Nursing
Director, Student Health Services
School of Health Sciences
Georgia College and State University
Milledgeville, Georgia
Case 17

Cheryl McKenzie, MN, RN, CS, FNP
Associate Professor
Department of Nursing
Northern Kentucky University
Northern Kentucky Family Health
   Centers, Inc.
Highland Heights, Kentucky
Cases 2, 13

Pat McMahon, MSN, NP-C
Associate Professor
Good Samaritan School of Nursing
Cincinnati, Ohio

Adult Nurse Practitioner
Cincinnati Arthritis Associates
Cincinnati, Ohio
Cases 6, 22

Denise L. Robinson, PhD, RN, FNP
Professor
Director, MSN Program
Northern Kentucky University
Highland Heights, Kentucky
Cases 1, 4, 8, 10, 11, 15, 16, 18, 23, 27, 30, 34, 35, 38, 39, 40, 41

Robin Schuckman
Case 1

Ann Stone, MSN, CNP
Nurse Practitioner, Internal Medicine
Internists of Fairfield
Fairfield, Ohio
Case 20

Becky Tackett, MSN, ANCC, AANP, ARNP
Nurse Practitioner
Summit Medical Group
Edgewood, Kentucky

Registered Nurse
St. Luke Hospital
Boone County, Kentucky
Case 21

Lynn Davis Waits, MSN, FNP
Assistant Professor
Georgia College and State University
Milledgeville, Georgia
Case 29

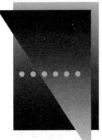

Preface

The purpose of this text is to help nurse practitioners (NPs) develop and refine the problem-solving skills needed to provide care for patients. In order to gain competence as nurse practitioners, students need to develop analytical skills. This text will help the nurse practitioner student, and newly practicing nurse practitioner in developing skills in problem solving and in making patient specific decisions.

The text was conceived when I was a nurse practitioner student. The faculty always tried to make sure each topic we talked about had clinical applicability. This was difficult since texts did not give enough detail or were not based on clinical application. Frequently, the cases used as examples were not detailed enough, and students ended up regurgitating information from their textbooks. As a class assignment, four nurse practitioner students were given the task of presenting content on depression. Luckily, one of our fellow students had developed, with another colleague, a problem focused self-directed modular learning method. We decided to use this technique for our presentation. As we developed the problem focused case study on depression, it became apparent to me that this format was a perfect method to assist nurse practitioner students in learning the diagnostic reasoning and clinical decision making skills that are so vital for nurse practitioners. The problem oriented method places the responsibility on the learners for mastery of the content and allows them to proceed at a pace which is appropriate for their learning style and speed of learning.

The cases in the text were chosen based on what the editor has seen in practice, and on the research done by Pickwell (1993) identifying what types of patients family nurse practitioners commonly see in practice. This was a difficult decision since there are so many different types of problems that NPs frequently encounter. It was very tempting to include many more diagnoses/problems in the text, however, the only most common problems were chosen for the text. These case studies reflect what is seen in practice, in other words, they are based on real patients with multiple physical and social problems. It seems in practice that rarely, if ever, is a typical "casebook" example seen. The real life perspective makes the cases more realistic and challenging, since it requires clinical judgment and critical thinking to sort through the large amount of data collected, and develop an appropriate and pertinent plan.

This text uses the problem oriented approach to therapy. This approach is used extensively by health care providers, and is a comprehensive and organized method for assessing and solving problems. The text utilizes the SOAP (S = subjective, O = objective, A = assessment and P = plan) format which is commonly seen in practice. Each case presents a brief scenario about a patient. The development of critical thinking skills is enhanced by the thought processes used to identify tentative differential diagnoses at this point in time. Even with very little data, the NP begins to identify the possible diagnoses that may be pertinent for the patient. The rest of the patient encounter revolves around the obtaining, sorting and organizing data to support or refute the potential differential diagnoses. Each case has questions to help identify questions needed at each level of data gathering, as well as more elaborate questions to help guide the NP in developing a thorough therapeutic plan of care.

The reader is encouraged to use a separate piece of paper to answer the questions for each patient. Writing the answers to each case will prove helpful in clinical decision making and to practice writing SOAP notes. Answer one section at a time, and then refer to the tutorial which provides the answers to the questions.

Information in the text may become incorrect as new discoveries or drugs become available. Based on personal interpretation, each reader may not agree with the actions taken by the authors. Each author was chosen for expertise in his/her field. Health care providers frequently argue over the best way to do things. There are several correct answers to clinical problems, with the answers dependent on the expertise and background of the person who is providing the care. At times this is difficult for students to learn—it is much easier when there is just one way to do things. It is important to develop the most patient specific plan by carefully utilizing all aspects of critical thinking and clinical judgment.

This text is appropriate for use by multiple audiences, including nurse practitioner students, NPs preparing for the certification examinations, and novice nurse practitioners. It could also serve as a review book for experienced nurse practitioners who might need to update knowledge in a particular area, or as they change from one job to another with a different patient population.

The first chapter in the text discusses the important issue of clinical decision making and critical thinking for nurse practitioners. Suggestions as to how the NP can learn and improve his/her own clinical judgments as well as how the text facilitates that process is presented. The remainder of the text consists of 41 case studies addressing patient issues/problems commonly seen by NPs in practice. Each case is presented using the SOAP format with appropriate questions. The tutorial presents the answers to each of the questions. References are provided to assist the reader with information provided in the answers.

This text has been designed to present patient scenarios. It is not meant to be a comprehensive textbook on the topics. Instead, it presents reality based learning, with "need-to-know" content. It has as its goal to facilitate the refinement of clinical decision making in nurse practitioners.

The first edition of *Clinical Decision Making for Nurse Practitioners* was found by readers to be helpful for its breadth, scope, depth and holism of the cases. This book uses those strengths and incorporates the suggestions of the nurse practitioner reviewers. The second edition has the following additional features:

- Cases which provide opportunity for the reader to solve. This book includes 16 complete cases demonstrating the problem-solving process. Twenty-five cases are provided for the reader to complete. This method will be useful to those programs that use the problem solving method.
- Increased use of lab tests—the reader is asked to identify why the tests are being performed and to interpret the results that are provided.
- Emphasis on RED FLAG conditions that cannot be missed in the diagnostic process
- Incorporation of more pathophysiology and etiology for the disease entity
- Using national guidelines as appropriate for the case—Internet links are identified
- Identification of resources that may assist both the NP and the patient
- Pictures as appropriate for the case—incorporating wet smears, microscope pictures, and skin disorders, thus giving the reader the opportunity to utilize their visual senses as well in the diagnostic process.

I think you will find this book encourages interaction on the part of both students and faculty. It will emphasize the critical thinking that is so much a part of what we as advanced practice nurses do. It will truly enhance your clinical decision making skills.

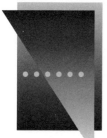

Acknowledgments

Development of this textbook has touched the lives of many people. I would like to give particular thanks to:

- Lisa Stead for recognizing the potential of the case studies format and acting on it
- The editors at Lippincott who facilitated the book's progress through the production phases
- Pamela Kidd and Kathleen Dorman Wagner who perfected the case study format in their own book
- All the expert practitioners who contributed real case studies for the book. It was especially exciting for me since a number of these writers are graduates from the Northern Kentucky University Primary Care Nurse Practitioner Program, and are now in practice.

*My family: John, Callie, Kristin, Mom, Robert, and Kim who once again were there for me when I needed them. I truly recognize and value the importance of my family in all that I am and do.

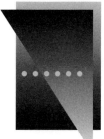

Contents

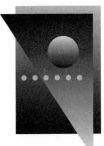

Clinical Decision Making

● THE USE OF CASE STUDIES TO DEVELOP CLINICAL DECISION MAKING

Clinical decision making (CDM) is the formulation and revision of hypotheses throughout a patient encounter (Barrows & Pickell, 1991). It is a dynamic activity in which the nurse practitioner (NP) builds a case in which hypotheses are accepted or rejected based on collected data. Flagler (2000) identifies a number of different processes that are used in CDM, such as searching, reasoning, prioritizing, and recognizing patterns. Experts in CDM can rapidly generate hypotheses from the beginning of the encounter (Thomas, 1997). They can test several hypotheses simultaneously and follow-up clues or hypotheses. Experts are able to generate better hypotheses and have a larger database of knowledge. An "expert" is an expert because he/she has seen it before. Experts are able to frame or structure the problem in a way that allows a solution strategy to be initiated. They have knowledge in long-term memory, and they have a set of rules that specify what action to take. Experts are able to make a distinction between strong and weak reasoning methods. This means being able to access and use the knowledge when the problem is familiar. Although student NPs are not expected to be experts, the ability of NPs to make sound clinical decisions is a vital outcome of any NP program.

The purpose of a case study is to apply acquired knowledge to a specific patient situation, using reflective thinking or thinking to a purpose (Graham & Uphold, 1997). Because the ultimate aim in NP education is learning how to apply knowledge in a clinical setting, the use of case studies seems an appropriate way to help students learn CDM skills. Students acquire scientific knowledge in the context in which it will be used (Allen, Duch, & Groh, 1996). Barrows and Pickell (1991) state that CDM can be thought of as the clinician's scientific method. Critical thinking skills are an integral part of CDM because the NP develops and examines decision alternatives, all components of critical thinking.

The characteristics of advanced practice (ambiguous issues that are poorly structured and require multilogical thinking, often requiring the perspectives of more than one paradigm) make it impossible to approach each case in the

1

same way with the same outcomes. Clinical decision making is the foundation of how an expert clinician can use prior knowledge and experience to draw conclusions and apply decision making skills and critical thinking in each new case. Research reveals that NPs who engage in successful CDM must have a comprehensive knowledge base, but the way they organize and understand their knowledge is even more important (Mandin, Jones, Woloschuk, & Harasym, 1997).

Educators, administrators, and experienced NPs often ask the question: How do I get professionals to actively think, rather than to passively accept what is observed? Getting others to think is difficult, but getting people to question the initial observations or conclusions often seems impossible (Bandman & Bandman, 1995). The goal of this chapter is to discuss critical thinking and CDM and then offer some methods for encouraging it in one's self or in others.

Although some people may not differentiate between critical thinking and CDM, there are some discernible differences (Bandman & Bandman, 1995). The terms are frequently used synonymously and, in that context, are intended to mean the same thing. In the role of the NP, not only is it important to differentiate the terms, but it also is logical to assume that the development of critical thinking should improve or lead to more appropriate CDM. Clinical decision making or critical clinical thinking is couched in the same assumptions used to support the teaching and enabling of critical thinking.

Critical Thinking

Some experts in the field of critical thinking make the point that without critical thinking, change (and thus progress) in our society would not/could not have occurred (Brookfield, 1987). Critical thinking by its very nature suggests questioning the how and why things are as they are and the development of methods for improvement for doing things differently. Brookfield identifies nine critical thinking themes. The first five themes deal with the identification of critical thinkers. These characteristics include critical thinking as a productive and positive activity; the context in which critical thinking occurs may change how critical thinking is seen; critical thinking may be positive or negative; emotions often are key to critical thinking; and critical thinking is a process (Brookfield). Although some of these themes are fairly common, two are of particular interest here. One is that critical thinking is productive and positive and it is an activity. This indicates that the critical thinker engages in a productive, positive activity. It is not passive; critical thinking involves doing something—a new way, a different way, a different stance or glance at a familiar methodology or assumption. Critical thinking is positive; it is not negating the organization or the facts but examining them in a different light or context. Critical thinking includes questioning the assumptions on which behavior, values, or action are based. The critical thinker asks the uncomfortable but necessary questions to understand how actions or decisions are made (Brookfield).

The second theme of interest is the notion that critical thinking involves emotions. Critical thinking often is seen as dispassionate, distant. and coldly logical. Thus, emotional value or concern is eliminated by the process of thinking critically. Brookfield (1987) believes that "emotions are central to the critical thinking process" (p.7). The fear of consequences from the consideration of alternatives to the "usual way" or the consequences of questioning authority are powerful fears. The thrill of coming out of a critical thinking process intact or even healthier also is a powerful feeling. Critical thinkers consider the emotional fallout of change or progress, rather than ignore it. Emotion is a part of the human experience and thus based on values and assumptions. It is as important to examine the emotional aspect of the critical thinking process as it is to look at the logically based assumptions (Brookfield).

Key to critical thinking is the thinker's ability to determine the assumptions that underlie beliefs, values, and attitudes. Once these assumptions are identified, the thinker has the opportunity and responsibility to examine them for appropriateness. Are the central assumptions culturally appropriate or logical? Are the assumptions based on current fact or fiction? Does the critical thinker see flaws in these assumptions? From this point, the critical thinker can make decisions and take action based on individual findings or beliefs about the assumptions. Again, this is a positive, productive activity because it examines long-held, culturally based beliefs that may no longer be appropriate. For example, one's assumption that a car will last 10 years may be rethought when the engine blows up and a new engine costs more than the car is worth. Rather than abiding by the original assumption, the owner may decide to purchase a different car because reexamination of the underlying assumptions reveals they are no longer appropriate in the current context. This kind of critical thinking occurs in the lives of adults on a regular basis and is critical for logical thinking. Simply assuming the underlying assumptions still hold true is not rational or appropriate. Rather, to question or understand underlying assumptions is the sign of mature, adult behavior. Figuring out what the underlying assumptions are is a step toward critical thinking. Examining these assumptions in the current context and determining what action to take is the basic process of critical thinking. Although it is rather simplistic as stated, it is a difficult, involved, time-consuming process. There is a certain amount of fear involved in critical thinking. The examination of long-held beliefs, values, and attitudes implies a self-examination that is both exciting and frightening. What if one finds one's long-held beliefs are not appropriate in the current culture? How does one go about replacing beliefs? How is a value system reordered? Of course, value systems are reordered frequently and often with little notice, but once in a while an individual feels the need to come to grips with some outmoded principles or values. As Brookfield points out, critical thinking can be stimulated by either positive or negative events in one's life or work (Bandman & Bandman, 1995; Brookfield, 1987; Chaffee, 1994; Meyers, 1986).

Once an individual has used the critical thinking process in one area of life or work, it is more likely the individual will use the process in other domains. If an individual consistently practices critical thinking, such thinking becomes a way of looking at the world and evaluating the context in which thoughts are generated. Getting people to think critically for the first time is a challenge.

Once done, it is more likely to continue. Meyers (1986) suggests use of a non-threatening, questioning approach. Rather than accepting parrot answers or superficial discussion, a questioning, quiet, nonchallenging approach circumvents the naturally defensive attitude one takes when one perceives one's beliefs and/or thought processes is being challenged or negated. Subtlety permits the learner of critical thinking to feel safe and secure while examining the assumptions that maintain an orderly world. Examination of those assumptions in a protected environment produces a confident, secure individual unafraid of change or doubt yet sensitive to the fear or concern of others engaging (perhaps for the first time) in the critical thinking process.

● CLINICAL DECISION MAKING

In the clinical arena, it is imperative for one to make the correct clinical decisions. The information presented in physical findings, history, and laboratory confirmation theoretically leads one to the correct decision. However, in some cases, differentiating one diagnosis from another is tedious and obscure. It is in this practice arena that accepting facts at face value may prolong the provision of proper treatment and care (Bandman & Bandman, 1995).

The nursing process is a well-known and well-used tool to promote both critical thinking and critical CDM. The steps of the nursing process are similar to the scientific method and a number of other problem-solving methodologies. The advantage of the nursing process for NPs is that most of them are familiar with it, and it encompasses the whole of nursing knowledge as a basis for treatment. By far the most important step of the process for the new practitioner is assessment—either a focused assessment for the apparently well individual with a specific complaint, or an in-depth complete assessment for the first-time patient or the patient with vague complaints, is necessary. The NP must make the decision on which assessment to begin and go from there. Of course, the NP may need to switch from one type of assessment to another, depending on what the data demonstrate.

As soon as a client offers some beginning complaint, the NP is quick to begin entertaining some diagnoses and eliminating others (Bandman & Bandman, 1995). As more information and physical findings become apparent, the NP begins to narrow the possibilities of diagnoses. Eventually, one or more diagnoses is determined, and the NP begins to formulate a treatment plan. The decision to accept or reject diagnoses is the point at which critical CDM becomes important.

● RELATIONSHIP OF CRITICAL THINKING AND CLINICAL DECISION MAKING

The relationship of critical thinking to CDM is convoluted. If the premise that critical thinking is a process that promotes skepticism, it is appropriate to assume that skepticism and continual examination of data in the diagnosis and treatment of illness also is a process. If the premise that processes can be learned is acceptable, then the assumption that the processes can be taught also is appropriate. But how does one teach these processes? Is it necessary to teach one before the other, or can they become concurrent learning experiences? Is it necessary to be a critical thinker in life to be a critical clinical decision maker, or can one think critically clinically and transfer that experience to life? As simplistic as it may seem, the two processes are transferable and can be promoted from either direction. Critical thinking of some form is the goal of most educational and higher degree programs (Brookfield, 1987). Thus, critical thinking can be taught and can be transferred by the learner to other aspects of life.

● TEACHING CRITICAL THINKING/CRITICAL CLINICAL DECISION MAKING

Again the question arises, how do educators, administrators, and experienced NPs encourage students to look beyond the obvious and question the common view of the data? It is not that the obvious may not be correct; it is that the less obvious may be more correct. Bates (1995) outlines a succinct method for clinical thinking. She recommends "clustering" symptoms and data to separate the data of concern from the normal or anticipated data. It is at the time of clustering that the critical thinking process needs to intersect the CDM process. This is the time at which the obvious and less obvious must be examined and accepted or rejected. Once the potential diagnoses have been critically examined, then data necessary to confirm, reject, or differentiate can be obtained. To not examine the data critically is a disservice to the client. As stated, it is important not to raise defenses and make defensiveness a barrier to learning (Meyers, 1986). Using a subtle approach and gently questioning how the NP reached a conclusion or diagnosis will promote critical thinking. Helping the NP develop a healthy skepticism toward the obvious conclusion will help the NP regard skepticism as a positive feeling or characteristic, rather than a negative one. Seeing the relationship between one's personal value system and one's professional decisions requires gentle nudging and care. For example, the NP who assumes recurrent head lice in a child is the result of an uncaring or lazy mother is making an assumption about the mother based not necessarily on fact but rather on illogical premises about mothers. This NP is not using all of the nursing knowledge available to critically evaluate why the child has a recurrent condition. When using all of that knowledge, the NP may discover that the mother is unaware of how head lice are transmitted and the importance of thorough bed/house cleaning in addition to the hair treatment. The NP's personal value system may have provoked the attitude that lazy, uncaring mothers do not treat the head lice in the first place. In this example, getting the NP to examine personal values will lead to reevaluation of the mother's knowledge base about head lice and their transfer.

Experienced critical thinkers routinely examine their thinking. One can view critical thinking as thinking about thinking in a way that improves one's thinking (Paul, 1995). To examine one's thinking requires a set of examination tools and a questioning attitude. Two tools proposed by Paul are elements of reasoning and universal intellectual standards. Let's examine how the NP can use these critical thinking tools in conjunction with the diagnostic reasoning process or CDM.

Elements of Reasoning

The elements of reasoning provide a framework for the NP to break apart thinking. These elements are purpose; question or issue; perspective or point of view; data; assumptions; concepts; inference; implication; and consequences.

When the NP applies the diagnostic reasoning process, he/she does so for a purpose. The overarching purpose for applying the process is to identify the basis for making diagnostic and treatment decisions about the patient. However, specific purposes for specific decision-making activities may vary. The purpose of the nurse's deliberations about diagnostic tests may be to rule out specific conditions from the differential diagnosis list, or the purpose for such deliberations about choice of test may be to maximize cost effectiveness for patient and/or provider. The NP frequently must reason from an economic perspective. Consider Marie, a 20-year-old woman with burning during urination. When prescribing antibiotics for Marie, the NP compares the daily cost of three equally effective drugs. Relevant questions that the NP asks of self might include:

1. What is my purpose for employing this diagnostic test?
2. Toward what end(s) am I considering this particular treatment option?

The questions or issues that arise during the diagnostic reasoning and treatment decision processes arise from data the NP gathers during the patient encounter. One may gather data from many perspectives: a nursing perspective, a medical or pathophysiologic perspective, a psychological perspective, or a cultural perspective. It's important for the NP to identify from what perspective or point of view the data are gathered. Sometimes it's more pertinent for the NP to gather data from the patient's perspective or from the family's perspective. Consider John, a 15-year-old boy who presents for his sports participation physical. John has freely offered information to the NP about his experimentation with marijuana and alcohol. When deciding what to do with this information, the NP must consider the confidence the patient has placed in the NP. That is, the patient apparently views his drug use as benign. The NP also must consider the possible implications or consequences of violating that confidence. The NP's initial perspective might be to view the drug use with concern. Pertinent questions to the NP's self-examined thinking include:

1. Are there other data that indicate the drug use may be serious?
2. What is the basis for my concern?

If there are not overt data to dispute the patient's perspective, the NP should strongly consider the patient's perspective before divulging this confidential information.

One reason the NP identifies multiple perspectives from which to interpret data is that each of these perspectives operates on inherent assumptions. As discussed earlier, assumptions represent an element of reasoning not often explicitly identified in clinical reasoning. However, assumptions can have a profound effect on treatment decisions and thus on outcomes and consequences. For example, the NP may base the concern for John's drug experimentation on the assumption that any substance use is inherently pathologic and requires direct intervention. Acting on this assumption might lead the NP to discuss John's marijuana use with his mother. If John's experimentation with marijuana was merely experimentation, John would not be very likely to confide in any health practitioner in the near future. It's important to do some thinking about what assumptions one holds when making a diagnosis or when making a treatment decision. Personal value assumptions may not always be compatible with client behavior. John's personal values or culture may condone experimentation with certain drugs, or it may be a part of normal teen growth and development.

Intellectual Standards

Universal intellectual standards provide another useful tool with which the NP can self-examine thinking. Intellectual standards include clarity and precision, depth, breadth, relevance, accuracy, and logicality. Clarity is a relevant standard at many points in the diagnostic reasoning process. Eliciting clear information from relevant data sources is crucial to the process. Clear communication of treatment decisions to the patient or other care givers may directly determine the success of the intervention(s). Key questions the NP asks of self during data collection might include:

1. Are the data clear?
2. Do I need to clarify certain cues with the patient or other informants?
3. Am I clearly communicating treatment options or procedures with the client?

Precision, in addition to clarity, often is necessary. For example, precise communication of medication regimen may determine the patient's understanding of and subsequent compliance with the regimen. The NP might instruct Marie, the 20-year-old woman with the urinary tract infection to take trimethoprim and sulfamethoxazole (TMP-SMZ) twice daily. The NP has been clear. However, precisely when and on what schedule should the patient take the antibiotics? With a 3-day course of antibiotics, it is important to maintain a serum level. To communicate precisely how such an outcome is achieved, the NP would advise the patient to take the antibiotic at the same time every 12 hours and to take the drug at least 1 hour before or 2 hours after a meal. With those instructions, the NP has been precise.

Depth and breadth are sometimes important standards for assessing one's thinking with regard to particularly ambiguous data sets. Questions to self might help the NP achieve depth and breadth when thinking through diagnostic or treatment decisions. Self- examination questions that promote depth and breadth, respectively, include:

1. Are there other important data elements that might support or refute my decision?
2. Are there other perspectives from which these data could be viewed?

It often is tempting to accept superficial data as relevant diagnostic indicators. If one accepts superficial, first-pass data as the most relevant in situations in which those data potentially represent a variety of diagnoses, that superficiality may cost the NP diagnostic accuracy.

To determine that the diagnosis is inaccurate may cost the NP and the patient profoundly in time, money, and even pain and suffering. In situations in which data are potentially ambiguous, NPs should ask themselves questions to assure that they base diagnoses on accurate and relevant data. Questions such as, "How could I check on the accuracy of these particular data?" might save valuable time in the long run.

The logic of a particular diagnoses is contained in the question, "Upon what cluster of data do I base this diagnosis?" In the case of differential diagnoses, the logic of a particular diagnosis may be contained in the answer to, "From what conditions may I differentiate my patient's condition based on particular clusters of data?" The dysuria that Marie experienced could result from several possible diagnoses. However, there were no cues to cluster with the dysuria to support any diagnosis other than a lower urinary tract infection. If the NP reflects upon the data underpinning particular diagnoses, and the data make sense with the diagnoses, the diagnosis probably is accurate.

● CASE STUDIES AS A TEACHING/LEARNING TOOL

Case studies are a terrific method to use to teach and learn critical thinking or CDM. Case studies provide guidance in learning the next step in the nursing process; the diagnostic tests necessary to differentiate, confirm, or reject diagnoses; the data findings and sorting of the data; and an opportunity to examine the underlying assumptions for both personal and professional values, beliefs, and attitudes. Case studies offer the opportunity for nonpersonal discussion because the threat of personalization is removed. Although the case study is based on and related to reality, it is not reality in the sense that the client is actually present in front of the NP. Case studies offer a wonderful opportunity for discussion without the potential for defensiveness or the fear of error.

Advantages to Using Case Studies to Promote CDM

Using case studies to teach CDM promotes learning as a process in which the learner actively constructs knowledge; it is student centered, rather than teacher centered. Students must identify their own learning needs, thus promoting principles of adult learning. The case study serves as reality; reality-based problems serve as the impetus for learning. The use of case studies for learning fosters critical thinking and the development of CDM because students must make and justify deductions and assumptions. Case studies promote guided reflection, knowledge discovery, and knowledge integration. The faculty facilitates the learning process by asking questions and mentoring the problem-solving process.

Case studies can be used to promote individual learning and data examination, as well as group discussion and learning. Sometimes, individuals feel less threatened in groups when discussing values because the individual does not have to defend personal values. The NP can listen and introspectively examine the context of personal values. Group discussion of diagnoses and differentiation is a rich environment for learning free from the pressures of the clinical arena. It provides data for the NP to consider in the privacy of her/his office and an opportunity to change without undue pressure or grief.

Principles of Learning That Are Emphasized in Case Studies

Learning is a constructive, not receptive process (Gijselaers, 1996). This means it is an active, not passive, experience. Knowledge is structured in semantic networks (networks of related concepts). These networks provide easy access to new information and are used to problem solve, recognize situations, or recall knowledge. These networks also influence how the information is interpreted and recalled. Activating existing knowledge to help with the processing of new information is a basic requirement of learning (Gijselaers).

Metacognition (self-monitoring skills) enhances learning. Metacognition includes the essential elements of goal setting, strategy selection, and goal evaluation. Faculty can encourage students to engage in deep processing; promote elaboration of new ideas; and stress understanding, rather than surface memory, as ways to promote the development of metacognition. Learning is quicker when students possess self-monitoring skills. Good students know when they do not understand and know when to use alternative strategies to help learn (Gijselaers, 1996).

Case studies teach how to use knowledge to solve real world problems in many ways. The use of complex and meaningful problem-solving situations makes the experience true to life but without the penalties of real life. Case study instruction focuses on metacognition skills and when to use them. Case studies encourage knowledge and skills taught from different perspectives and applied in many different situations. Because the case studies are used in collaborative learning situations, students are exposed to beliefs held by other students, as well as how others might solve the cases. In addition, case studies provide an opportunity to see how experts (faculty or guest speakers) analyze problems. Analysis of case studies provides feedback on the students' own actions and enables them to get suggestions during the process. Clinical decision making skills go beyond simple knowledge and comprehension. Synthesis and analysis are integral components of CDM.

Characteristics of Effective Cases

In an effective case study real patients serve as the basis for the case. They represent a real situation experienced by the NP author. Because it is a real case, the information is presented as the patient would present it—not always as neatly packaged as we would like. In fact, "disinformation" may be included as perceived from the patient's perspective, such as ambiguity or conflicting or inadequate data (Graham & Uphold, 1997). Effective cases also provide a wide gamut of acute, relatively innocuous cases to serious or potentially serious cases. The cases address implications for prevention/health promotion. The case introduces "new knowledge" that can be integrated with previous learning.

There are numerous strategies for making case studies as effective as possible.

- Faculty must be comfortable with the content presented.
- Faculty must define objectives and expected outcomes.
- Students must have done sufficient background reading.
- Cases must be both straightforward and ambiguous.
- The ability to identify problems is also a skill, so initial problem identification should be included.
- Problems can not be too simple or have only one acceptable solution and strategy for reaching it; they should reflect the complexity of life, including social, political, legal, divergent, and financial ramifications.

The suggested process for case analysis is as follows:

- Develop a working hypothesis.
- Gather data (identify possible learning issues).
- Rule out hypotheses using data.
- Identify other possible learning issues.
- Develop a treatment based on final diagnosis, including financial, social, etc., issues.
- Report knowledge gained in process.

Figure 1-1 shows a schematic of how CDM might look if diagrammed.

● CONCLUSIONS

Elements of reasoning and universal intellectual standards are but one way to view critical thinking and its relation to diagnostic reasoning and CDM. Clinical decision making embodies knowledge, experience, level of cognitive development, and a number of specific competencies and attitudes (Benner, 1984; Kataoka-Yahiro & Saylor, 1994; Schon, 1983). Developing CDM abilities requires time and commitment from the NP. However, maintaining a questioning, skeptical attitude will assist the NP in developing CDM skills.

The use of case studies to promote individual and/or group examination of assumptions underlying assessments and diagnosis is a nonthreatening and effective method for teaching and learning critical thinking and CDM. Case studies are liked by faculty and students, and based on theories of learning seem appropriate for teaching NPs CDM skills.

The use of subtle, gentle questioning and prodding in combination with

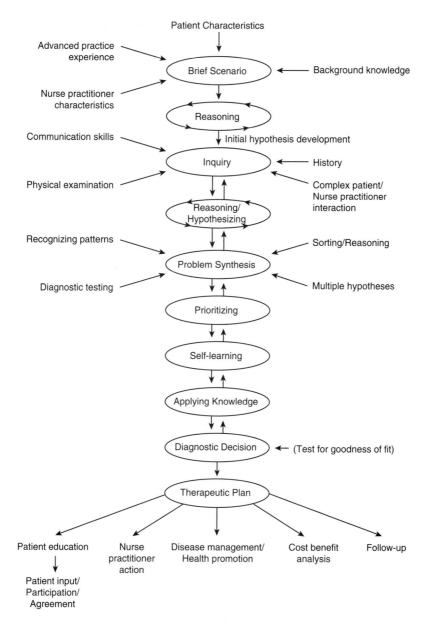

FIGURE 1–1. *Schematic of clinical decision making.* Figure adapted from: Carnavali, Mitchell, Woods, Tanner, (1984). *Diagnostic reasoning in nursing,* Philadelphia: Lippincott; Flagler, S. (2000). Recognizing the thinking processes behind clincial decision making. In K. Crabtree (Ed). *Teaching clinical decision making in advanced nursing practice.* Washington, DC: NONPF., 7–16; Mandin, H., Jones, A., Woloschuk, W., Harasym, P. (1997). Helping students learn to think like experts when solving clinical problems. *Academic Medicine, 72*(3), 173–179; Rendas, A., Pinto, P., & Gamboa, T. (1999). A computer simulation designed for problem based learning. *Medical Education, 33,* 47–54; White, J., Nativio, D., Kobert, S., Engberg, S (1992). Content and process in clinical decision making by nurse practitioners. *Image, 24*(2), 153–158.

case studies offers the opportunity for growth without defensiveness and wariness on the part of the NP. Learning to think critically is a difficult process that requires encouragement and support. Once the basic components are learned, the transfer of the CDM process to personal or professional worlds becomes easier and less fear producing and, over time, becomes an integral, natural part of patient care.

REFERENCES

Albanese, M., & Mitchell, S. (1993). Problem based learning: A review of literature on its outcomes and implementation issues. *Academic Medicine, 68,* 52–81.

Allen, D., Duch, B., & Groh, S. (1996). The power of problem based learning in teaching introductory science courses. *New Directions for Teaching and Learning, 68,* 6–13.

Amos, E., & White, M. (1998). Teaching tools: PBL. *Nurse Educator, 23*(2), 11–14.

Andrews, M., & Jones, P. (1996). PBL in an undergraduate nursing programme: A case study. *Journal of Advanced Nursing, 23,* 257–265.

Bandman, E. L., & Bandman, B. (1995). *Critical thinking in nursing* (2nd ed.). Norwalk, CT: Appleton & Lange.

Barrows, H., & Pickell, G. (1991). *Developing clinical problem solving skills: A guide to more effective diagnosis and treatment.* New York: W.W. Norton.

Bates, B. (1995). *A guide to clinical thinking.* Philadelphia: J. B. Lippincott Co.

Benner, P. (1984). *From novice to expert: Excellence and power in clinical practice.* Menlo Park, CA: Addison-Wesley.

Bernstein, P., Tipping, J., Bercovitz, K., & Skinner, H. (1995). Shifting students and faculty to a PBL curriculum: Attitudes changed and lessons learned. *Academic Medicine, 70,* 245–247.

Boud, D., & Feletti, G. (1991). *The challenge of PBL.* London: Kogan Page.

Brandon, J., & Majumdar, B. (1997). An introduction and evaluation of PBL in health professions education. *Family and Community Health, 20*(1), 1–15.

Brookfield, S. D. (1987). *Developing critical thinkers.* San Francisco: Jossey-Bass Publishers, 1987.

Carnevali, D., & Thomas, M. (1993). *Diagnostic reasoning and treatment decision making in nursing.* Philadelphia: J. B. Lippincott Co.

Chaffee, J. (1994). Teaching for critical thinking. *National Vision, 2*(1), 24–25.

Crabtree, K. (2000). *Teaching clinical decision making in advanced nursing practice.* Washington, DC: National Organization of Nurse Practitioner Faculty.

Creedy, D., & Hand, B. (1994). The implementation of PBL: Changing pedagogy in nursing education. *Journal of Advanced Nursing, 20,* 696–702.

Crowe, M. (1994). PBL: A model for graduate transition in nursing. *Contemporary Nurses: A Journal for the Australian Nursing Profession, 3*(3), 105–109.

Dailey, M. (1992). Developing case studies. *Nurse Educator, 17*(3), 8–11.

Flagler, S. (2000). Recognizing the thinking processes behind clinical decision making. In K. Crabtree (Ed.), *Teaching clinical decision making in advanced nursing practice* (pp. 7–16). Washington, DC: National Organization of Nurse Practitioner Faculty.

Frost, M. (1996). An analysis of the scope and value of PBL in the education of health care professionals. *Journal of Advanced Nursing, 24,* 1047–1053.

Gijselaers, S. (1996). Connecting problem based practices with educational theory. *New Directions for Teaching and Learning, 68,* 13–21.

Graham, M., & Uphold, C. (1997). Using the case method: An effective strategy for nurse practitioner educators. *Clinical Excellence for Nurse Practitioners, 1,* 191–197.

Kataoka-Yahiro, M., & Saylor, C. (1994). A critical thinking model for nursing judgment. *Journal of Nursing Education, 33,* 351–356.

Mandin, H., Jones, A., Woloschuk, W., & Harasym, P. (1997). Helping students learn to think like experts when solving clinical problems. *Academic Medicine, 72*(3), 173–179.

Meyers, C. (1986). *Teaching students to think critically.* San Francisco: Jossey-Bass Publishers.

Orme, L., & Maggs, C. (1993). Decision making in clinical practice: How do expert nurses, midwives, and health visitors make decisions today? *Nurse Education Today, 13*(4), 270–276.

Paul, R. (1995). *Critical thinking: How to prepare students for a rapidly changing world.* Santa Rosa, CA: The Foundation for Critical Thinking.

Ryan-Wenger, N., & Lee, J. (1997). The clinical reasoning case study: A powerful teaching tool. *Nurse Practitioner, 22*(5), 66–70, 76–79.

Schon, D. (1983). *The reflective practitioner.* New York: Basic Books.

Thomas, R. (1997). Problem based learning: Measuring outcomes. *Medical Education, 31,* 320–329.

Vernon, D., & Blake, R. (1993). Does PBL work? A meta analysis of evaluative research. *Academic Medicine, 68,* 550–563.

White, J., Nativio, D., Kober, S., & Engberg, S. (1992). Content and process in clinical decision making by nurse practitioners. *Image, 24*(2), 153–158.

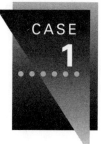

A 16-year-old boy with sore throat and fever

SCENARIO

Jack is a 16-year-old Egyptian boy who comes to the office today with his mother because he has a persistent sore throat, head congestion, teeth pain, low-grade fever, and fatigue. He was seen 1 week ago for headache and sinus congestion and was prescribed a 10-day course of cefuroxime axetil (Ceftin) 250 mg BID and pseudoephedrine (Sudafed) QID, which he continues to take.

● TENTATIVE DIAGNOSES

Based on the information given, what are your tentative diagnoses? What are **red flag** *diagnoses that you cannot miss?*

● HISTORY

What are significant questions in the history for Jack? What are the key points to cover in the review of systems?

● PHYSICAL EXAMINATION

What are the significant portions of the physical examination that should be completed for Jack? Include your rationale for each part of the physical exam.

● DIFFERENTIAL DIAGNOSES

What are the significant positive and negative data that support or refute your diagnoses for Jack?

● DIAGNOSTIC TESTS

Based on the history and physical exam, what, if any, diagnostic testing should be done? Include rationale and interpretation of the tests obtained.

● DIAGNOSIS

What diagnosis(es) do you determine as being appropriate for Jack? Identify the data supporting this diagnosis and the pathophysiology of the condition.

● THERAPEUTIC PLAN

1. *What were the main goals of therapy for Jack's condition?*
2. *What growth and development considerations were pertinent to the patient's care?*
3. *What education needs to be provided for the patient and the family?*
4. *How did the method of payment for health care affect the plan selected?*
5. *What are the specific elements of the plan of care?*
6. *How soon should Jack return for follow-up?*
7. *Describe the need for consultation/collaboration in this case.*

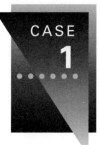

TUTORIAL

A 16-year-old boy with sore throat and fever

SCENARIO

Jack is a 16-year-old Egyptian boy who comes to the office today with his mother because he has a persistent sore throat, head congestion, teeth pain, low-grade fever, and fatigue. He was seen 1 week ago for headache and sinus congestion and was prescribed a 10-day course of cefuroxime axetil (Ceftin) 250 mg BID and pseudoephedrine (Sudafed) QID, which he continues to take.

● TENTATIVE DIAGNOSES

Based on the information provided, what are your tentative diagnoses? What are **red flag** *diagnoses that you cannot miss?*

DIAGNOSIS	RATIONALE
Persistent sinusitis	A sore throat, head congestion, teeth pain, and fatigue often accompany sinusitis (Robinson, Kidd, & Rogers, 2000).
Infectious mononucleosis	C/o a gradual onset of sore throat, low-grade temperature, cervical adenopathy, and pronounced fatigue are commonly seen with mono (Dains, Baumann, & Scheibel, 1998). Red flag due to possibility of splenic rupture with activity.
Viral pharyngitis	Sore throat, malaise, fever, headache, cough, and fatigue are common symptoms of viral pharyngitis (Dains et al., 1998).
Cold/viral syndrome	A low-grade fever, nasal congestion, mild sore throat, and small amounts of clear to yellow sputum production are common symptoms of a viral upper respiratory infection (Dains et al., 1998).
Dental abscess	Teeth pain.

● HISTORY

What are significant questions in the history for Jack? What are the key points to cover in the review of systems?

REQUESTED DATA   DATA ANSWER

Allergies	NKDA.
Medications	Cefuroxime axetil (Ceftin), 250 mg BID; pseudoephedrine (Sudafed), BID PRN; ibuprofen (Advil) 1–2 every 4 hours PRN.
History of upper respiratory illnesses or sinusitis	Averages 1–2 sore throats each year. Was treated for strep pharyngitis in April 2000. No previous history of mononucleosis.
Dental history	Exam every 6 months. Last exam was 2 months ago and included X-rays with no problems noted.
Childhood illnesses	Chicken pox.
Immunizations	Childhood immunizations up to date. Last DT, 1993.
Surgery	None.
Hospitalizations	None.
Outside activities	Is a junior in high school; works part time at Tristate Pools; plays recreational soccer.
Substance abuse	Denies tobacco, alcohol, or recreational drug use.
Onset and duration of symptoms	Ten days ago started with headache, fever, sinus congestion, facial tenderness. Was given a prescription for Ceftin and Sudafed, which he has continued to take. Throat is still sore; he is very fatigued; teeth still hurt; no cough.
Fever, cough, and color of nasal discharge?	Temperature has not gone over 100 °F. Denies any cough. Small amount of yellowish nasal discharge.
Has this illness interfered with activities?	Has missed a couple days of school; has not worked since being seen 1 week ago; did not play soccer this past weekend.
Does anything help the sore throat?	Advil offers some relief, but the sore throat returns after a few hours.
Are any other family members or close friends sick?	No other family members or acquaintances are sick.

● PHYSICAL EXAMINATION

What are the significant portions of the physical examination that should be completed for Jack?

SYSTEM	FINDINGS	RATIONALE
Vital signs	BP: 108/78 mm Hg; P, 78; RR, 16; T, 97.1 ° F.	Baseline information.
HEENT	Sclera without injection or jaundice.	Screening of eye for jaundice
	TMs: normal with good light reflex.	Make sure there is no ear infection.
	Nares: + erythema, no edema.	Resolving sinusitis.
	OP: tonsillar hypertrophy and erythema with small amount of exudate.	Tonsillar hypertrophy with exudates is commonly seen in patients with mononucleosis.
	Lymph nodes: + submandibular, anterior and posterior lymphadenopathy.	LA is common in patients with mononucleosis.
	Maxillary sinuses tender to palpation.	Tenderness of maxillary sinuses is common in maxillary sinusitis.
Chest	CTA.	Rule out pneumonia or other chest infections.
Heart	RRR. No MRG.	Baseline screening.
Abdomen	Active bowel sounds; no masses or tenderness; no organomegaly.	Hepatomegaly is present in 50% of patients, and splenomegaly is found in 75% of patients with mononucleosis (Robinson et al., 2000).

● DIFFERENTIAL DIAGNOSES

What are the significant positive and negative data that support or refute your diagnoses for Jack?

DIAGNOSIS	POSITIVE DATA	NEGATIVE DATA
Persistent sinusitis	Head congestion, teeth pain, maxillary sinus tenderness despite 1-week treatment with antibiotics.	None.
Infectious mononucleosis	Low-grade temperature; tonsillar hypertrophy and erythema with exudates; cervical lymphadenopathy; and pronounced fatigue are all common symptoms of mono.	None.
Viral pharyngitis	Sore throat, malaise, fever, cough, headache, and fatigue.	No cough.
Cold/viral syndrome	Low-grade fever, nasal congestion, mild sore throat, and small amounts of clear to yellow sputum production.	No sputum production or cough.
Dental abscess	Teeth pain.	Normal dental exam with x-rays 2 months ago.

● DIAGNOSTIC TESTS

Based on the history and physical exam, what, if any diagnostic testing should be done? Include the rationale for testing and interpretation of the test results obtained.

TEST	RATIONALE	RESULTS	INTERPRETATION
CBC with differential	Identifies the extent of the infection and is diagnostic of mono if CBC reveals > 50% lymphocytosis.	WBC, 12,000/mm^3 RBC, 4.76 Hgb, 14.5 g/dL. HCT, 42%. Segs, 33%. Lymphocytes, 56%.	Increased WBC and lymphocytosis > 50% indicates mono.
Epstein-Barr viral titer (IgM anti-VCA) [Immunoglobulin M antibody to viral capsid antigen]	EB virus is the causative organism of mono in 90% of cases. An elevated IgM is indicative of an acute episode. An elevated IgG is indicative of a	IgG, > 170 mg/dL. IgM, > 140 mg/dL.	Elevated levels IGM anti-VCA appear early in primary infection and disappear within 3–6 months. A rising titer during the first few weeks of clinical illness

(continued)

TEST	RATIONALE	RESULTS	INTERPRETATION
	recent or past infection.		is the most useful and generally the most easily available serologic evidence of recent primary infection. IgG anti-VCA appears slightly later than IgM and remains detectable for life.
Heterophile agglutins (serum); mono spot test	A screening test for mono and other viral illnesses. It is positive 3–10 days after infection, peaks within 3 weeks, and can remain elevated up to 1 year.	Positive.	Indicates presence of an antigen (such as for mono, cytomegalovirus, serum sickness, and toxoplasmosis).
Rapid strep test/throat culture	25% of patients with mono have strep. All patients should be screened for strep.	Negative.	Indicates that Jack does not have strep throat.

● DIAGNOSIS

Infectious Mononucleosis

Data Support

- History and physical findings supporting this diagnosis include persistent sore throat for 1 week; tonsillar hypertrophy with erythema and exudates; low-grade fever; submandibular, anterior, and posterior cervical lymphadenopathy; congestion; and fatigue.
- Diagnostic laboratory findings that support this diagnosis include CBC findings of lymphocytosis and Epstein-Barr viral titers, which show an IgM of >140 mg/dL, which is diagnostic of an acute Epstein-Barr infection.

Pathophysiology

- Infectious mononucleosis is caused by the Epstein-Barr virus. It is an acute febrile illness that usually affects primarily teen-agers and young adults between 15 and 25 years. The virus is spread by oral contact, first affecting the throat, then B-lymphocytes generate a T-cell response that results in atypical lymphocytosis.

● THERAPEUTIC PLAN

1. What were the main goals of therapy for Jack's infectious mononucleosis?

Goals of therapy include

- Rest
- Adequate hydration
- Prevention of superimposed infection
- Avoidance of splenic rupture
- Prevention of recurrent symptoms, and
- Return to normal activity.

2. What growth and development considerations were pertinent to the patient's care?

Teenagers do not always recognize what is best for them as far as recovering from an illness. It is important to include a parent when advising the teen of therapeutic measures to be followed for recovery.

3. What education needs to be provided for the patient and the family?

In the case of mononucleosis, it is important Jack understands he should not play soccer for at least 1 month and should not take gym class to avoid the possibility of splenic rupture. In addition, rest is essential for the timely, complete recovery from an acute episode with mononucleosis.

Jack was advised that he could go to school, for half days or whole days, depending on how he felt. If he went half days, he was advised to alternate morning and afternoon sessions to help him keep up with his classes equally. He was given a work excuse for 1 week so that he could come home from school and rest, keep up with his homework, and get adequate rest at night. He and his mother were advised that mononucleosis is spread through direct contact with saliva, which meant intimate contact, including kissing and sharing glasses or eating utensils, should be avoided.

In addition, Jack and the family should be aware that any sharp, brief, sudden abdominal pain should be taken seriously because of the possibility of splenic rupture, and emergency care should be sought if such pain occurs.

4. How did the method of payment for health care affect the plan selected?

This family had PPO insurance, which required a $10 copayment for each office visit. Laboratory tests were covered by the insurance, and prescriptions cost the family $10 per prescription. In this case, the method of payment for health care did not influence the plan for care.

5. Elements of the therapeutic plan

Pharmaceutical therapy includes ibuprofen for the sore throat and headache. Jack was advised to continue taking the cefuroxime axetil (Ceftin), which had been prescribed 1 week earlier for a sinus infection. Because mononucleosis is a viral infection, antibiotic therapy is not necessary unless, as in this case, there is an underlying bacterial infection. Although it was not a factor in this case, amoxicillin should be avoided in patients with mononucleosis because the drug may cause a rash in 80% of such patients treated (Robinson et al., 2000).

Nonpharmaceutical therapy includes limited activity as long as Jack experiences the fatigue; adequate fluid intake; anesthetic throat lozenges for pain relief; and salt water or half-strength mouth wash gargles for comfort.

Diet should be soft, with plenty of fluids to prevent constipation, which could develop because of the decrease in exercise and activity during the recovery period.

Activity restrictions include no contact sports or gym class for a period of at least 1 month to avoid splenic rupture, which could occur because of splenomegaly, which is commonly found in patients with mononucleosis. A work excuse was given for 1 week so that Jack could go to school as he was able, come home to rest, keep up with his studies, and get plenty of rest at night.

Jack and his mother were reassured that mononucleosis is self-limiting, and isolation is not necessary. The virus is spread by direct contact with the saliva of the infected person. Thus, sharing of utensils or drinking from the same glass should be avoided, as should direct contact with saliva through kissing or other intimate contact.

6. *How soon should the patient return for follow-up?*
Jack was advised to return to the office for follow-up within the next 10 days to 2 weeks, unless his symptoms worsened. Worsening symptoms that would need to be checked before this time period would include difficulty swallowing because of throat swelling or severe throat congestion, nausea, inability to eat, or abdominal pain or discomfort. Severe pharyngitis may require the use of corticosteroids (40–60 mg of prednisone for 7 days) to help prevent impending airway obstruction.

The purpose of the follow-up visit is to check for hepatosplenomegaly and determine Jack's level of fatigue and activity. Resumption of normal activities, including sports, will be decided based on the findings at his follow-up visit. If there is any question of organomegaly or other GI symptoms, including anorexia, nausea, or abdominal discomfort, a blood test for liver studies should be ordered.

7. *Describe the need for consultation/collaboration in this case.*
It is appropriate for nurse practitioners to treat patients with persistent upper respiratory symptoms and mononucleosis. If complications, such as marked splenomegaly, respiratory compromise, excessively enlarged tonsils and difficulty swallowing, jaundice, or hyperbilirubinemia, develop, referral to another health care provider would be appropriate. The development of any of these complications probably would be able to be treated by the nurse practitioner in collaboration with a primary care provider unless the patient required hospitalization. It would be appropriate for the nurse practitioner to follow up with this patient as recommended in 10 days to 2 weeks.

There probably is no need for community resources for this patient. However, a note to the school regarding the expected recovery time for Jack might be appropriate so that his teachers could get his assignments together for him, lessening some of the stress of making up work while he is recovering.

REFERENCES

Bailey, R. E. (1992). Diagnosis and treatment of infectious mononucleosis. *American Family Physician, 49*(4), 879–888.

Cecchini, J. A. (1996). Streptococcus 'A' screens. *Nurse Practitioner, 21,* 152–153.

Dains, J., Baumann, L, & Scheibel, P. (1998). *Advanced health assessment and clinical diagnosis in primary care.* St. Louis: Mosby, Inc.

Ganzel, T., Goldman, J., & Padhya, T. (1996). Otolaryngologic clinical patterns in pediatric infectious mononucleosis. *American Journal of Otolaryngology, 17,* 397–400.

Godshall, S. E., & Kirchner, J. T. (2000). Infectious mononucleosis: Complexities of a common syndrome. *Postgraduate Medicine, 107*(7), 175–179, 183–184, 186.

Gray, J. J., Caldwell, J., & Sillis, M. (1992). The rapid serologic diagnosis of infectious mononucleosis. *Journal of Infection, 25*(1), 39–46.

Greenslade, R. A. (2000). Presumed infectious mononucleosis in a college basketball player. *Physician and Sportsmedicine, 28*(6), 79–80, 85–86.

Hickey, S. M., & Strasburger, V. C. (1997). What every pediatrician should know about infectious mononucleosis in adolescents. *Pediatric Clinics of North America, 44,* 1541–1556.

Infections in children and adolescents. (1999). [A photo essay.] *Consultant, 39*(9), 2572, 2574–2577, 2581–2582.

Jenson, H. (2000). Acute complications of Epstein-Barr virus infectious mononucleosis. *Current Opinions in Pediatrics, 12,* 263–268.

Lajo, A., Borque, C., Del Castillo, F., & Martin-Ancel, A. (1994). Mononucleosis caused by Epstein-Barr virus and cytomegalovirus in children: A comparative study of 124 cases. *Pediatric Infectious Disease Journal, 13*(1), 56–60.

Leiner, S. (2000). Case report. Acute pharyngitis with lifelong implications. *Nurse Practitioner: American Journal of Primary Health Care, 25*(4), 119–120, 122.

Leung, A. K. C., & Pinto-Rojas, A. (2000). Double take: An intriguing diagnosis. Infectious mononucleosis. *Consultant, 40*(1), 134–136.

Miuscari, M. E. (1999). Adolescent health. Rising above 'soar' throats. *American Journal of Nursing, 99*(3), 18, 20.

Robinson, D. (1998). Clinical decision making for nurse practitioners: A case study approach. Philadelphia: Lippincott-Raven.

Robinson, D., Kidd, P., & Rogers, K. (2000). Primary care across the lifespan. St. Louis: Mosby, Inc.

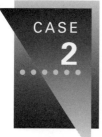

A 25-year-old woman requesting a checkup

SCENARIO

Kate Martin presents to the health center for a checkup. She is a new patient; she lives with a boyfriend of 6 months. She works full-time as a waitress but recently missed work because of "personal reasons". She is usually in good health. She had her annual Papanicolaou smear within the past year by a gynecologist.

● TENTATIVE DIAGNOSES

*Based on the information provided, what are the potential diagnoses you have identified? Make sure you include any vital **red flag** diagnoses that cannot be missed.*

● HISTORY

What are significant questions in the history for Kate?

● PHYSICAL ASSESSMENT

What are the significant portions of the physical examination that should be completed for Kate?

● DIFFERENTIAL DIAGNOSES

What are the significant positive and negative findings that support or refute your diagnoses for Kate?

● DIAGNOSTIC TESTS

Based on the history and physical examination, what, if any, diagnostic testing would you obtain?

25

● DIAGNOSES

What diagnoses do you determine as being appropriate after a review of the subjective and objective data?

● THERAPEUTIC PLAN

1. *What are some issues Kate may be dealing with regarding a new boyfriend?*
2. *What could be the "personal reasons" she has missed work recently?*
3. *What are some specific questions that need to be addressed during this first visit?*
4. *What are some warning signs of victims of domestic violence?*
5. *What specific information is needed to determine Kate's risks for being in a dangerous situation?*
6. *When should Kate return for follow-up?*

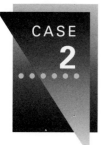

TUTORIAL

A 25-year-old woman requesting a checkup

SCENARIO

Kate Martin presents to the health center for a checkup. She is a new patient; she lives with a boyfriend of 6 months. She works full-time as a waitress but recently has missed work because of "personal reasons." She usually is in good health. She had her annual Papanicolaou smear within the past year by a gynecologist.

● TENTATIVE DIAGNOSIS

Based on the information provided, what are the potential diagnoses you have identified? Make sure you include any vital red flag diagnoses that cannot be missed.

DIAGNOSIS	RATIONALE
Depression	Diagnosis of elimination that presents with depressed mood, loss of interest in activities, weight loss/gain, as well as fatigue. Victims of domestic violence often have depression and other emotional problems related to problems with self-esteem. Screening for depression is an important part of a checkup.
Annual exam	The well exam is an important time to address other health maintenance issues.
Domestic violence	Patients do not always volunteer information regarding partner abuse. They may present for routine care or other vague health problems. They may begin to miss work because of the abuse. All female patients should be asked about domestic violence.

(continued)

DIAGNOSIS   *RATIONALE*

Substance/alcohol abuse

Patients do not always disclose information about drug and alcohol use. They may use drugs or alcohol to cope with the situation. They may begin to miss work, which is an early warning sign of substance abuse.

● HISTORY

What are significant questions in the history for Kate?

REQUESTED DATA   *DATA ANSWER*

Allergies	NKA.
Current medications	Ortho Tri-Cyclen (oral contraceptive).
Medical history	Chickenpox. Received all childhood immunizations; last MMR at age 12. Last well care visit at age 15. Completed Hepatitis B vaccine series and had tetanus-diphtheria toxoid.
Surgery/transfusions	None
Gyn history	Menarche: age 13; periods usually last 5–6 days; cycles of approximately 30 days; light flow; no cramping. LNMP: 2 weeks ago, no problems. Last pelvic: within a year. GPA: Gravida 0. Contraception: Has been taking Ortho Tri-Cyclen for three years. No problems; does not use condoms with present partner of 6 months.
Appetite	Eats a lot of fast food, junk food. No change in appetite.
24-hour diet recall	B: coffee. L: Mountain Dew, roast beef sandwich. D: fast food: burrito, chips, Coke.
Sleeping	7 hours; feels tired most of the time.
Sexuality	Relationship with boyfriend is strained. He wants to have sex more than she does, and she feels forced into having sex with him. He likes to have sex after they argue.
Family history	Mother: age 45, good health. Father: age 50, alcoholism. Brother: age 22, good health.

(continued)

REQUESTED DATA DATA ANSWER

Work/finances	Kate is a high school graduate; she works full time as a waitress. She has health insurance through work. Her boyfriend works at a car wash; he dropped out of school at the age of 17.
Home	Lives in an apartment, 15 minutes from work.
Relationship with boyfriend	They argue frequently about money. Boyfriend does not help with any housekeeping. Believes that it's "woman's work." He is very jealous and doesn't want her to talk with her friends on the phone or go out with them, unless he is with her. He has been showing up at her work site, just to check up on her. Denies he has ever hit her; he becomes very mean when drinking alcohol. He drinks a six-pack every day.
Relationship with family	Kate's mother and father live 100 miles away. They divorced when she was 10. They argued all the time. Kate's father was always yelling at her mother, and he would "slap her around" whenever he was drinking.
What do you do when you are stressed? How do you manage stress? Medications for stress?	I cannot afford to call my Mom, because it is long-distance. My brother is away at college. My friends are afraid of my boyfriend. I smoke cigarettes to decrease my stress. I do not take medication for stress.
Do you ever think about hurting yourself?	No
Where do see yourself in 10 years?	I want to go to college so I can get a better job. My boyfriend thinks college is a waste of time.
Any complaints or change in health?	Denies any recent changes in health; no complaints.
Safety	Wears seat belts when she drives; has smoke detectors.
Exercise	Does not exercise.

● PHYSICAL ASSESSMENT

What are the significant portions of the physical examination that should be completed for Kate?

SYSTEM	RATIONALE	FINDINGS
Vital signs	Provides baselines data.	BP, 120/80 mm Hg; P, 80; RR, 20; T, 98.6 °F.

(continued)

SYSTEM	RATIONALE	FINDINGS
General appearance/skin	Overall view of patient. Assess for new bruises and bruises that are in the healing stage.	Appears thin and stated age. Skin is pale, warm, and dry; no ecchymosis; nails are neatly trimmed.
HEENT	Assess for any signs of trauma; need to check for thyroid enlargement during annual exam.	No signs of trauma, no thyromegaly.
Lungs	Baseline information.	CTA.
Heart	Baseline information.	S1, S2 normal; no murmur.
Neurological assessment	Important to do as basic screening, especially because of concerns related to depression.	Alert and oriented, poor eye contact. Screening neuro: strength/sensation intact, DTRs 2+.
Extremities	Baseline screening. Look for signs of abuse	No edema, no ecchymosis.

● DIFFERENTIAL DIAGNOSES

What are the significant positive and negative findings that support or refute your diagnoses for Kate?

DIAGNOSIS	POSITIVE DATA	NEGATIVE DATA
Depression	Has missed work recently. Parents and sibling live out of town; has lost contact with friends. Has no other support systems. Has decreased eye contact.	Denies suicidal ideation. Negative screening for depression.
Poor dietary habits	History revealed no breakfast; high-fat, fast foods; and increased caffeine intake.	
Domestic violence	Boyfriend is jealous of friends; forces her to have sex; does not want her to pursue college education. They argue, and he becomes mean when he drinks alcohol. He drinks every day.	

(continued)

DIAGNOSIS	POSITIVE DATA	NEGATIVE DATA
Altered health maintenance	Not had well care, with exception of Gyn exam, since age 16.	

● DIAGNOSTIC TESTS

Based on the history and physical examination, what, if any, diagnostic testing would you obtain?

DIAGNOSTIC TEST	RATIONALE	RESULTS	INTERPRETATION
Beck Self-Report Depression Scale	Can help identify depression. Kate can complete while waiting for exam.	Denies suicidal ideas, sleeps OK; no change in appetite. At times feels hopeless in relationship with boyfriend.	Normal.
Electrolytes, liver function test, renal function, cholesterol	Baseline labs for general health status. Cholesterol testing is appropriate because it has never been done.	Na, 138 mEq/L; K, 4.3 mEq/L; Cl, 98 mEq/L; CO_2, 30 mEq/L; BUN, 11 mg/dL; creatinine, 0.7 mg/dL; cholesterol, 196 mg/dL; alkaline phosphatase, 102 U/L; ALT, 10 U/L; AST, 14 U/L; albumin, 4.0 g/dL; protein, total 6.7 g/dL; bilirubin, total 0.3 mg/dL.	WNL.
X-ray series	If abuse is suspected, could determine if there are healed fractures.	Not done, denies physical abuse.	N/A.

● DIAGNOSES

What diagnoses do you determine as being appropriate after a review of the subjective and objective data? Domestic violence, well history and physical

Domestic Violence is defined as a "pattern of coercive control and terror that one person uses over another," (Poirier, 1997). The control may or may not involve actual physical injury and includes psychological (verbal assaults and criticisms) and economic abuse (the creation of economic dependence) (Poirier).

Assessment of Victims of Abuse or Violence

TARGET AREAS FOR ASSESSMENT	SPECIFIC ACTIONS
Take a domestic violence history	Past history of domestic violence events. Past history of sexual assault.
Send important supportive messages to the client	You are not alone. You are not to blame. There is help available. You do not deserve to be treated this way.
Assess client's immediate safety	Are you afraid to go home? Have there been threats of homicide or suicide? Are there weapons present? Can you stay with family or friends? Do you need access to a shelter? Do you want police intervention?
Make referrals and assure follow-up visits	Involve social workers if available. Provide lists of shelters, resources, and hotline numbers. Schedule a follow-up appointment.
Document all findings clearly	Use the client's own words regarding the injury or abuse. Document time, place, and order of events leading to the injury. Legally document all injuries using a body map. Take photographs of injuries.

From: Cromwell, S., & Kish, C. (2001). Domestic violence. In D. Robinson & C. Kish (Eds.), *Core concepts of advance practice (pp. 547–564).* St. Louis: Mosby.

Other areas that need to be targeted in plan of care includes:
• Altered health maintenance
• Poor dietary habits

- Tobacco abuse
- Potential for depression

● THERAPEUTIC PLAN

1. *What are some issues Kate may be dealing with regarding a new boyfriend?*
   She is a victim of domestic violence. Her boyfriend is controlling, and he abuses alcohol. The abuse may escalate at any time because when the abuser is drinking alcohol, the situation is more unpredictable.

2. *What could be the "personal reasons" she has missed work recently?*
   Kate may be missing work because of depression about her job and home situation. Although she denies substance abuse and physical abuse, she is a victim of domestic violence. Chronic absenteeism can be a clue that someone is a victim of abuse (Farella, 2000). Women need to know that abuse is not their fault. They need to talk with someone about the situation.

3. *What are some specific questions that need to be addressed during this first visit?*
   Women need to be screened for domestic violence at any health maintenance visit and most interval visits (Poirier, 1997). Women tend to disclose abuse during an interview rather than by self-report methods (Poirier). Kate may be more likely to disclose abuse if she feels she can trust the primary care provider. A good screening question is, "Are you safe at home?" (Farella, 2000).

4. *What are some warning signs of victims of domestic violence?*
   Women may present with frequent physical complaints, such as insomnia, irritability, chest pain, abdominal pain, and headache. They also may present with symptoms of depression. (Poirier, 1997).

5. *What specific information is needed to determine Kate's risks for being in a dangerous situation?*
   Kate needs to realize that the abuse is more unpredictable because of her boyfriend's use of alcohol. It also IS important to know if the abuser has ever used a weapon or threatened to kill her (Poirier, 1997). She needs education about the cycle of abuse and how to protect herself from a potentially dangerous situation. Give her information about domestic violence along with the telephone number of the local women's shelter. Make sure she knows what documents to have available if the situation becomes volatile. Most women's crisis centers can provide this information.

6. *When should Kate return for follow-up?*
   Kate needs close follow-up because of the potential for danger. The provider can plan to have Kate keep in contact by telephone. She may be willing to share more information at a follow-up visit in 1 month.

Altered Health Maintenance

Kate needs to have exams along with the Papanicolaou smear. She also would benefit from regular exercise. Regular exercise may make her feel more energetic.

Consider giving her a tetanus booster because it has been 9 years since she got her last one.

Poor Dietary Habits

Review the food pyramid with Kate to educate her about a balanced diet. Encourage Kate to incorporate more fruits, vegetables, and fiber into her diet.

Tobacco Dependence

It will be important to determine if Kate is interested in smoking cessation. If not, continue to discuss it with her at each visit. It may not be a good time at this visit because she has indicated that it is a stress reliever. Let her know you are available to discuss the specifics of smoking cessation when she is ready.

Potential for Depression

Most communities have resources that could be of help if Kate feels she is becoming more depressed. Make sure you give her information and a crisis hotline number in case she becomes suicidal.

Web Resources

Nurse Advocate website *http://www.nursadvocate.org*

National Domestic Violence Hotline
1-800-799-SAFE (7233)
1-800-787-3224 (TDD)

The National Domestic Violence Hotline is staffed 24 hours a day by trained counselors who can provides crisis assistance and information about shelters, legal advocacy, health care centers, and counseling.

RAINN Hotline, 1-800-656-HOPE
The Rape, Abuse, Incest National Network will automatically transfer you to the rape crisis center nearest you, anywhere in the nation. It can be used as a last resort if people cannot find a domestic violence shelter.

Visit the US Department of Justice Violence Against Women Office for information on regional information and other resources, including government press releases and statements. Other shelter information can be found on our Sexual Assault Resources page.

Safe Horizon
Domestic Violence Shelter Tour
http://www.dvsheltertour.org

Feminist Majority's Domestic Violence Information Center
http://www.feminist.org/911/crisis.html

Family Violence Prevention Fund
383 Rhode Island Street, Suite 304
San Francisco, CA 94103-5133
Phone: 415-252-8900
FAX: 415-252-8991

National Coalition Against Domestic Violence
Policy Office
PO Box 34103
Washington, DC 20043-4103
Phone: 703-765-0339
FAX: 202-628-4899
http://www.ncadv.org

National Coalition Against Domestic Violence
PO Box 18749
Denver, CO 80218
Phone: 303-839-1852
FAX: 303-831-9251

National Battered Women's Law Project
275 7th Avenue, Suite 1206
New York, NY 10001
Phone: 212-741-9480
FAX: 212-741-6438

Victim Services
Domestic Violence Shelter Tour
2 Lafayette Street
New York, NY 10007
Phone: 212-577-7700
Fax: 212-385-0331
24-hour hotline: 800-621-HOPE (4673)

National Resource Center On DV
Pennsylvania Coalition Against Domestic Violence
6400 Flank Drive, Suite 1300
Harrisburg, PA 17112
Phone: 800-537-2238
FAX: 717-545-9456

Health Resource Center on Domestic Violence
Family Violence Prevention Fund
383 Rhode Island Street, Suite 304
San Francisco, CA 94103-5133
Phone: 800-313-1310
FAX: 415-252-8991

Battered Women's Justice Project
Minnesota Program Development, Inc.
4032 Chicago Avenue South
Minneapolis, MN 55407
TOLL-FREE: 800-903-0111 Ext: 1
Phone: 612-824-8768
FAX: 612-824-8965

Resource Center on Domestic Violence, Child Protection, and Custody
NCJFCJ
PO Box 8970
Reno, NV 89507
Phone: 800-527-3223
FAX: 775-784-6160
They are a resource center for professionals and agencies.

Battered Women's Justice Project
c/o National Clearinghouse for the Defense of Battered Women
125 South 9th Street, Suite 302
Philadelphia, PA 19107
TOLL-FREE: 800-903-0111 ext. 3
Phone: 215-351-0010
FAX: 215-351-0779
National Clearinghouse is a national resource and advocacy center providing assistance to women defendants, their defense attorneys, and other members of their defense teams in an effort to insure justice for battered women charged with crimes.

National Clearinghouse on Marital and Date Rape
2325 Oak Street
Berkeley, CA 94708
Phone: 510-524-1582

Center for the Prevention of Sexual and Domestic Violence
936 North 34th Street, Suite 200
Seattle, WA 98103
Phone: 206-634-1903
FAX: 206-634-0115

National Network to End Domestic Violence, Administrative Office
c/o Texas Council on Family Violence
PO Box 161810
Austin, TX 78716
Phone: 512-794-1133
FAX: 512-794-1199

National Network to End Domestic Violence
666 Pennsylvania Avenue SE, Suite 303
Washington, DC 20003
Phone: 202-543-5566
FAX: 202-543-5626

REFERENCES

Abbott, J. (1997). Injuries and illnesses of domestic violence. *Annals of Emergency Medicine. 29,* 781–785.

Campbell, J, & Humphreys, J. (1993). *Nursing care of survivors of family violence* (2nd ed.). St. Louis: Mosby-Year Book.

Campbell, J. C. (1998). *Empowering survivors of abuse: Health care for battered women and their families.* Thousand Oaks, CA: Sage Publications.

Carlson, B. (2000). Children exposed to intimate partner violence: Research findings and implications for intervention. *Trauma, Violence, & Abuse, 1*(4), 321–342.

Chalk, R., & King, P. (Eds.) (1998). *Violence in families: Assessing prevention and treatment programs.* Washington DC: National Academy Press.

Count, D., Brown, J., & Campbell, J. (1999). *To have to hit: Cultural perspectives on wife beating.* Champaign, IL: University of Illinois Press.

Dearwater, S. R., Coben, J. H., Campbell, J. C., Nah, G., Glass, N., McLoughlin, E., & Bekemeier, B. (1998). Prevalence of intimate partner abuse in women treated at community hospital emergency departments. *Journal of the American Medical Association, 280,* 433–438.

Dutton, M. A., Mitchell, B., & Haywood, Y. (1996). The emergency department as a violence prevention center. *Journal of American Medical Womens Association, 51,* 92–95.

Farella, C. (2000). Love shouldn't hurt: Understanding domestic violence. *Nursing Spectrum, 1*(1), 14–16.

Feldhaus, K. M., Koziol-McLain, J., Amsbury, H. L., Norton, I. M., Lowenstein, S. R., & Abbott, J. T. (1997). Accuracy of 3 brief screening questions for detecting partner violence in the emergency department. *Journal of the American Medical Association, 277,* 1357–1361.

Fishwick, N. (1995). Getting to the heart of the matter: Nursing assessment and interventions with battered women in psychiatric mental health settings. *Journal of the American Psychiatric Nursing Association, 1,* 48–54.

Furbee, P. M., Sikora, R., Williams, J. M., & Derk, S. J. (1998). Comparison of domestic violence screening methods: A pilot study. *Annals of Emergency Medicine, 31,* 495–501.

Gagan, M. (1996). Correlates of nurse practitioner diagnosis and intervention performance for domestic violence. Unpublished Doctoral Dissertation, University of Iowa, Iowa City.

Gremillion, D. H., & Kanof, E. P. (1996). Overcoming barriers to physician involvement in identifying and referring victims of domestic violence. *Annals in Emergency Medicine, 27,* 769–773.

Hoff, L. A., & Rosenbaum, L. (1994). A victimization assessment tool: Instrument development and clinical implications. *Journal of Advanced Nursing, 20,* 627–634.

Isaac, N. E., & Sanchez, R. (1999). Emergency department response to battered women in Massachusetts. *Annals of Emergency Medicine, 23,* 855–858.

Larkin, G. L., Hyman, K. B., Mathias, S. R., D'Amico, F., & MacLeod, B. A. (1999). Universal screening for intimate partner violence in the emergency department: Importance of patient and provider factors. *Annals of Emergency Medicine, 33,* 669–675.

Mayer, B. (2000). Female domestic violence victims: Perspectives on emergency care. *Nursing Science Quarterly, 13*(4), 340–346.

McCoy, M. (1996). Domestic violence: Clues to victimization. *Annals in Emergency Medicine, 27,* 764–765.

McFarlane, J., Greenberg, L., Weltge, A., & Watson, M. (1995). Identification of abuse in emergency departments: Effectiveness of a two-question screening tool. *Journal of Emergency Nursing, 21,* 391–394.

McFarlane, J., Parker, B., Soeken, K., & Bullock, L. (1992). Assessing for abuse during pregnancy: Severity and frequency of injuries and associated entry into prenatal care. *Journal of American Medical Association, 267,* 3176–3178.

McGrath, M. E., Bettacchi, A., Duffy, S. J., Peipert, J. F., Becker, B. M., & St. Angelo, L. (1997). Violence against women: Provider barriers to intervention in emergency departments. *Academic Emergency Medicine, 4,* 297–300.

McLeer, S. V., Anwar, R. A., Herman, S., & Maquiling, K. (1989). Education is not enough: A systems failure in protecting battered women. *Annals in Emergency Medicine, 18,* 651–653

Muelleman, R. L., & Liewer, J. D. (1998). How often do women in the emergency departments without intimate violence injuries return with such injuries? *Academic Emergency Medicine, 5*(10), 982–985.

Norton, L. B., Peipert, J. F., Zierler, S., Lima, B., & Hume, L. (1995). Battering in pregnancy: An assessment of two screening methods. *Obstetrics and Gynecology Clinics of North America, 85,* 321–325.

Olson, C., Anctil, C., Fullerton, L., Brillman, J., Arbuckle, J., & Sklar, D. (1996). Increasing emergency physician recognition of domestic violence. *Annals of Emergency Medicine, 27,* 741–746.

Parker, B., & McFarlane, J. (1991). Identifying and helping battered pregnant women. *American Journal of Maternal Child Nursing, 16,* 161–164.

Poirier, L. (1997). The importance of screening for domestic violence in all women. *The Nurse Practitioner, 22*(5), 105–121.

Quillian, J. P. (1996). Screening for spousal or partner abuse in a community health setting. *Journal of the American Academy of Nurse Practitioners, 8,* 155–160.

Roberts, A., & Burman, S. (1998). Crisis intervention and cognitive problem-solving therapy with battered women: A national survey and practice model. In A. Roberts (Ed.), *Helping battered women: New perspectives and remedies* (pp. 13–70). New York: Oxford University Press.

Rodriguez, M. A., Bauer, H. M., McLoughlin, E., & Grumbach, K. (1999). Screening and intervention for intimate partner abuse: Practices and attitudes of primary care physicians. *Journal of the American Medical Association, 282,* 468–474.

Soeken, K. L., McFarlane, J., Parker, B., & Lominack, M. C. (1998). The Abuse Assessment Screen: A clinical instrument to measure frequency, severity, and perpetration of abuse against women. In J. C. Campbell (Ed.), *Empowering survivors of abuse: Health care for battered women and their children* (pp. 195–203). Newbury Park, CA: Sage.

Steen, M. (2000). Developing midwifery responses to women in their care who are living with violent men. *Midwifery Digest, 10*(3), 313–317

Sugg, N. K., & Inui, T. (1992). Primary care physicians' response to domestic violence: Opening Pandora's box. *Journal of the American Medical Association, 267,* 3157–3160.

Sugg, N. K., Thompson, R. S., Thompson, D. C., Maiuro, R., & Rivara, F. P. (1999). Domestic violence and primary care: Attitudes, practices, and beliefs. *Archives of Family Medicine, 8,* 301–306.

Thompson, R. S., Meyer, B. A., Smith-DiJulio, K., Caplow, M., Maiuro, R., Thompson, D., Sugg, N., & Rivera, F. (1998). A training program to improve domestic violence identification and management in primary care: Preliminary results. *Violence Victim, 13,* 395–410.

Tilden, V., & Limansdri, B. (1994). Factors that influence clinicians' assessment and management of family violence. *American Journal of Public Health, 84,* 628–633.

Waller, A. E., Hohenhaus, S. M., Shah, P. J., & Stem, E. A. (1996). Development and validation of an emergency department screening and referral protocol for victims of domestic violence. *Annals of Emergency Medicine, 27,* 754–760.

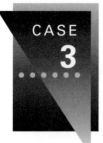

A 38-year-old man with headaches

SCENARIO

Joseph Randall presents to the clinic with a history of reoccurring "excruciating" headaches. He is a computer programmer; he is divorced with two teen-aged children.

● TENTATIVE DIAGNOSES

Based on the information provided, what are potential differential diagnoses? What are red flag diagnoses that cannot be missed?

DIAGNOSIS	RATIONALE
1	
2	
3	
4	
5	
6	

● HISTORY

As the nurse practitioner, what questions do you want to ask Joseph? Are there any important questions which are not included here?

REQUESTED DATA   DATA ANSWER

REQUESTED DATA	DATA ANSWER
Allergies	NKA.
Medications	OTC vitamins; OTC ibuprofen for pain.
Surgery/transfusion	Tonsillectomy at 6 y/o, no transfusion.
Medical history	Chicken pox, mumps, and hospitalized for measles as a child.
Family history	Mother: age 60, HTN.
Social history	Tobacco: 1½ packs per day for 23 years. Alcohol: 1–2 beers nightly since divorce, more on the weekend; not specific with amount. Caffeine: 2–5 cups of coffee daily.
Appetite/weight changes	No change in appetite; weight stable since his 20s.
History of current illness	Headaches occasionally occur after a night of heavy drinking. He was drinking heavily last weekend. Had this a few times before over the years, but it goes away. He has not had one in months (10). This episode has been every day for the last week and has been lasting about 1–2 hours each time. It has awakened him nightly for the past week. Nothing seems to make it better, but will take up to 3 or 4 OTC NSAIDs at a time to reduce the pain, repeating this every 2 hours. Pain is on one side but may switch. Denies radiation. It is a burning or stabbing quality. Score of 10 (scale 1–10). Accompanying complaints include ptosis, miosis, eyelid redness, and lacrimation on the affected side. C/o nasal congestion, rhinorrhea. Denies nausea, vomiting, photophobia, or phonophobia. Denies pain at this time.
Stress management	Doesn't feel very stressed. Sometimes finds that he gets angry easily; drinking beers seems to help relieve stress.

● PHYSICAL ASSESSMENT

What areas of the physical examination are most important for Joseph? Determine which of the systems identified below you would exam and why.

SYSTEM	RATIONALE	FINDINGS
Vital signs		BP, 134/85 mm Hg left arm sitting; HR, 84 bpm; RR, 20; T, 98.7 °F; Ht, 5' 11"; Wt, 165 lb.
General appearance/skin		Alert, appears tired; skin warm and dry; no areas of ecchymosis; no spider angioma; no pallor, cyanosis, or jaundice.
HEENT		Normocephalic, no sinus tenderness, + transillumination. No tenderness or bruit noted over temporal artery. Snellen OU 20/20; no ptosis; conjunctiva clear; sclera white; EIOM; normal confrontation; +Horner's syndrome. Discs flat with flat margins, no AV nicking; no exudate or hemorrhage; macula with even color. TMs gray and WNL; Weber/Rinne WNL. Nose pink, moist, with septum midline, no drainage. Oral mucosa moist and pink.
Lungs		Clear to auscultation throughout all fields.
Cardiac		S1, S2 WNL; no MRG. Alert and oriented ×3.
Neurological assessment		CN II–XII intact. Strength/sensation intact bilaterally. Gait steady—Romberg. Intact tandem walk, heel/toe. DTRs, 2+.

● DIFFERENTIAL DIAGNOSES

What are the pertinent positives and negative data items that support or refute your tentative diagnosis for Joseph?

DIAGNOSIS	POSITIVE DATA	NEGATIVE DATA
1		
2		

(continued)

DIAGNOSIS	POSITIVE DATA	NEGATIVE DATA
3		
4		
5		
6		
7		
8		
9		
10		
11		
12		
13		
14		

● DIAGNOSTIC TESTS

Based on your findings from the history and examination, what diagnostic tests are appropriate, if any? Identify the tests you would order. Interpret the tests that have been done.

DIAGNOSTIC TEST	RATIONALE	RESULTS	INTERPRETATION
CBC with differential		WBC, 5,900/mm^3; RBC, 5.02 million/mm^3; Hgb, 15.8 g/dL;	

(continued)

DIAGNOSTIC TEST	RATIONALE	RESULTS	INTERPRETATION
		HCT, 46.8%; MCV, 92.1 μm^3; Platelet count, 236,000 /mm^3; Absolute neutrophils, 3,098 cells/μL; Lymphocytes, 2,100 cells/μL; Monocytes, 2,100 cells/μL; Eosinophils, 130 cells/μL; Basophils, 183 cells/μL.	
Erythrocyte sedimentation rate		25 mm/hr	
Electrolytes, renal		Na, 139 mEq/L; K, 4.0 mEq/L; Cl, 101 mEq/L; CO_2, 30 mEq/L; Glucose, 81 mg/dL; BUN, 8 mg/dL; Creatinine, 0.7 mg/dL.	
Lumbar puncture		No blood present in CSF; no xanthochromia present.	
Sinus films		Not done.	
Cervical spine x-rays		Not done.	
Neuroimaging		CT unremarkable.	
Electroencephalogram		Not done.	
Cerebral angiography		Not done.	

● DIAGNOSIS

What diagnosis(es) do you determine is appropriate for Joseph?

1.

2.

Identify the data supporting the diagnosis(es):

● PATHOPHYSIOLOGY

● THERAPEUTIC PLAN

1. What information does Joseph need about his diagnosis?

2. What lifestyle changes are recommended for Joseph?

3. What are the treatment options for Joseph?

4. What additional education does Joseph need about his medication and management plan?

5. What support sources can the nurse practitioner recommend for Joseph?

6. When should Joseph return for follow-up?

REFERENCES

Brandes, J. L. (2000). *Differential diagnosis of migraine.* www.medscape.com.
Dubose, C., & Cutlip. W. (1995).Migraines and other headaches: An approach to diag-

nosis and classification. *American Family Physician, 54:* 1498–1504. www.medscape.com/PCI/headaches/headaches.ch05/headaches.ch05-01.html.

International Headache Society. (1998). Classification and diagnostic criteria for headache disorders, cranial neuralgias and facial pain. *Cephalgia, 8*(Suppl. 7): 1–96.

Kunkel, R. (2000). Managing primary headache. *Patient Care, 34*(2), 100–103, 107–110, 115–117.

Loder, W. (1998). Migraine management: an overview of nonpharmacologic and pharmacologic interventions. *Postgraduate Medicine, 102,* 13–19.

Moore, K., & Noble, S. (1997). Drug treatment of migraine: Part I. Acute therapy and drug-rebound headache. *American Family Physician, 56:* 2039–2048.

National Institute of Neurological Disorders and Stroke. (1997). *Headache: Hope through research.* Washington, DC: U.S. Government Printing Office. www.ninds.nih.gov.

Noble, S., & Moore, K., (1997). Drug treatment of migraine. Part II. Preventive therapy. *American Family Physician,* 56, 2279–2286.

Nurse Practitioner's Clinical Companion. (1999). Springhouse, PA: Springhouse.

Pagana, K., & Pagana, T., (1998). *Mosby's manual of diagnostic and laboratory tests.* St. Louis, MO: Mosby.

Patient Information. (2000). Comparison of treatment results for cluster headaches. www.mayfieldclinic.com.

Singleton, J., Sandowski, S., Green-Hernandez,C., Horvath,T., DiGregorio,R., Holzemer, S., (1999). *Primary Care.* New York, NY: Lippincott.

Smetana, G. (2000). The diagnostic value of historical features in primary headache syndromes: A comprehensive review. *Archives in Internal Medicine, 160* (18), 2729–2737.

Tepper, S. (1998). Recent advances in antimigraine therapy: a clinical overview of zolmitriptan's efficacy and tolerability. *Postgraduate Medicine, 102,* 1–26.

Tierney, L., McPhee, S., Papadakis, M., (Eds.). (1999). *Current medical diagnosis & treatment 1999.* (38th ed.). Stamford,CT: Appleton & Lange.

Uphold, C., & Graham, M. (1998). *Clinical guidelines for family practice* (3rd Ed.). Gainesville, FL: Barmarrae Books.

Walling, A. (1993). Cluster headache. *American Family Physician, 47:* 1457–1463.

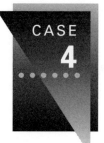

CASE

4

A 5-year-old girl for a kindergarten physical

SCENARIO:

Callie is a 5-year-old girl who presents to your office for a 5-year physical. She is 5 years, 2 months old. Her mother wants to determine if she is ready for kindergarten in the fall.

● TENTATIVE DIAGNOSES

What are the potential diagnoses you have identified based on the scenario presented?

● HISTORY

What are significant questions in the history for a school-age child?
What are important questions to ask related to safety for Callie?
What are the key points on the review of systems?
What are questions you need to review with Callie's mother in terms of her development?

● PHYSICAL ASSESSMENT

What are the significant portions of the physical examination that should be completed for Callie?
What developmental assessment should be included in the exam?

● DIFFERENTIAL DIAGNOSES

What are the significant positive and negative findings that support or refute your diagnoses for Callie?

● DIAGNOSTIC TESTS

Based on the history and physical examination, what, if any, diagnostic testing would you obtain?

● DIAGNOSES

What diagnoses do you determine as being appropriate after a review of the subjective and objective data?

● THERAPEUTIC PLAN

1. *What immunizations does Callie need today?*
2. *What recommendations would you make for Callie's readiness for kindergarten?*
3. *What anticipatory guidance issues would you discuss with Callie's mother?*
4. *What treatment options do you have for pinworms?*
5. *What recommendations will you share with Callie and her Mother to prevent the occurrence of pinworms in the future?*
6. *How will the diagnosis of pinworms affect the rest of the family?*
7. *Does Callie need follow-up for the pinworms?*
8. *When should Callie return for another well-exam?*

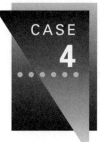

TUTORIAL

A 5-year-old girl for a kindergarten physical

SCENARIO

Callie is a 5-year-old girl who presents to your office for a 5-year physical. She is 5 years, 2 months old. Her mother wants to determine if she is ready for kindergarten in the fall.

● TENTATIVE DIAGNOSES

What are the potential diagnoses you have identified based on the scenario presented?

DIAGNOSIS	RATIONALE
Not applicable at this time	Well visit. When reviewing this case, keep in mind that the school physical exam may be the only health maintenance visit for a school-age child.

● HISTORY

What are significant questions in the history for a school-age child?

REQUESTED DATA	DATA ANSWER
Allergies	NKA.
Current medications	None.

(continued)

REQUESTED DATA   DATA ANSWER

Birth history

Planned pregnancy. Had complete prenatal care, including amniocentesis. Born full term; induced vaginal delivery. Mother had mildly elevated BP shortly before delivery. Birth wt., 9 lbs. 5½ oz; length, 21½". Content newborn; happy temperament.

Childhood illnesses

Chickenpox.
Strep throat 2 times/this season.

Immunizations

Completed Hep B series, 4 DTAP, 4 Hib, 3 IPV, 1 MMR.

Surgery

Pneumatic ear tubes inserted May 1992.

Medical history and hospitalizations/ fractures/injuries/ accidents

Multiple otitis media episodes, with mild hearing loss noted. PE tubes inserted; no subsequent episodes.

Last complete PE

Last well-child PE at age 4

Appetite

Good; mother notes patient snacks frequently.

24-Hour diet recall

No special diet.
B: dry cereal with water.
L: eats at day care, example, pizza, applesauce, milk.
D: Chili, salad, milk, fruit, dessert.
S: Popsicle.

Sleeping

Sleeps approximately 12 hours per night, no naps.

Social history

Active child, inventive imagination.
Sister, 14, recently went to Texas to live with father.

Family history

Father: 40, arthritis, back problems, smokes 1½ packs a day.
Mother: 42, HTN.
Sister: 14, living and well, ADHD.
PGF and MGF died at age 51 with MI.
MGM, 63 HTN. PGM, 66, living and well.

What are important questions to ask related to safety for Callie?

REQUESTED DATA   DATA ANSWER

Seat belts

Wears every time she is in the car.

Guns in house

Yes; locked in gun cabinet in basement.

Hot water temperature

Set at 120°.

(continued)

REQUESTED DATA   DATA ANSWER

Bike helmets	Yes, also wears pads for in-line skating.
Water safety	Knows she can not go swimming by herself.
Call 911	Knows number to call.
Strangers	Knows about strangers; would seek help.
Pedestrian safety	Knows to look both ways; not allowed to cross street by herself.
Sun exposure	Has pale skin, blue eyes, and freckles. Wears sunscreen when outside for prolonged periods. Mom cautious about sun exposure.
Noise	Mom monitors use and volume of headphones and loud music.

What are the key points on the review of systems?

SYSTEM REVIEWED   DATA ANSWER

General	Mother feels Callie is doing well; no problems, no concerns.
HEENT	No problems. Callie has not lost any teeth yet. None appear to be loose. She brushes her teeth morning and before bed. Callie has gone to the dentist two or three times, and uses fluoride toothpaste.
Respiratory	Able to do activities she wants; runs and plays with no difficulty. Denies SOB or cough.
Elimination	Had recent bout of fever with N/V and diarrhea. Resolved on its own. No problems usually with constipation, diarrhea, or dark stools. Complains of rectal itching in past week or so. Urination QS. No problems with bedwetting or incontinence.

What are questions you need to review with Callie's mother in terms of Callie's development?

DEVELOPMENTAL AREA	MOTHER'S REPORT
Speech	No difficulties. No lisps. Very large vocabulary. Asks mother about what different words mean.
Emotional development	Callie seems very competent to manage daily routine. She picks out her clothes each day and seems to like the interaction of day care.
Intellectual development	Enjoys learning; can count to 110; can even add some numbers. Enjoys puzzles, drawing, using markers. Sings songs; able to remember words to songs with little difficulty.
Work/home responsibilities	Has own responsibilities to take care of: feed fish, keep room clean, and set/clear table. Usually will do tasks with little argument. Gets along with mother and father. Older sister teases her a lot. They do not get along well.
Social development	Has many friends. Plays with other girls in day care. Has neighbor boy (7 y/o) who she plays with occasionally. Seems to have difficulty agreeing on play activities with him. Instruments such as the ABC Inventory to Assess Kindergarten and School Readiness can be used to help assess school readiness.

● PHYSICAL ASSESSMENT

What are the significant portions of the physical examination that should be completed for Callie?

SYSTEM	FINDINGS
Vital signs	BP, 92/64 mm Hg; P, 92; RR, 18; T, 97.8 °F; Wt, 43 lbs; Ht, 48″.
General appearance/skin	Alert, interactive, playing. Body appears proportionate with appropriate muscle development. Good eye-to-eye contact. Participates in answering questions. Skin: no excessive bruises or burns. Has some bruises noted on anterior surface of legs.

(continued)

SYSTEM	FINDINGS
HEENT	Equal tracking of eyes. WNL cover/uncover test. Ears: TMs with scarring; no erythema. Teeth in good repair. None missing. Throat with slight erythema. No exudate. Neck supple.
Lungs	CTA.
Heart	S1, S2 WNL; no murmurs.
Breasts	Appropriate for age. Extra nipple in MCL on right.
Abdomen	BS+, soft, no tenderness.
Genitalia	No erythema, irritation, discharge. Rectal area excoriated. No worms visualized.
Neurological/ musculoskeletal assessment	Strength appropriate for age. Negative for scoliosis.

What developmental assessment should be included in the exam?

DEVELOPMENTAL AREA	FINDINGS
Coordination	Able to hop, skip, jump; able to walk on tiptoe. Can do duck walk; heel-and-toe walk. Able to balance on one foot for 5 seconds.
Fine motor skills	Able to draw triangle, circle, square. Able to complete a stick figure drawing of man, including clothing.
Language development	Able to define nine words. Understands meanings of opposites. Able to identify words that rhyme. Able to recite alphabet.
Safety	Knows telephone number but not address.

● DIFFERENTIAL DIAGNOSES

What are the significant positive and negative findings that support or refute your diagnoses for Callie?

DIAGNOSIS	POSITIVE DATA	NEGATIVE DATA
Well-child exam	Appropriate growth and development. Attainment of developmental milestones.	None.
Pinworms	C/o rectal itching; excoriated rectal area.	No pinworms visualized.

● DIAGNOSTIC TESTS

Based on the history and physical examination, what, if any, diagnostic testing would you obtain?

DIAGNOSTIC TEST	RATIONALE	RESULTS
Visual acuity	Provides baseline to determine if additional evaluation is needed.	OS, 20/30; OD, 20/30.
Hearing screen	Provides indication if additional workup is needed.	L/R 20 dB: 500, 1000, 2000, 4000 Hz.
Tympanogram	Indicates functioning of TM and presence of middle ear effusion. Not invasive, relatively inexpensive test. Can be done in office	Not done because hearing WNL and no complaints of ear problems
PPD	Required on admission to school.	0 mm reaction.
Hgb	Recommended once annually.	Hgb, 14.2 g/dL.
U/A	Recommended once between 3–6 years.	U/A WNL.
Tape test (see Figure 4-1)	Test permits visualization of ova under microscope.	Ova visible.

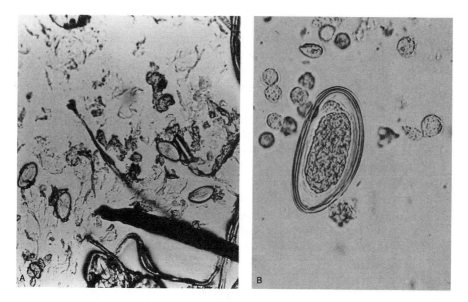

Figure 4–1. Pinworm ova (A) 100× (B) 400×. From Robinson, D., & McKenzie, C. (2000). *Procedures for primary care providers* (p. 8). Philadelphia: Lippincott Williams & Wilkins.

● DIAGNOSES

What diagnoses do you determine as being appropriate after a review of the subjective and objective data?

- Well 5-year-old exam
- Pinworms
- Immunizations

● THERAPEUTIC PLAN

1. *What immunizations does Callie need today?*
   Callie needs:

   - DtaP (acellular is recommended)
   - IPV
   - MMR

2. *What recommendations would you make for Callie's readiness for kindergarten?*
   Callie appears ready for school. She does not have any gross or fine motor dysfunction. Her language, speech, and behavior appear age appropriate (Shapiro, 1999). Callie is currently attending day care, so she is able to spend time away from home, and she interacts with adults other than her parents. She is able to accept behavior-control expectations. In addition, she has sufficient self-esteem to be able to carry on independent activity (Stephens, 1994).

3. *What anticipatory guidance issues would you discuss with Callie's mother?*
   A. *Injury prevention.* Discuss with Mom the area of most likely occurring injuries: burns, falls, use of car seat belts, toxic substance ingestions, safety around mowers and tools, guns should be kept locked up; supervision needed when playing around streets. Need to review stranger safety practices. Callie should know her address, phone number, and how and when to dial 911. Her mother should be reminded about bike safety and the wearing of a bike helmet at all times.
   B. *Good parenting practices/discipline.* The use of time out for behavior modification should be discussed. The use of corporal punishment should be discouraged. Callie's ability to assume some responsibilities around home should be discussed, as should her ability to begin simple money management with an allowance. Encourage the parents to interact with Callie and act as role model for reading and decreased TV watching.
   C. *Sleep.* Reinforce a regular bedtime for Callie. Napping is dependent on behavior seen.
   D. *Dental health.* Encourage brushing at least two times a day. Callie may begin using floss at this time. Encourage twice-yearly preventive exams.

4. *What treatment options do you have for pinworms?*
   The recommended treatment for pinworms is mebendazole (Vermox) 100 mg, 1 chewable tablet now and repeated in 2 weeks. Sitz baths may be helpful for rectal irritation. Desitin may be of assistance for rectal excoriation.

5. *What recommendations will you share with Callie and her mother to prevent the recurrence of pinworms?*
   Callie should bathe daily. She should wash her hands after toileting and before eating. She should wear tight underpants during the treatment phase. She should change her underpants in the morning and at bedtime. She should have her bedding changed nightly. Recurrences are common.

6. *How will the diagnosis of pinworms affect the rest of the family?*
   The rest of the family may need to be treated simultaneously with mebendazole (Vermox). Handwashing will need to be emphasized because communicability is high. Towels, linens, and clothing need to be washed in hot water.

7. *Does Callie need follow-up for the pinworms?*
   Follow-up generally is not indicated. If symptoms are not gone in 3 weeks, Callie will need to return to the office or be in contact with the office.

8. *When should Callie return for another well-child exam?*
   Callie should return for a 6-year well visit.

REFERENCES

(1994). A checklist. School readiness for parents. *School Nurse News, 11*(4), 5.

Advisory Committee on Immunization Practices (2000). Recommended Childhood Immunization Schedule. Chicago, IL: American Academy of Pediatrics, and American Academy of Family Practice Physicians.

Boyton, R., Dunn, E., & Stephens, G. (1998). *Manual of ambulatory pediatrics* (4th ed.). Philadelphia: Lippincott.

Byrd, R. (1998). School readiness: More than a summer's work. *Contemporary Pediatrics, 15*(5), 39–40, 42, 44.

Byrd, R. (1999). Adherence to AAP guidelines for well child care under managed care. *Pediatrics, 104*(24), 536–540.

Cheng, T. (2000). Teaching prevention in pediatrics. *Academic Medicine, 75*(7 Suppl), S66–S71.

Davidson, R. (1993). Common intestinal parasites in American medical practice . . . part I. *Hospital Medicine, 29*(8), 43–50, 85–87.

Dershewitz, R. (1999). *Ambulatory pediatric care* (3rd ed.). Philadelphia: Lippincott.

Deutchman, M., Brayden, R., Siegel, C., Beaty, B., & Crane, L. (2000). Childhood immunization in rural family and general practices: Current practices, perceived barriers and strategies for improvement. *Ambulatory Child Health, 6*(3), 181–189.

Grossman, D. (2000). Firearm safety counseling in primary care pediatrics: A randomized, controlled trial. *Pediatrics, 106*(1), 22–26.

High, P. (2000). Literacy promotion in primary care pediatrics: Can we make a difference? *Pediatrics, 105*(4), 927–934.

LeBaron, C., Rodewald, L., & Humiston, S. (1999). How much time is spent on well child care and vaccination? *Archives in Pediatric Adolescent Medicine, 153*(11), 1154–1159.

Powell, E. (2000). Injury prevention using pictorial information. *Pediatrics, 105*(1), 16.

Robinson, D., Kidd, P., & Rogers, K. (2000). *Primary care across the lifespan.* St. Louis: Mosby.

Ronsaville, D., & Hakim, R. (2000). Well child care in the United States: racial differences in compliance with guidelines. *American Journal of Public Health, 90*(9), 1436–1443.

Shapiro, B. (1999). School readiness. In R. Dershewitz (Ed.), *Ambulatory pediatric care,* (3rd ed.). Philadelphia: Lippincott.

Stephens, G. (1994). Well child care. In R. Boyton, E. Dunn, & G. Stephens (Eds.), *Manual of ambulatory pediatrics* (3rd ed.). Philadelphia: Lippincott.

Wilson, D., & Knudtson, M. (1992). Assessing school readiness through the school-entry screening. *Nurse Practitioner: American Journal of Primary Health Care, 17*(9), 24, 26, 29.

Wright, C., Diener, M., & Kay, S. (2000). School readiness of low-income children at risk for school failure. *Journal of Children and Poverty, 6*(2), 99–117.

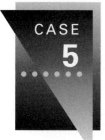

A 72-year-old man requesting an annual exam

SCENARIO

John Michaels is a 72-year-old African-American man who presents to the office for the first time to become an established patient of the practice. He has a history of mild hypertension, for which he takes hydrochloro-thiazide 25 mg/day, and hyperlipidemia, for which he takes atorvastatin (Lipitor) 20 mg/day. There are no other known health problems.

● TENTATIVE DIAGNOSES

Based on the information provided, what are the actual and potential diagnoses?

DIAGNOSIS	RATIONALE
1	
2	
3	

● HISTORY

What are significant questions to be addressed in John's history? Are there other questions or data that are important to know?

REQUESTED DATA   DATA ANSWER

REQUESTED DATA	DATA ANSWER
Allergies	None.
Current prescription and OTC medications	HCTZ, 25 mg/day. Atorvastatin calcium (Lipitor) 20 mg/day. Ibuprofen, 200 mg prn arthritis pain. Multivitamin.
Surgery/hospitalizations/ transfusions/trauma	None.
Immunizations	Up to date on all immunizations, tetanus, and flu shots. No pneumococcal vaccine or PPD.
Medical history	Reports history of usual childhood illnesses. Diagnosed with mild hypertension 15 years ago; well controlled for the past "several" years. Elevated cholesterol diagnosed 5 years ago and controlled with medication.
Adult illnesses	Walking pneumonia at age 55.
Family history	Father: died at 62 of cancer, "prostate or colon." Mother: died at 88, "old age." Brother: 68, alive with hypertension. Sister: 65, good health. Son: 43, hyperlipidemia. Daughter: 40, good health.
Personal/social history	Two grown children, a son and daughter. Retired electrical engineer with adequate income for comfortable retirement. Both wife and he have Medicare and supplemental insurance. Live in 2-bedroom apartment in an assisted living complex. Smoked 1 pack a day for 15 years; quit more than 40 years ago; occasional cocktail/beer/cola. No illicit drug use. Tries to walk around the complex (1/2 mile) at least 3 times a week. Participates in complex's activities with wife/others.
Appetite	Good; weight steady. Watches fat/salt intake.
24-hour dietary recall	B: cereal with banana, milk, artificial sweetener, orange juice, 2 cups coffee. L: turkey sandwich on bagel, salad, yogurt. D: grilled chicken breast, baked potato with low-fat margarine, broccoli, fruit compote.
Sleep patterns	Sleeps well, except gets up 2–3 times a night to urinate.

(continued)

REQUESTED DATA *DATA ANSWER*

Relationship with spouse	Married for 45 years; monogamous. Loving relationship with satisfactory sexual/intimate relationship.
Relationship with family	Recently moved to be closer to daughter, son-in-law, and grandchildren. Good relationship with son who lives approximately 1,000 miles away, see him 1–2 times a year.
Have you ever experienced chest pain, jaw/arm aching, diaphoresis, N & V, SOB?	Denies any cardiac symptoms. Has home BP monitoring kit; usually WNL.
Have there been any other urinary symptoms, other than nocturia, such as hesitancy, dribbling, incomplete emptying, urgency, dysuria?	Some hesitancy, incomplete emptying, dribbling. No dysuria, urgency.
Have you ever had PSA?	No.
Have you ever had a sigmoidoscopy/ colonoscopy?	No to both.
Last dental and eye exams?	Last eye exam 2 years ago; wears bifocals. Last dental exam 1 year ago.
Safety measures?	Grab bars in bathroom, bathtub seat, handheld shower, CO and smoke detectors, wall-to-wall carpet, daily check by complex staff, no guns. Wears seat belts 100% time.
Other difficulties that I should be made aware of?	None.

● PHYSICAL ASSESSMENT

What are the significant portions of the physical examination that should be completed for John? Identify the portions of the exam that you would do, along with the rationale for examining that system.

SYSTEM	RATIONALE	FINDINGS
Vital signs		BP, 142/82; HR, 84 bpm regular; Ht, 68 inches; Wt, 175 lbs.
General appearance		Well-nourished, well developed African-American man who appears his stated age and in no apparent distress. Alert and oriented ×3, affect appropriate.
Skin		Warm and dry w/o lesions.
HEENT		Normocephalic; external canals clear; TMs WNL; Rinne/Weber WNL. Vision 20/20 OU (corrected); EOMI. Disc margins sharp; no AV nicking or arterial narrowing. No sinus tenderness; buccal mucosa pink; dentition in good repair with multiple fillings noted.
Neck		No thyroid enlargement; no LA; no carotid bruits or JVD.
Cardiopulmonary		Cardiac: regular rate and rhythm @ 84; no S3 or S4; Gr II/VI midsystolic murmur w/o radiation. Lungs: Clear breath sounds with no added sounds.
Abdomen		Soft, flat, BS+; no HSM, masses, tenderness, bruits.
GU		Circumcised male; scrotum w/o lesions or masses.
Rectum		Prostate smooth, symmetrical, slightly enlarged, hemoccult negative. Neuromuscular DTRs 2+ bilaterally, and oriented ×3, strength/sensation intact. FROM; gait WNL; crepitus both knees.
Extremities		Peripheral pulses 2+; no edema.

● DIFFERENTIAL DIAGNOSES

What are the significant positive and negative data to support or refute your diagnoses for John?

DIAGNOSIS	POSITIVE DATA	NEGATIVE DATA
1		
2		
3		

● DIAGNOSTIC TESTS

Based on the history, physical exam, and your tentative diagnoses, what lab tests would you order? Identify the rationale for the tests that you would do, and interpret the tests done.

TEST	RATIONALE	RESULTS	INTERPRETATION
Coronary risk profile		Total cholesterol, 212 mg/dL; LDL, 140 mg/dL; HDL, 45 mg/dL; Triglycerides, 155 mg/dL; cholesterol/HDL ratio, 4.77.	
Electrolytes, renal, LFT's,		Glucose, 112 mg/dL; BUN, 17 mg/dL; creatinine, 1.3 mg/dL; Na, 143 mEq/L; K, 4.4 mEq/L; Cl, 101 mEq/L; CO_2, 27 mEq/L; total protein, 8.4 g/dL; albumin, 4.7 g/dL; Globulin, 3.9 g/dL; total bilirubin, 1.3 mg/dL; alkaline phosphatase, 89 U/L; AST, 42 U/L; ALT, 48 U/L.	
Electrocardiogram		Rate 72; PR, 12; QSR, 0.8.	
U/A		Leuk: negative. Nitrites: negative. Specific gravity: 1.020. Glucose: negative. Protein: negative. Urobilinogen: negative. pH: 5.2. Ketones: negative. Blood: negative.	
TSH		2.5 μU/mL.	
CBC		WBC, $5.9 \times 10^3/\mu L$; RBC, $5.03 \times 10^6/\mu L$; Hgb, 15.8 g/dL; HCT, 46%; MCV, 92.1 μm^3; Platelet count, 236,000/mm³;	

(continued)

TEST	*RATIONALE*	*RESULTS*	*INTERPRETATION*
		Neutrophils, 52.5%; Lymphocytes, 35.6%; Monocytes, 6.6%; Eosinophils, 2.2%; Basophils, 3.1%.	
Hemoccult		Negative.	
PSA		PSA, 2.5 ng/mL	
IPSS		16.	
Urinary flow, post void residual urine, urodynamics		Not done at this time.	

● DIAGNOSES

Identify the pathophysiology and data that support each diagnosis:
1.
2.
3.
4.

● THERAPEUTIC PLAN

1. *What plan will you develop for John related to his hypertension?*

2. *What plan will you develop for John related to his hyperlipidemia?*

3. *What plan will you develop for John related to his enlarged prostate?*

4. *What health promotion/disease prevention suggestions would you make for John?*

5. *How often should John be seen for follow-up?*

6. *What recommendations can you make to John and his family related to his diagnoses?*

7. *What community resources might be of assistance to John and his family?*

REFERENCES

Andel, G., Visser, A., Voogt, E., Kurth, E., & Goodkin, K. (2000). The influence of psychosocial factors on the measured quality of life (QoL) in patients suffering from benign prostate hyperplasia (BPH) and patients with prostate cancer. *Prostate Cancer and Prostatic Diseases, 3*(Suppl 1), 41–49.

Arai, Y, Aoki, Y., Okubo, K., Maeda, H., Terada, N., Matsuta, Y., Maekawa, S., & Ogura, K. (2000). Impact of interventional therapy for benign prostatic hyperplasia on quality of life and sexual function: A prospective study. *Journal of Urology, 164*(4), 1206–1211.

Bates, B. (1999). *Bates' guide to physical examination and history taking.*

Blanker, M., Bohnen, A., Groeneveld, F., Bersin, R., Prins, A., & Ruud, B. (2000). Normal voiding patterns and determinants of increased diurnal and nocturnal voiding frequency in elderly men. *Journal of Urology, 164*(4), 1201–1205.

Cookson, M. S., & Smith, J. A. (2000). PSA testing: Update on diagnostic tools. *Consultant, 40*(4), 670–676.

Heil, B. J. (1999). Treatment of benign prostatic hyperplasia. *Journal of American Academy of Nurse Practitioners, 11,* 303–310.

National Cholesterol Education Program. (1993, January). *Report of the expert panel on detection, evaluation, and treatment of high blood cholesterol in adults.* NIH Publication No. 89-2925. Bethesda, MD: US Government Printing Office. US Department of Health and Human Services, Public Health Service, National Institute of Health, National Heart, Lung, and Blood Institute.

National High Blood Pressure Education Program. (1997). *The sixth report of the Joint National Committee on Detection, Evaluation, and Treatment of High Blood Pressure.* NIH Publication No. 98-4080. Bethesda, MD: US Government Printing Office. US Department of Health and Human Services, Public Health Service, National Institute of Health, National Heart and Lung, and Blood Institute.

Report of the US Preventive Services Task Force. (1996). *Guide to clinical preventive services* (2nd ed.). Alexandria, VA: xxviii–xx, 89–99.

Stutzman, R. E. (1999). Bladder outlet obstruction. In L. R. Barker, J. R. Burton, & P. D. Zieve (Eds.). *Principles of ambulatory medicine* (pp. 605–615). Baltimore: Williams & Wilkins.

Uphold, C. R., & Graham, M. V. (1998). *Clinical guidelines in family practice* (3rd ed.). Gainesville, FL: 156–164, 464–471, 576–580.

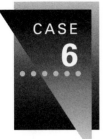

A 35-year-old woman with diffuse joint pain

SCENARIO

Sally Short presents to the office with diffuse joint pain that started a few months ago and has steadily gotten worse. She is having difficulty getting ready for work in the morning because of stiffness and is very tired by the end of the day. She has swelling in both hands and feet. She is married and has one child. She works part time as a nurse.

● TENTATIVE DIAGNOSIS

Based on the information provided, what are the potential diagnoses?

● HISTORY

What are significant questions in the history for Sally? What are the key areas to cover on the review of systems?

● PHYSICAL ASSESSMENT

What are the significant areas of the physical exam that should be covered?

● DIFFERENTIAL DIAGNOSES

What are the significant positive and negative data that support or refute your diagnoses for Sally?

● DIAGNOSTIC TESTS

Based on the history and physical assessment, what, if any, diagnostic tests would you do? Include your rationale for the tests.

● DIAGNOSIS

What diagnoses do you determine as being appropriate for Sally?

● THERAPEUTIC PLAN

What criteria are used to make the diagnosis?

What is the management plan?

Why is early aggressive treatment so critical?

What medications are available for treatment, and how do they work?

What impact does this disease have on function?

What is the role of exercise in the treatment?

What patient education should you provide to Sally?

When should Sally return for follow-up?

What referral criteria will you use?

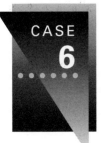

TUTORIAL

A 35-year-old woman with diffuse joint pain

SCENARIO

Sally Short presents to the office with diffuse joint pain that started a few months ago and has steadily gotten worse. She is having difficulty getting ready for work in the morning because of stiffness and is very tired by the end of the day. She has swelling in both hands and feet. She is married and has one child. She works part time as a nurse.

● TENTATIVE DIAGNOSES

What are the potential diagnoses you have identified based on this scenario?

DIAGNOSIS	RATIONALE
Viral infection	Acute polyarthritis may be a sequel to a viral infection, especially in a young woman. Although self-limited, viral arthropathies present with AM stiffness and systemic involvement of hands and wrists. Possible viral-induced etiologies include rubella, human parovirus B19, acute hepatitis B, HIV, and some enteroviruses.
Septic arthritis	This is a possible diagnosis that can not be missed. A missed diagnosis could lead to permanent disability. It usually presents with a single swollen, hot joint, but about 20% of adults have two or more large joints involved. Red flag.
Rheumatoid arthritis	Sally is a woman of child-bearing age, which fits the demographics. She presents with diffuse joint pain during a period of several months. She c/o of early AM stiffness and evening fatigue. Additional symptoms include bilateral, symmetrical joint swelling of the hands and feet. These symptoms fit the major criteria for the diagnosis of rheumatoid arthritis set by the American College of Rheumatology (ACR).

(continued)

DIAGNOSIS	RATIONALE
Psoriatic arthritis	Sally presents with pain and swelling of multiple joints. Often the arthritis symptoms can precede the onset of psoriasis. Self and family history of psoriasis is unknown. Additional symptoms could include psoriatic plaques, nail pitting, DIP joint involvement and spondylitis.
Systemic lupus erythematosus	Sally has a polyarticular presentation and complaint of fatigue. Would expect more symptoms of multisystem involvement, such as malar rash, fever, alopecia, pleurisy, or Raynaud's syndrome.
Fibromyalgia	More prevalent in women especially under age 50. Fatigue is a major complaint. It often is difficult to distinguish joint pain from muscle pain. Major criteria for diagnosis set by the American Rheumatism Society include fatigue, poor sleep, and 11 of 18 tender points.
Lyme disease	Likely diagnosis with a presentation of diffuse joint pain and swelling over a few weeks. We need to know if symptoms occurred after outdoor activities. There is greater suspicion if there was a tick bite, followed by a bulls-eye rash.
Bacterial endocarditis	May present with arthralgia. Should suspect if accompanied by symptoms of fever, heart murmur, and positive blood cultures.
Hypothyroidism	A possibility because fatigue is a presenting symptom. More common in women. Other symptoms include weight gain, irregular menses, dry skin, cold intolerance, and constipation.
Depression	Diagnosis of exclusion, which presents with depressed mood, loss of interest in usual activities, fatigue, and change in weight. Often it is difficult to determine if a symptom of depression or depression is secondary to the symptoms of a chronic disease.

● HISTORY

What are significant questions in the history for Sally?

REQUESTED DATA	DATA ANSWER
Allergies	PCN.
Current medications	BCP, MVI qd, and Advil every 4 hr for joint pain.
Surgery/transfusions	C-section x 1, no transfusions.

(continued)

REQUESTED DATA   DATA ANSWER

REQUESTED DATA	DATA ANSWER
Medical history and hospitalizations/ fractures/injuries/ accidents	Chicken pox, mumps, measles as a child. MVA 1 year ago, whiplash injury of neck.
OB/GYN history	LNMP 1 week ago; normal flow and duration. G1P1A0. Menarche, age 13. Last pelvic: 6 months ago, WNL. Mammogram: none. Sexually active, HX 3 partners—used barrier method. Monogamous relationship with husband, no barrier method used. Denies vaginal dryness, discharge, odor, or dyspareunia.
Appetite/weight change 24-hour recall	No changes in appetite. Loss of 10 lbs in last 2 months. B: Toast and coffee with milk. L: Turkey sandwich, fruit, coffee with cream. D: Meat, vegetable, starch, pop. S: Ice cream.
Family history	Father: age 60, good health. Mother: age 58, RA since age 45. HX osteoporosis. Sisters: 2, ages 31 and 33. Good health. Spouse: 36, good health Child: daughter, age 4, in good health. No family history of psoriasis, inflammatory bowel disease, or iritis.
Social history	No tobacco use. Drinks ETOH socially; wine 1–2 ×/wk. No recreational drugs. 2–3 cups of coffee/day. 2–3 colas. No regular exercise. Married 5 yrs; 1 child, 4 yrs old Immediate family assisting with child care since illness. Works part time as RN on cardiac unit.
Spirituality	Attends services regularly at a Catholic church.
Income/insurance/home	Husband works as mortgage loan originator, salary based on commission. Medical and dental insurance through husband's job. Own home, 2 story.
Stress management	Occasionally walks. Prayer. Enjoys crafts.
Functional status	Has difficulty with fine hand movement because of stiffness and swelling. Decreased strength makes opening jars and picking up child difficult. Dressing child and self becoming more difficult. Painful to walk distances, which has

(continued)

REQUESTED DATA   DATA ANSWER

	restricted activities, such as leisurely walks and shopping. Unable to do crafts because of pain. Fatigue alters energy level; too tired after work to do activities with child. Tries to make up time on days off. Naps 1–2 hr qd late afternoon. No libido related to fatigue. Family helping with housework and child care.
History of symptoms	Joint pain started a few months ago. Pain in 2nd, 3rd, and 4th MCP and PIP joints at intensity of "6–8" on a 1–10 pain scale. Has noticed swelling in the hands. Morning stiffness lasts up to 2 hours, relieved by hot shower in AM. Takes Advil every 4 hrs with minimal relief. Also has pain in the balls of both feet aggravated by walking. Some relief with rubbing them. Only wears flats; pain aggravated by heels. Rates pain at "8" on scale with pressure. Symptoms have gotten steadily worse over last several months. Starting to interfere with ADLs and lifestyle.
Recent travel	None. No camping, hiking or gardening.
Exposures	Minimal exposure to needles at work. Hospital switched to needleless system a few years ago.
ENT	Last eye exam: 1 year ago. No dryness, inflammation, or infection of eyes. Wears contacts; denies photosensitivity. Denies dysphagia, dry mouth, or oral lesions.
Skin	Dry, no rashes, lesions, or bits. No heat or cold intolerance.
Chest	Denies SOB, cough, or pain.
Cardiac	Denies chest pain or recent viral infections.
GU	No history of infections. Denies frequency, dysuria. Color of urine is yellow.
GI	No c/o of constipation or diarrhea. BM pattern once qd, formed, soft brown stool, and no blood.
Musculoskeletal	Pain and swelling in hands, wrists, elbows, and feet. No deformities. Decreased strength in hands. Decreased fine motor movement. Unable to walk distances because of pain in feet.
Neurological	No H/A, loss of memory. Denies tingling or numbness in extremities.
No recent sickness in family	

● PHYSICAL ASSESSMENT

What are the significant areas of the physical examination that should be completed for Sally?

SYSTEM	RATIONALE	FINDINGS
Vital signs	Baseline data. Elevated temp could indicate recent infection or inflammation.	T 98.6° F, HR, 60 regular, RR, 16; BP 100/60 rt. arm, sitting; Ht. 5′ 10″; Wt. 145 lbs.
General appearance/skin	Gives indication of overall status. Also can indicate nutritional status. Skin assessment can help to indicate specific rheumatic diseases.	Thin woman. Alert and oriented × 3. NAD. Skin warm and dry; color natural. No rashes, lesions, bites, or scratches. No pallor or jaundice. Nail beds: no clubbing or splinter hemorrhages.
HEENT	Dryness of eyes and oral cavity could indicate Sicca syndrome. It is important to check for lymphadenopathy to rule out viral infection or inflammatory disease	Eyes: No dryness, conjunctivitis, or infection. Hair: thick and evenly distributed. Throat: Positive gag reflex. MM pink and moist. No lesions. No lymphadenopathy. Thyroid nonpalpable, no masses.
Lungs	To rule out pulmonary problems, which can be a systemic manifestation of RA or SLE.	Chest symmetrical. No costochondral tenderness upon palpation. LCTA.
Cardiac	Quick screen for bacterial endocarditis or systemic manifestations of RA or SLE.	S1, S2 normal. No MRG. Apical pulse 60 and regular.
Abdomen	Quick screen because possible diagnosis is viral infection (hepatitis).	Flat, soft. BS all 4 quadrants. No hepatosplenomegaly. No tenderness or masses.
Musculoskeletal	C/o diffuse joint pain requires a complete musculoskeletal assessment.	Full ROM of neck and spine. No pain upon palpation of tender points (occiput, low cervical, trapezius, supraspinatus, 2nd rib, lateral epicondyle, gluteal, greater trochanter, or knee). Positive synovitis 2nd, 3rd, and 4th MCPs and PIPs bilaterally, warm and tender to palpation. No deformities. Decreased grip strength, R>L. Positive synovitis bilateral wrists, elbows, tender to palpation. Decreased extension 20 degrees both elbows.

(continued)

SYSTEM	RATIONALE	FINDINGS
		Full ROM shoulders, hips, knees, and ankles. No synovitis. Tender MTPs bilateral. Positive hallux valgus bilaterally. No nodules. Pulses 2+.
Neurological	Important to do for screening. Some diseases may present with neurological deficits, such as hypothyroidism or entrapment syndrome from joint swelling.	Alert and oriented. Gait, mild limp. Sensation intact. DTRs 2+. No asterexsis, negative Phalen's and Tinel's sign. See motor under musculoskeletal.
Rectal	Since c/o of fatigue should check stool for occult blood.	Sphincter tone firm, no masses or hemorrhoids. Light brown stool, guiac negative.

● DIFFERENTIAL DIAGNOSES

What are the significant positive and negative findings that support or refute your diagnoses for Sally?

DIAGNOSIS	POSITIVE DATA	NEGATIVE DATA
Viral-induced: hepatitis	Polyarthritis, AM stiffness involving hands and wrists. RN high-risk occupation.	No known exposure. Afebrile, no dyspnea, jaundice, hepatosplenomegaly or spider angiomata. Not preceded by an urticarial rash.
Viral-induced: HIV	Fatigue. High-risk occupation, sexually active, no barrier method. Arthralgias and wt. loss	No known exposure. No fever, night sweats, skin rashes/lesions, diarrhea, lymphadenopathy, or oral lesions. Negative candidiasis, cough, or SOB.
Viral-induced: parovirus B19	Polyarthralgias, symmetric involvement of MCP, PIP, and wrist joints. Morning stiffness.	Joint symptoms usually self-limited. No known exposure.
Septic arthritis	Swollen and warm joints (20% involve more than one joint). Joint pain worsened by palpation and movement.	Onset not acute, knees most commonly involved. No known risk factors of advanced age, coexistent joint disease, joint surgery, prosthetic joints, or IV drug use. No history of preexisting rheumatic disease. Not immunosuppressed. Highly unlikely.

(continued)

DIAGNOSIS	POSITIVE DATA	NEGATIVE DATA
Rheumatoid arthritis	Family history; female of child-bearing age. Symptoms for several months. C/o AM stiffness, fatigue, pain and swelling of hands and feet. Positive gelling, 10 lb. wt. loss in 2 months. Both passive and active range of joint motion limited; restricted movement through all ranges. Pain interferes with ADLs and lifestyle. Positive synovitis in 3 or more joints. Symmetrical presentation. Decreased grip strength, decreased extension of elbows. Tender MTPs, positive hallux valgus. Meets ACR criteria.	No deformities or rheumatoid nodules. Afebrile. Negative synovitis shoulders; knees, hips, and ankles with full ROM.
Psoriatic arthritis	Peak age of onset 30–55 yrs. Caucasian female. Pain and swelling in multiple joints, insidious onset, symmetrical, involves small joints of hands, wrists, elbows, and feet. Arthritis can precede the onset of psoriasis.	No personal or family HX of psoriasis. No DIP arthralgia, nail pitting, or onycholysis. Negative psoriatic lesions or claw or paddle deformities of hands. Negative enthesitis or dactylitis of a digit or toe (sausage appearance).
Systemic lupus erythematous	Tenderness of 2 or more peripheral joints, swelling, fatigue, and wt. loss. Female, age 35. SLE can present with only arthritis.	No family history. No malar (butterfly) rash or discoid rash; negative photosensitivity. No multisystem symptoms such as pleuritic pain, pericardial rub, seizures, and renal problems. Negative alopecia, lymphadenopathy, splenomagaly. Sensation intact.
Fibromyalgia	Female, age 35, whiplash injury 1 year ago. Has diffuse pain both sides of the body and above and below the waist. Fatigue is a major c/o.	No tender points upon exam; no axial skeletal pain or proximal pain. Symptoms present for less than 3 months; no wt. gain.
Lyme disease	In early disease c/o of fatigue and arthralgias. Late disease has polyarthrialgia.	Not living in endemic area, no recent travel or exposure, and no recall of tick bites. No recent camping, hiking, or gardening. Negative erythema migrans, negative neuropathy with sensation intact.

(continued)

DIAGNOSIS	POSITIVE DATA	NEGATIVE DATA
		No lymphadenopathy, cardiac, or neurological symptoms.
Bacterial endocarditis	C/o arthralgias.	No fever, back pain, heart murmur, or splinter hemorrhages in nail beds.
Primary hypothyroidism	Female, c/o fatigue, stiffness, and decreased libido.	Negative cold intolerance, dry skin, hair loss, or constipation. Normal menses and no wt. gain. Thyroid nonpalpable. Age younger than 40.
Depression	Fatigue, decreased libido, and wt. loss.	No self or family history of depression. Continues to have interest in activities; no episodes of crying or sadness. Denies change in appetite. No recent crisis.

● DIAGNOSTIC TESTS

Based on the history and physical exam, what, if any, diagnostic tests would you obtain? Interpret test results.

DIAGNOSTIC TEST	RATIONALE	RESULTS	INTERPRETATION
CBC with differential	Provides information regarding hematocrit and hemoglobin (H&H) for anemia, as well as WBC for information about possible infection. H&H will be low with anemia, and WBC will be elevated with infection.	Hgb, 11.0 g/dL. Hct, 33%. MCH, 30. WBC, 6,800 /mm^3. RBC, 4.4 million/mm^3	H&H are low, and MCH is normal. This indicates a normocytic anemia, which often is seen in a chronic inflammatory disease. The WBC is normal, so there is no infection or immunosuppression, and no viral infection.
Erythrocyte sedimentation rate (ESR)	Increased in inflammation. Not a definitive test but will indicate inflammation. Level correlates with the	ESR, 80 mm/HR.	Indicates some inflammation is present.

(continued)

DIAGNOSTIC TEST	RATIONALE	RESULTS	INTERPRETATION
	degree of synovial inflammation. Useful in following the course of inflammatory activity and evaluating effectiveness of treatment.		
C-reactive protein (CRP)	A nonspecific, acute-phase reactant. Diagnoses infectious diseases and inflammatory disorders, such as acute rheumatic fever and RA. Levels do not consistently rise with viral infections. A more rapid and sensitive indicator than the ESR of acute inflammatory change.	CRP, 1.2 μg/mL.	Indicates some inflammation is present.
Rheumatoid factor (RF)	Order when RA is suspected. Does not establish diagnosis of RA; can be positive with SLE, bacterial endocarditis, or viral infection. Is found in 70%–80% of those with RA. The higher the titer, the more likely the diagnosis of RA.	RF, 1:300.	Does not establish the diagnosis of RA, but a high level gives high suspicion.
Antinuclear antibody (ANA)	Used to diagnose SLE. Positive results occur in 95% of those with SLE, but many other rheumatic diseases are associated with positive ANA.	Negative.	A negative ANA excludes diagnosis of SLE.
Thyroid screen	Elevated TSH with hypothyroidism. Free T4 will be low in hypothyroidism.	TSH, 4.0 μU/L. T4, 1.8 μg/dL.	WNL.

(continued)

DIAGNOSTIC TEST	RATIONALE	RESULTS	INTERPRETATION
Creatinine	Elevation could indicate multisystem disease such as SLE. Also done to check renal function before treatment with NSAIDs.	CR, 0.8.	WNL.
Urinalysis	Order if multisystem disease is suspected. Can be done to assess organ dysfunction caused by comorbid disease before starting drug therapy.	Not done.	
Hepatitis B & C serology	Order if abnormal results of liver function tests, symptom of splenomegaly.	Not done.	
Parovirus serology	Only if high suspicion of viral disease	Not done.	
Lyme serology	Only if high suspicion of Lyme disease.	Not done.	
Liver function tests	To rule out hepatitis. Also to get baseline before starting drug therapy, especially DMARDs.	ALT, 25 IU/L. AST, 15 IU/mL.	WNL.
Alkaline phosphatase	Get if weakness or muscle pain is present.	102.	WNL.
Albumin	Does have weight loss as a symptom; can help to determine nutritional status. Only 10 lb. loss in 2 months.	Not done.	
HIV	To rule out HIV infection. High-risk job and previous multiple partners.	Negative.	
Synovial fluid analysis	Do if effusion is present. Usually used to evaluate monoarthritis or febrile patient with established arthritis.	Not done.	

(continued)

DIAGNOSTIC TEST	RATIONALE	RESULTS	INTERPRETATION
Radiographs	Not helpful if new diagnosis of RA or SLE because earliest changes are nonspecific. May see only tissue swelling and periarticular osteoporosis, which are absent on initial presentation. Symptoms for less than a year.	Not done.	
Stool guiac	H&H low. Rule out GI disease.	Negative.	No loss of blood through GI tract.

● DIAGNOSIS

What diagnoses do you determine to be appropriate after a review of the subjective and objective data?

The data support the diagnosis of rheumatoid arthritis (RA), which is a systemic, inflammatory disorder characterized by a symmetrical polyarthritis, as presented here. Sally fits the demographics of a person with RA: female, age 35 years. RA affects 2 to 3 times more females than males. A positive family history of Sally's mother having RA supports the possible genetic predisposition to the disease. "It is estimated that the first degree relative of a person with RA has about a 16-fold increased risk over the general population" (Klippel, Weyand, & Wortmann, 1997, p. 155).

RA is an autoimmune disease in which some areas of the immune system are overactive. Lymphocytes gather in the lining of the affected joints, resulting in inflammation, which contributes to cartilage damage and bone erosion. Certain cytokines, tumor necrosis factor (TNF), and interleukin-1 (IL-1) have been identified as key players in the inflammatory response and disease progression.

The etiology remains unknown. The possibility of a bacterial or viral cause has been vigorously pursued, especially after several infectious agents, such as Parovirus, Rubella virus, and Lyme virus, were found to induce chronic arthropathy as a symptom. "All efforts to associate an infectious agent with RA by isolation, electron microscopy, or molecular biology have failed. It is possible that there is no single primary cause of RA and that different mechanisms may lead to the initial tissue injury and precipitate synovial inflammation" (Kippel et al., 1997, p.156). The cause is most likely a complex interaction between genetic and environmental factors.

The subjective and objective data support the diagnostic criteria of the American College of Rheumatology (ACR). These include the following: joint pain for > 3 months, morning stiffness for > 60 minutes, symmetrical presentation, synovitis in > 3 joints, extra-articular manifestations of weight loss and fatigue, and a positive result of rheumatoid factor test. The lab data of increased ESR, positive RF, and mild hypochromic-microcytic anemia are not diagnostic but are supportive of the diagnosis of RA.

● THERAPEUTIC PLAN

1. What criteria are used to make the diagnosis of RA?

CRITERION	DEFINITION
1. Morning stiffness	Morning stiffness in and around the joints, lasting at least one hour before maximal improvement.
2. Arthritis of 3 or more joint areas	At least 3 joint areas simultaneously have had soft tissue swelling or fluid (not bony overgrowth alone). The 14 possible areas are right or left PIP, MCP, wrist, elbow, knee, ankle, and MTP joints.
3. Arthritis of hand joints	At least one area swollen (as defined above) in a wrist, MCP, or PIP joint.
4. Symmetric arthritis	Simultaneous involvement of the same joint areas (as defined in 2) on both sides of the body (bilateral involvement of PIPs, MCPs, or MTPs is acceptable without absolute symmetry).
5. Subcutaneous nodules	Subcutaneous nodules over bony prominences, or extensor surfaces, or in juxtaarticular regions.
6. Serum rheumatoid factor	Demonstration of abnormal amounts of serum rheumatoid factor by any method for which the result has been positive in <5% of normal control subjects.
7. Radiographic changes	Radiographic changes typical of rheumatoid arthritis on posteroanterior hand and wrist radiographs, which must include erosions or unequivocal bony calcifications localized in or most marked adjacent to the involved joints (osteoarthritis changes alone do not qualify).

[Reprinted from Arnett, F.C., Edworthy, S.M., Bloch, D.A., et al. (1988). The American Rheumatism Association 1987 revised criteria for the classification of rheumatism arthritis. *Arthritis and Rheumatism, 31,* 313–324. Reprinted with the permission of the American College of Rheumatology.]

For classification purposes, a person shall be said to have RA if he/she has satisfied at least four of these seven criteria. Criteria 1 through 4 must have been present for at least 6 weeks. Patients with 2 clinical diagnoses are not excluded. A designation of classic, definite, or probable RA is not to be made.

2. *What is the management plan for Sally's diagnosis?*
   The goals of therapy are to relieve pain, control inflammation, preserve function, and prevent joint destruction. The clinician needs to determine the severity of disease activity and synovitis, structural damage, and impact on functional and psychological status. Sally's disease is early Stage I, so the initial treatment should be a NSAID and possible systemic oral steroid therapy. The oral steroid can help to confirm the diagnosis if swelling responds immediately and also can act as a bridge therapy until the NSAID takes effect. The choice of NSAID is based on patient's medication history, other existing disease, and age. NSAIDs inhibit the synthesis of pro-inflammatory prostaglandins, thus controlling inflammation and pain. There is no evidence they alter the course of the disease. A common practice is to try several different NSAIDs during a 3- to 4-week period to find one that gives the best results with the fewest adverse effects. GI and renal toxicity are of concern, so complete blood cell counts, liver and renal function tests, and stool guiac analysis should be done every 4 months.

   Cox 2 inhibitors, a new class of drug on the market, can be used if the patient is at high risk of GI complications. The Cox 2 inhibitors work by inhibiting cyclooxygenase-2 without affecting cyclooxygenase-1, an enzyme that primarily protects the stomach lining. The main advantage of the Cox 2 inhibitors is they are less likely to cause GI problems, such as ulcers and bleeding. In addition, a disease-modifying antirheumatic drug (DMARD), which does change the course of the disease, can be administered. Start with a medication with low toxicity, such as hydroxychloroquine or sulfasalazine.

   Patient education should begin early. Pamphlets are available from the Arthritis Foundation. Because Sally is having some difficulty with her activities of daily living, an occupation therapy (OT) and physical therapy (PT) consultation can be helpful. An occupational therapist can show Sally different ways to do daily activities to protect her joints; make splints to relieve inflammation, decrease joint trauma, and improve alignment; and provide adaptive equipment, as needed. A physical therapist can provide Sally with an exercise routine to help her maintain joint mobility, strength, and flexibility; water exercise is especially useful in such a program because it puts little stress on the joints.

3. *Why is early aggressive treatment so critical?*
   Joint destruction occurs early, especially within the first year of diagnosis. Within 3 years, 70% of patients show radiographic damage. "Rheumatoid arthritis is one of the most common causes of disability. After 12 years of disease, more than 80% of patients with RA are partially disabled, and 16% are completely disabled" (Matteson, 2000). Because joint destruction contributes to this disability and is most pronounced within the first year, early aggressive therapy with DMARDs is essential for preventing severe disability. The PCP or NP often is the patient's first contact with the medical system, so

such clinicians must understand the importance of early diagnosis and immediate aggressive treatment.

4. *What medications are available for treatment, and how do they work?*
There are now five classes of medications used in the treatment of RA. They include NSAIDs, Cox 2 inhibitors, steroids, DMARDs, and biologic response modifiers. The NSAIDs are the cornerstone of therapy. They have an anti-inflammatory and analgesic effect, but there is no evidence they alter the course of the disease. The Cox 2 inhibitor drug Celebrex can be used instead of an NSAID if the patient has GI side effects or is at high risk for GI complications.

Steroids are recommended for short-term therapy during a flare-up or as bridge therapy until the DMARDs start to work, usually within 4 to 6 weeks. Most studies have failed to demonstrate that systemic steroids alter the natural history of RA. They should be used with extreme caution because of their multiple side effects. Intraarticular steroids can be used if one or two isolated joints are inflamed. Local injections to the joint should be limited to three a year to prevent joint destruction.

The optimum time to start treatment with DMARDs remains a matter of controversy. It is recommended to start early because these agents have been shown to improve function; decrease synovial inflammation; and slow, prevent, or heal structural joint damage. Hydroxychloroquine, methotrexate, and sulfasalazine were most commonly viewed by a surveyed group of 200 rheumatologists as "appropriate" initial DMARDs. In this same survey, 64% of the rheumatologists chose methotrexate as first-line therapy. The ACR recommends that patients with early RA be evaluated for treatment with DMARDs. Treatment should not be delayed beyond 3 months in any patient with an established diagnosis who continues to have the symptoms of joint pain, morning stiffness, fatigue, and active synovitis despite treatment with NSAIDs.

In recent years, several new agents have been introduced for the treatment of RA. Leflunomide (Arava), etanercept (Enbrel), and infliximab (Remicade) recently were approved by the United States Food and Drug Administration for the treatment of RA. Leflunomide inhibits the pathway for synthesis of pyrimidines and interferes with the cell cycle progression in immune cells. It is taken by mouth daily. A loading dose of 100 mg 3 times a day is begun, then 20 mg every day. Etanercept and infliximab both interfere with tumor necrosis factor (TNF), which is a potent proinflammatory cytokine implicated in the pathogenesis of RA. Etanercept 25 mg is given 2 times a week by subcutaneous injection, and infliximab 3 mg/kg is given by intravenous injection in an initial dose and repeated at 2 weeks and 6 weeks and then every 8 weeks. The drawbacks to the use of these drugs is that symptoms may resurface if drug therapy is discontinued, and these agents are expensive.

5. *What impact does this disease have on function, and what are the criteria for classification of functional status?*
Pain, morning stiffness and fatigue all can contribute to decreased function. Timing of activities is critical to promote improved function. De-

creased strength can make simple tasks, such as holding a cup, pouring coffee, opening jars, or lifting a child, difficult. Decreased range of joint motion, depending on the joint involved, can make dressing, reaching, or fine motor movements a challenge. Sally had no joint deformities, which also can contribute to decreased function. The American College of Rheumatology set revised criteria for classification of functional status in RA in 1991.

The criteria for classification of functional status are as follows:

"Class I: Completely able to perform usual activities of daily living (self-care, vocational, and avocational)

Class II: Able to perform usual self-care and vocational activities, but limited in avocational activities.

Class III: Able to perform usual self-care activities, but limited in vocational and avocational activities.

Class IV: Limited in ability to perform usual self-care, vocational, and avocational activities"

Usual self-care activities include dressing, feeding, bathing, grooming, and toileting. Avocational (recreational and/or leisure), and vocational (work, school, homemakimg) activities are patient desired and age and gender specific. [Hochberg MC, Chang RW, Dwosh I, Lindsey, S., Pincus, T., & Wolfe, E. (1992). The American College of Rheumatology 1991 revised criteria for the classification of global functional status in rheumatoid arthritis. Arthritis and Rheumatism, 35, 498–502.

6. *What is the role of exercise in the treatment of RA?*
   The role of exercise is very important. Exercise can help decrease weight or maintain ideal body weight to take the strain off weight-bearing joints. A mere 10-lb weight loss can relieve the stress on the knee joints. Weight-bearing exercises should be encouraged to prevent osteoporosis for this population that is at high risk. A regular exercise program that includes flexibility, strengthening, and aerobic exercises lessens fatigue, builds stronger muscles and bones, increases flexibility, improves stamina, and improves general health and sense of well being. After 2 to 3 months of exercise, most patients report less pain, anxiety, and depression. Strong muscles help to support the joints by improving stability and absorbing shock. Range of joint motion improves circulation and provides nutrition to the joint. Improved flexibility reduces the risk of sprains and strains. During a flare-up, it is recommended to rest more and protect the inflamed joints, but after the flare-up is over, exercise should be resumed. It is recommended that patients plan their exercise routines with their physician or NP.

7. *What education should you provide to Sally?*
   The education should include knowledge about the disease, medications and their side effects, lab follow-up, exercise program, maintaining or losing weight, pain management, joint protection, energy conservation, relaxation techniques, risk factors, the use of calcium supplements to prevent osteoporosis, and psychological support.

8. *When should Sally return for follow-up?*
   Sally should follow up in several weeks because it usually takes several weeks for the NSAID to produce maximal effect. She will need to have lab work done every 2 months because she is taking a DMARD. It takes several months for a DMARD to work, so a steroid can be given as a bridge medication.

9. *What referral criteria will you use?*
   Referral criteria would include the following:

   suspected septic arthritis
   undiagnosed multisystem or systemic rheumatic disease
   musculoskeletal pain undiagnosed after 6 weeks
   musculoskeletal pain not adequately controlled with treatment
   progressive loss of function
   suspect active tendon/muscle rupture
   pregnant or post-partum patient
   undiagnosed synovitis
   consider steroid or immunosuppressive therapy

10. *What community resources are available for the NP and Sally?*
    The Arthritis Foundation offers many programs, such as:

    support groups,
    PALS program,
    arthritis self-help course,
    exercise programs, such as People with Arthritis Can Exercise (PACE)
        and swim programs at the YMCA and local swimming pools

The Arthritis Foundation also offers pamphlets on the disease, medications, and management of the disease. The group offers many resources for health care professionals, such as educational programs. The group's website is *www.arthritis.org.*

REFERENCES

American College of Rheumatology Ad Hoc Committee on Clinical Guidelines. (1996). Guidelines for the initial evaluation of the adult patient with acute musculoskeletal symptoms. *Arthritis and Rheumatism, 39,* 1–8.

American College of Rheumatology Ad Hoc Committee on Clinical Guidelines. (1996). Guidelines for the management of rheumatoid arthritis. *Arthritis and Rheumatism, 39,* 713–722.

American College of Rheumatology Ad Hoc Committee on Clinical Guidelines. (1996). Guidelines for monitoring drug therapy in rheumatoid arthritis. *Arthritis and Rheumatism, 39,* 723–731.

Barker, L.R., Burton, J.R., & Zieve, P.D. (1999). *Principles of ambulatory medicine* (5th ed.). Baltimore: Williams & Wilkins.

Ensworth, S. (2000). Rheumatology: 1. Is it arthritis? *Canadian Medical Association Journal 162*(7), 1011–1016.

Goldring, S. R. (2000). A 55-year-old woman with arthritis. *Journal of the American Medical Association, 283,* 524–531.

Klinkhoff, A. (2000). Rheumatology: 5. diagnosis and management of inflammatory polyarthritis. *Canadian Medical Association Journal, 162,* 1833–1838.

Klippel, J. H., Weyand, C. M., & Wortmann, R. L. (1997). *Primer on the rheumatic diseases* (11th ed.). Atlanta: Arthritis Foundation.

Lorig, K., & Fries, J. F. (2000). *The arthritis helpbook* (5th ed). Cambridge: Perseus Books.

Matteson, E. L. (2000). Current treatment strategies for rheumatoid arthritis. *Mayo Clinic Proceedings, 75,* 69–74.

Mikuls, T. R., & O'Dell, J. (2000). The changing face of rheumatoid arthritis therapy: Results of serial surveys. *Arthritis and Rheumatism, 43,* 464–467.

Pagana, K. D., & Pagana, T. J. (1999). *Mosby's diagnostic and laboratory test reference* (4th ed.). St. Louis: Mosby.

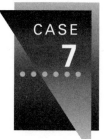

A 5-year-old girl presenting with fatigue, pallor, and fever

SCENARIO

Grace Matthews presented to the NP in the middle of January with complaints of fever and ear pain, at which time she received a diagnosis of OM and was placed on a 10-day course of amoxicillin/ clavulanic acid (Augmentin). On January 27, Grace returned the NP for continued complaints of ear pain and was referred to an ENT. The ENT placed Grace on Gantrisin for 2 months. On February 23, Grace returned to the NP because of fever, pallor and fatigue.

● TENTATIVE DIAGNOSES

What are the potential diagnoses you have identified based on the scenario provided?

DIAGNOSIS	RATIONALE
1	
2	
3	
4	

● HISTORY

What are significant questions in the history for Grace? Are any important data missing?

REQUESTED DATA   DATA ANSWER

REQUESTED DATA	DATA ANSWER
Allergies	NKDA.
Immunizations	Up to date.
Current medications	Gantrisin for OM. Occasionally acetaminophen (Tylenol) or ibuprofen (Motrin) for fever, ear pain.
Surgeries/transfusions	None.
Medical history and hospitalizations/ fractures/injuries/ accidents	Chicken pox at 3 years of age. No hospitalizations, fractures, injuries, or accidents. Normally healthy with a history of 6 OM infections.
Prenatal history	39-week gestation. Normal vaginal delivery. No complications.
Appetite/weight changes	No change in weight. Appetite a little less than baseline.
Family history	Father: 39 years, good health. Mother: 33 years, good health. Sisters: 8 years, good health; 15 years, good health. Brother: 2 years, good health. No family history of anemia, cancer.
Diet history	Eats a good variety of foods, especially fruits and vegetables.
Social history	Usually active, playful. Involved in soccer.
Length of symptoms	History of fever on and off during past 1–2 months. History of OM, with referral to ENT at the end of first month secondary to continued complaints of ear pain and history of 6 OM infections. Grace was started on Gantrisin for resolution of OM and prophylactically per ENT. Approximately 2–3 weeks later, Grace returned to their private medical doctor with complaints of fever plus fatigue and pallor that had increased during the past 2 weeks.
How have symptoms affected ADLs?	During febrile periods, decreased activity and appetite. During past few weeks, decreased play activity secondary to fatigue.

(continued)

REQUESTED DATA   DATA ANSWER

Any evidence of blood loss (epistaxis, stool, urine, bleeding gums)?	No history of epistaxis, bleeding gums, or blood in urine or stool.
Any increase in bruising or any rash? Jaundice?	No increase in bruising. No rash. No jaundice.
Any recent illness with family members?	None.

● PHYSICAL ASSESSMENT

What are the significant portions of the PE that should be completed for Grace?

SYSTEM   RATIONALE   FINDINGS

SYSTEM	RATIONALE	FINDINGS
Vital signs		T (oral), 99.6 °F; BP, 103/70 mm Hg RUE; HR, 82 bpm; RR, 24; Ht, 44 inches; Wt, 40 lbs.
General appearance/skin		Alert, tired-appearing, NAD. Skin warm and dry. Color pale pink. No jaundice noted. Petechial rash noted to posterior area of lower legs bilaterally. No ecchymosis noted.
HEENT		Normocephalic. No sinus tenderness. Neck supple; no LA. Eyes sclera and conjunctiva clear bilaterally. Dark circles noted under eyes bilaterally. TMs pearly gray and WNL. Nose pink with septum midline. Mouth with oral mucosa moist, pink and intact. Posterior pharynx without erythema, exudate, or sores/lesions. Uvula midline.
Lungs		CTA bilaterally with good aeration noted throughout.
CV		RRR, S1, S2 WNL, no murmur.
Abdomen		BS × 4 quadrants, soft, NT, ND. No HSM noted. No LA noted.
Extremities		MAE × 4. Pedal pulses 2 + bilaterally. Cap. refill < 2 sec. No edema noted.
GU		No LA or obvious bleeding noted. Perirectal area intact, without erythema or sores noted.
Neurological assessment		Alert, oriented. Gait steady. DTRs 2 + bilaterally.

● DIFFERENTIAL DIAGNOSES

What are the significant positive and negative findings that support or refute your diagnoses for Grace?

DIAGNOSIS	POSITIVE DATA	NEGATIVE DATA
1		
2		
3		
4		
5		
6		
7		

● DIAGNOSTIC TESTS

Based on the history and physical exam, what, if any, diagnostic testing would you obtain?

TEST	RATIONALE	RESULTS	INTERPRETATION
CBC with differential		2/23 results: WBC, 2.7 × 10³/µL; Hgb, 9.5 g/dL; HCT, 26.5%; platelets, 117,000/mm³; RBC, 3.19 × 10⁶/µL; MVC, normal; MCH, normal; MCHC, 35.8 g/dL; 41% neutrophils; 23% bands; 45% lymphocytes; 5% monocytes; 9% eosonophils; 0.1% basophils.	

(continued)

TEST	RATIONALE	RESULTS	INTERPRETATION
Electrolytes, renal panel, liver function test		Na, 142 mEq/L; K, 4.2 mEq/L; Cl, 100 mEq/L; CO_2, 25 mEq/L; glucose, 75 mg/dL; BUN, 8 mg/dL; creatinine, 0.5 mg/dL; AST, 18 U/L; ALT, 20 U/L; alkaline phosphatase, 108 U/L.	
Monospot		Negative.	
Iron studies (Fe, ferritin, and TIBC)		Not done.	
CXR		Not done.	
Hep BsAg		Not done.	
HIV		Not done.	
Bone marrow aspiration and biopsy		Not done.	

● DIAGNOSIS

What diagnosis do you determine as being appropriate after a review of the subjective and objective data? What data support your diagnosis(es)? Discuss the pathophysiology pertaining to the diagnosis.

● THERAPEUTIC PLAN

1. When should Grace be followed up again?

2. Are there any limitations on Grace's activities?

3. What education should the parents have regarding Grace and the potential for this to occur in the future?

4. What are medications that can depress the CBC?

REFERENCES

Abramson, N., & Melton, B. (2000). Leukocytosis: Basics of clinical assessment. *American Family Physician, 63.* Available online: http://www.aafp.org/afp/20001101/2053.html.

Bates, B., Bickley, L. S., & Hoekelman, R. A. (1995). *A guide to: Physical examination and history taking* (6th ed.). Philadelphia: J. B. Lippincott Company.

Cook, L. S. (2000). A simple case of anemia: Pathophysiology of a common disease. *Journal of Intravenous Nursing, 23*(5), 271–281

Deglin, J. H., & Vallerand, A. H. (Eds.). (1998). *Nurse's med deck* (6th ed.). Philadelphia: F. A. Davis Company.

Fox, J. A. (Ed.). (1997). *Primary health care of children.* St. Louis: Mosby.

Greene, H., Johnson, W., & Lemcke D. (1998). *Decision making in medicine* (2nd ed.). St. Louis: Mosby.

Mayo Clinic. (2000). Anemia. *Mayo Clinic Health Letter, 18*(9), 4–5.

Mitus, A., & Rosenthal, D. (1995). History and physical examination of relevance to the hematologist. In R. Handlin, S. Lux, & T. Stossel (Eds.), *Blood: Principles and practice of hematology.* Philadelphia: Lippincott.

Phipps, W. J., Long, B. C., Woods, N. F., & Cassmeyer, V. L. (Eds.). (1991). *Medical-surgical nursing: Concepts and clinical practice* (4th ed.). St. Louis: Mosby Year Book.

Robinson, D., Kidd, P., & Rogers, K. (2000). *Primary care across the lifespan.* St. Louis: Mosby.

Shapiro, M. F., & Greenfield, S. (1987). The complete blood count and leukocyte differential count. An approach to their rational application. *Annals of Internal Medicine, 106,* 65–74.

Thomas, C. L. (Ed.). (1993). *Taber's cyclopedic medical dictionary* (17th ed.). Philadelphia: F. A. Davis Company.

Uphold, C. R., & Graham, M. V. (Eds.). (1998). *Clinical guidelines in family practice* (3rd ed.). Gainesville, FL: Barmarrae Books.

Young, G., Toretsky, J., Campbell, A., & Eskenazi, A. (2000). Recognition of common childhood malignancies. *American Journal of Family Practice, 63.* Available online: http:// www.aafp.org/afp/20000401/2144.html.

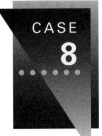

A 75-year-old woman with confusion and incontinence

SCENARIO

Mrs. Emmitt is a 75-year-old Native American woman who presents with recent confusion. She is accompanied by her daughter. Mrs. Emmitt is neatly dressed in her "Sunday best" dress. She is pleasant, talkative, and easily distracted. She relates she is not having much trouble with her HTN medicines and says she believes it is important to take them. When engaged in small talk about current events, Mrs. Emmitt states, "I don't pay much attention to those things anymore." When asked who is the current president, she responds "there was no one like Ike. Those were the good old days." She states she doesn't get out much anymore. She stopped driving "because of the traffic" and got lost in town on more than one occasion. Her daughter reports that she used to play bridge but had lost interest in that, in part because club members had complained about her not being able to keep up with the game. Mrs. Emmitt admits to feeling lonely. Her daughter has helped with the shopping ("My arthritis really has been acting up" for the last years) and does the bills ("my eyes aren't as good as they used to be"). The daughter says her mother usually has a great memory and can remember things way back but has a tendency to repeat stories from years ago. The daughter adds lately her mother seems more confused; for example, she has been calling her in the middle of the night talking about a long-dead relative. This morning, when her daughter went to check on her, she discovered that her mother was incontinent, with soiled clothing and bed linens. This had not happened before.

● TENTATIVE DIAGNOSIS

Based on the information provided, what are potential differential diagnoses? What are possible differential diagnoses for changes in cognitive status?

● HISTORY

What are significant questions in the history for Mrs. Emmitt and her daughter? What are the key points to cover on the review of systems?

● PHYSICAL ASSESSMENT

What are the significant portions of the physical examination that should be completed for Mrs. Emmitt?

● DIFFERENTIAL DIAGNOSES

What are the significant positive and negative data that support or refute your diagnoses for Mrs. Emmitt?

● DIAGNOSTIC TESTS

Based on the history and physical assessment, what, if any, diagnostic testing would you do. Include your rationale for the testing.

● DIAGNOSIS

What diagnoses do you determine as being appropriate for Mrs. Emmitt?

● THERAPEUTIC PLAN

1. *What might be the family's response to the diagnosis of Alzheimer's disease?*
2. *What treatments are available for dementia?*
3. *What are suggestions the NP could make in terms of family support for on-going care?*
4. *What are home safety issues that need to be discussed?*
5. *At what point will Mrs. Emmitt's family know she is unable to care for herself?*
6. *What suggestions can you make so Mrs. Emmitt does not feel so lonely?*
7. *What community resources might be helpful to the NP and Mrs. Emmitt and her family?*
8. *Discuss how the plan of care might need to be readjusted and revised as the dementia progresses.*

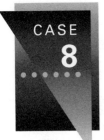

TUTORIAL

A 75-year-old woman with confusion and incontinence

SCENARIO

Mrs. Emmitt is a 75-year-old Native American woman who presents with recent confusion. She is accompanied by her daughter. Mrs. Emmitt is neatly dressed in her "Sunday best" dress. She is pleasant, talkative, and easily distracted. She relates she is not having much trouble with her HTN medicines and says she believes it is important to take them. When engaged in small talk about current events, Mrs. Emmitt states, "I don't pay much attention to those things anymore." When asked who is the current president, she responds "there was no one like Ike. Those were the good old days." She states she doesn't get out much anymore. She stopped driving "because of the traffic" and got lost in town on more than one occasion. Her daughter reports that she used to play bridge but had lost interest in that, in part because club members had complained about her not being able to keep up with the game. She admits to feeling lonely. Her daughter has helped with the shopping ("my arthritis really has been acting up for the last years") and does the bills ("my eyes aren't as good as they used to be"). The daughter says her mother usually has a great memory and can remember things way back but has a tendency to repeat stories from years ago. The daughter adds lately her mother seems more confused; for example, she has been calling her in the middle of the night talking about a long-dead relative. This morning, when her daughter went to check on her, she discovered that her mother was incontinent with soiled clothing and bed linens. This had not happened before.

● TENTATIVE DIAGNOSIS

What are the potential diagnoses you have identified based on the scenario provided?

DIAGNOSIS   RATIONALE

DIAGNOSIS	RATIONALE
Change in cognitive status: dementia	Dementia is a change in mental status characterized not only by declining memory but also by declining functional capabilities, visual-spatial difficulties, and/or language impairment (AHCPR, 1996). Patient presents a history of getting lost, vague answers, and dodges specific information, especially about recent events. Long-term memory can be preserved for some time as a dementing process continues. Note the change in level of functioning before this onset of acute confusion. Caregivers can be the best source of information about the functional and mental status of the patient. The transfer of ADLs can occur gradually, and the extent of this transfer may not be fully realized by the caregiver. The reason this transfer has occurred can be blamed on arthritis, diminished vision, etc.
Change in cognitive status: delirium	Abrupt onset of change in mental status, abrupt onset of confusion, and urinary incontinence are clues to a delirium. By definition, delirium is an abrupt change in mental status characterized by inattention, disorganized thinking, an altered level of awareness and a fluctuating course. Delirium has many causes or precipitating events, including infections, cardiac events, transient ischemic attack, medication side effects, electrolyte imbalance, alcohol intoxication, and other medical problems.
Change in cognitive status: depression	Loss of friends or loss of independence may be causes for a dysphoric or depressed state. Depression can present itself as a state of less alertness or apathy or even as a change in the mental status of an elder.
HTN	By history.

What are possible differential diagnoses for changes in cognitive status?

DIFFERENTIAL DIAGNOSES   RATIONALE

DIFFERENTIAL DIAGNOSES	RATIONALE
Dementia: Alzheimer vs vascular type	80% of dementias are thought to be Alzheimer type, whereas about 10% are thought to be of a vascular type (Geldmacher & Whitehouse, 1996). The clinical presentation can be very similar, both having a progressive decline. Some types of dementia may be partially reversed, for example those caused by polypharmacy. Even in irreversible dementias, the problematic symptoms such as wandering can be treated with some success (AHCPR, 1996)

(continued)

DIFFERENTIAL DIAGNOSES	RATIONALE
Delirium: Hyper/hypothyroidism	Hyper/hypothyroidism are common findings in the elderly. They may present as a change in mental status or loss of interest in usual activities.
Delirium re: nutritional deficiencies	Eating alone and the changes in the ability to taste and chew food may result in inadequate nutrition. Prolonged nutritional deficiencies may affect cognition.
Delirium re: anemia	Changes in mental status may indicate an anemia. Mrs. Emmitt states she has arthritis. If she is taking OTC NSAIDS for her arthritis pain she may have an asymptomatic GI bleed.
Delirium re: electrolyte imbalance	Changes in mental status can be triggered by electrolyte imbalances. Her anti-HTN medicine may cause electrolyte imbalances
Delirium re: UTI	Sudden changes in mental status may indicate an infectious process. UTIs are common in elderly women for a variety of reasons. The sudden incontinence may reflect a deteriorating mental status but also may reflect the presence of an UTI. Certainly, dehydration, change in hormonal levels, and inattention to personal hygiene may contribute to the likelihood of an UTI.
Delirium re: cardiac event	Abrupt changes in mental status and functioning may indicate a cardiac event such as a MI, CHF, or arrhythmia. The patient may be unable to describe events surrounding such an event.
Delirium re: neurological event	Abrupt changes in mental status and functioning may indicate a neurological event, such as a transient ischemic attack or CVA.
Delirium re: Medication side effects	Multiple medications, complicated dosing schedules, and continuing medications beyond therapeutic necessity all contribute to medication errors, drug interactions, and increased side effects.

● HISTORY

1. What are significant questions in the history for Mrs. Emmett?

REQUESTED DATA	DATA ANSWER
Allergies	Sulfa breaks out in hives per daughter.

(continued)

REQUESTED DATA *DATA ANSWER*

REQUESTED DATA	DATA ANSWER
Current medications	HCTZ, 25 mg QD. BenGay analgesic rub. Multivitamin (Centrum Silver) per daughter.
Surgery/transfusions	Cataract surgery, 1992. Hysterectomy, 1950s reason unknown. No transfusions.
Medical history and hospitalizations/ fractures/injuries/ accidents	Hospitalized for hysterectomy. Pneumonia, 1960s. No fractures, injuries.
Adult illness	HTN; diverticulosis; cataracts.
Ob/Gyn history	G1P1A0. Never used hormones. Unknown last Papanicolaou smear or pelvic exam. Never had mammogram; doesn't examine breasts.
Appetite	Usually about 140 lbs, wore size 12. Has lost 10 lbs during last 6 months. Appetite decreased; food doesn't taste as good anymore.
24-hour diet recall	"Oh, you know—the usual."
Typical day	Up at 7; light breakfast; "putters around the house" rest of day.
Social history	Finished high school, had one year of secretarial school. Worked as housewife and mother. Now lives alone; daughter lives in town. Lives in single-story home, 5 steps. Never used tobacco or alcohol. Three cups of coffee ("good strong coffee") a day.
Family history	Father: died when she was young. Mother: died of old age. Older brother: fine (daughter states in nursing home with Alzheimer's). Health of younger siblings is unknown. "I think they are in California." Daughter: fine.
Relationship with spouse, children, lifelong friends	Widow "for a while now." Feels close to daughter and grandchildren. Doesn't see old friends as often as she used to.
Prevention/ immunizations, sigmoid, exercise, diet, eye, hearing, dentist	Can't state last physical, mammogram, or pelvic exam. Not sure if she took the flu shot last year. Gets "plenty of exercise house cleaning." Had dentures and glasses for a "long time."

(continued)

REQUESTED DATA   DATA ANSWER

ADLs and IADLs	Set the stove on fire last week making coffee. Dresses, bathes, toilets self (usually, until the crises of yesterday). Ambulates independently. For the last several years, daughter helps with meal planning, shopping, paying the bills, and arranging transportation.

2. What are the key points on the review of systems?

SYSTEM REVIEWED   DATA ANSWER

General	Acute confusion, agitation noticed yesterday: did not know day. Agitated; reassurance helped, but essentially the same today.
Cardiac	No SOB, chest pain, or pressure.
Neurological assessment	"Memory pretty good for my age." No H/A, dizziness, LOC, or syncope. Tripped once and fell, no injury.
GU	Some burning, and frequency—started yesterday. Hasn't felt well for a while. Denies previous incontinence or UTIs.
Musculoskeletal	"Good days and bad days—doesn't everyone?"
Sensory	Unable to further clarify.

● PHYSICAL ASSESSMENT

What are the significant portions of the physical examination that should be completed for Mrs. Emmitt?

SYSTEM	RATIONALE	FINDINGS
Vital signs	Provide baseline data	BP 180/74 mm Hg sitting; HR, 80 bpm; RR, 20; T, 98.8 °F; Wt, 112 lb; Ht, 5'4".
General appearance/skin	A complete exam is warranted for Mrs. Emmitt due to the complexity of the symptoms, their interrelatedness, and the fact that patient is a poor historian.	Pale scattered keratosis; bruise left forearm; skin looks fragile.

(continued)

SYSTEM	RATIONALE	FINDINGS
HEENT	Observe for neuro deficits; factors that would indicate nutritional deficiencies; factors indicating problems with eating; general state of hydration; and factors that can be addressed, ie, poor vision/cataracts so orientation can be facilitated.	Ear: TMs opalescent. Funduscopy: Unable to visualize due to cataracts. VA: can read magazine. Peripheral vision via confrontation: deferred, unable to follow instructions. Mouth: mucosa dry, no lesions. Edentulous. Neck: no NVD, supple.
Lungs	Observe for presence of adventitious lung sounds that may indicate acute or chronic disease that may influence oxygenation and therefore delirium, such as pneumonia.	CTA.
Heart	Observe for rhythm disturbance, rate abnormalities, cardiomegaly, and new murmurs. Recent changes may cause delirium, for example, atrial fibrillation with slow rate may cause syncope, etc.	Regular rate and rhythm. S1, S2 WNL. 2/6 systolic murmur at the sternal border radiating to the right, heard best sitting. No carotid bruits.
Breast	Done as part of general survey. Breast cancers may metastasize to the brain but would most likely show as a focal neurological deficit, rather than dementia/ delirium seen here.	Symmetrical, no masses, no axillary nodes, no d/c.
Abdomen	New complaints of urinary incontinence, questionable hydration and food intake, unreliable historian means a complete abdominal exam should be done.	BS+, soft, nondistended, slight suprapubic tenderness, no masses, no rebound tenderness, no HSM.
Pelvic	A complete exam is warranted because of the urinary incontinence.	Atrophic vaginal tissues, no d/c or urine leakage with exam. Urine strong smelling. No lesions, pale cervix, stenosed os, no adnexae tenderness.

(continued)

SYSTEM	RATIONALE	FINDINGS
Rectal	Part of a general exam to observe for hydration, constipation, hemoccult for signs of GI bleeding (taking OTC NSAIDs).	Tight sphincter, hard stool in vault, no masses, hemorrhoidal tags.
Extremities	Observe for signs of impaired circulation, injury, ability to care for nails.	Pulses 2+, no edema, no varicosity.
Neurological assessment	A complete exam is warranted to rule out focal neurological deficits, gait abnormalities, neuropathies related to circulatory or nutritional deficits.	CN I–XII intact, gait wide based, small steps, decreased step height, hand grasp equal bilaterally. General muscle strength +3/5 upper and lower extremities. Unable to lift bag of groceries (approx. 10 lb). Sensation intact; unable to determine joint position sense or vibratory sense. DTRs 3+ bilaterally. Babinski negative bilaterally.
Mental	A complete exam is warranted to identify mental status deficits (more than merely deficits in orientation) (Strub & Black, 1993).	Folstein minimental exam: 19/30. Deficits in short-term memory, orientation, attention, and calculation.

● DIFFERENTIAL DIAGNOSES

What are the significant positive and negative findings that support or refute your diagnoses for Mrs. Emmitt?

DIAGNOSIS	POSITIVE DATA	NEGATIVE DATA
Delirium	Sudden increase in confusion as exhibited by incontinence, inattention.	May be a progression of dementia.
Dementia	+FH of Alzheimer's, progressive inability to do IADLs, vague answers, Folstein score.	None. UTI symptoms may exaggerate the presentation of cognitive deficits, but the presence of these deficits precedes the new complaint of urinary problems.

(continued)

DIAGNOSIS	POSITIVE DATA	NEGATIVE DATA
Depression	Loss of companionship, lack of interest in life and food.	Assessment colored by illness presentation.
UTI	Sudden incontinence, foul-smelling urine, increased frequency and burning, suprapubic tenderness, constipated.	Afebrile
HTN	Elevated systolic blood pressure, +FH of heart problems, unknown daily BP control, SEM.	Unknown daily BP; may have "white coat" HTN.
Cardiac event/failure	Long history HTN.	RRR, lungs clear, no SOB, no HSM, no NVD, no edema.
Transient ischemic attack	Sudden confusion, HTN, episode not directly observed, unreliable historian.	No focal deficits.
Nutritional deficiencies, dehydration	Dry skin and oral mucosa, unknown food and fluid intake patterns. HCTZ, unknown time frame for weight loss.	
Hyper/hypothyroidism	Dry skin, decreased appetite, age, female, agitation.	VS, DTRs normal.
Medication side effects	HCTZ prescribed, unknown compliance patterns.	Taking HCTZ for years.

● DIAGNOSTIC TESTS

Based on the history and physical examination, what, if any, diagnostic testing would you obtain?

It is unlikely that any laboratory result or other diagnostic procedure will identify correctable causes of dementia. Thus, although these tests generally are to be ordered for demented persons, the likelihood of a positive result is less than 10% (Geldmacher & Whitehouse, 1996). Obviously, Mrs. Emmitt has other physiological illnesses that make these tests advisable.

DIAGNOSTIC TEST	RATIONALE	RESULTS	INTERPRETATION
U/A	Good choice to determine UTI. May consider C & S, but since that is not recurrent, may choose to empirically treat with nonsulfa drug.	Color: dark yellow. Leukocytes: large. Nitrites: positive. Bilirubin: negative. Blood: moderate. pH: 4.5. Protein: negative. SG: 1.030.	Indicates the presence of a urinary tract infection.
Electrolytes, renal, liver (multichem analysis)	Because nutritional intake is essentially unknown and electrolyte imbalances can cause a change in mental status, a good choice. Mrs. Emmitt is taking a K-depleting diuretic, although in unknown frequencies and amounts.	Na, 135 mEq/L; K+, 3.4 mEq/L; Cl, 108 mEq/L; CO_2, 25 mEq/L; BUN, 25 mg/dL; creatinine, 1.3 mg/dL; ALT, 35 U/L; AST, 27 U/L; alkaline phosphatase, 40 U/L; glucose, 76 mg/dL.	Slightly low K+. All others normal.
CBC with differential	Good choice. Mrs. Emmitt is pale and has some degree of peripheral neuropathy. This test would show anemia may be contributing to their present state. In addition, if an infection is present, you might see changes in the WBC count.	RBC, 5.2 million/mm^3; Hgb, 14 g/dL; MCV, 85 fl; MCH, 1.75 fmol; MCHC, 37%; WBC, 11,000/mm^3; Segs, 60%; Basos, 0; Bands, 4%; Eos, 2%; Monos, 4%; Lymphs, 28%; Platelets, 220,000 /mm^3.	Elevated WBC possibly related to her incontinence and UTI symptoms.

(continued)

DIAGNOSTIC TEST	RATIONALE	RESULTS	INTERPRETATION
B_{12} and RBC folate	Good choice for determining nutritional status and the presence of pernicious anemia.	Folate, 320 ng/mL; B_{12}, 500 pg/mL.	WNL.
TSH, thyroid panel	Hypothyroidism in the elderly may present as a cloudiness of sensorium without the usual signs seen in younger people. Since TSH is the most sensitive test, the thyroid panel would be ordered only if the TSH is low.	TSH, 4.0 mU/L; T4, 8.0 g/dL; T3, 158 ng/dL; Free thyroxine index, 10.0.	WNL.
CT or MRI of head	Expensive but can show any lesions, areas of infarction, presence of subdural hematoma that may explain the changes in mental status, especially if the changes are abrupt. The MRI may better identify areas of ischemia not detected by the CT. MRI may be used when the individual has a focul neurological deficit.	No areas of infarction can be seen. No ischemia noted; brain atrophy, no focal lesions.	Early Alzheimer's disease may show temporal lobe atrophy on CT scan or MRI, but cerebral atrophy correlated more with advancing age than mental status decline.

(continued)

DIAGNOSTIC TEST	RATIONALE	RESULTS	INTERPRETATION
Geriatric Depression Scale	Good choice to quantify and open discussion of feelings. Suggest this done after mental status returns to baseline. Depression can make the dementia seem worse.	13/30 on scale.	Mild depression. This test may be delayed until present delirium lifts.
Neurocognitive testing	May more precisely define areas of deficits, especially judgment, visual spatial, construction, and intelligence.	Not done at this time. Will plan to do once acute illness has improved. (Test shows decline in visual spatial skills, judgment and abstraction.)	
CXR	Will help determine the size of her heart, presence of pulmonary lesions or tumors, CHF or pneumonia.	Slight cardiomegaly, atherosclerosis of aorta, osteoporosis, no masses, no acute disease.	WNL.
Rapid plasma reagin	Latent syphilis may present as dementia	Nonreactive.	WNL. This test may not be covered by insurance carriers.
HIV	Dementia is not a common presenting symptom in HIV infection, but there is an HIV dementia. Mrs. Emmitt does not have any known risk factors.	Not done.	N/A.

(continued)

DIAGNOSTIC TEST	RATIONALE	RESULTS	INTERPRETATION
EEG Electroen-cephalogram	Not routinely ordered for dementia but may be helpful in identifying coexisting seizure disorder.	Not done.	N/A.
Genetic testing (apollipoprotein E4)	May be available, but because its value as a diagnostic or predictive test has not been established, do not recommend its use in general practice now (Geldmacher & Whitehouse, 1996).	Not done.	N/A.

● DIAGNOSES

What diagnoses do you determine as being appropriate after a review of the subjective and objective data?

- Delirium, most likely related to UTI
- Dementia, type not determined but probably Alzheimer type or multi-infarct

Data Supporting the Diagnosis

Delirium: The description of incontinence, supra-pubic tenderness, foul smelling urine in addition to positive U/A suggests an acute delirium related to UTI. Clearing the infection may return Mrs. Emmitt to or near her baseline demented state.

Dementia: The Folstein mini-mental ADL suggests a dementing process that has been progressing slowly over the years. Mrs. Emmitt has a cognitive decline greater than merely memory loss. She is unable to care for herself, take care of financial obligations, or drive. The reasons given for stopping these activities should be carefully ascertained. Positive FH and gradual progression of the illness support the tentative diagnosis of Alzheimer's disease, but given Mrs. Emmitt's long-standing history of HTN, she may have a multi-infarct type of illness. Alzheimer's accounts for 70% of dementia, with multi-infarct or vascular dementia accounting for 10% to 20% of dementia (Geldmacher & Whitehouse, 1996). This diagnosis can be made only after other causes of dementia have been excluded, such as alcohol abuse, AIDS, neurosyphilis, previous head trauma, or other medical problems.

● THERAPEUTIC PLAN

1. What might the family's response be to the diagnosis of Alzheimer's disease?
At first the family may deny that the confusion seen is a continuation of an ongoing dementia. They may deny that this is true or cry at the loss of their mother as they knew her. It is frightening to project to the future knowing that their mother/grandmother may not recognize them and to the real possibility of her inability to care for herself in the future.

2. What treatments are available for dementia?
The drugs tacrine (Cognex) and donepezil (Aricept) have shown some efficacy in the treatment of mild to moderate Alzheimer's disease. These drugs do not change the fundamental brain deterioration that is taking place but enhance cognitive function in a percentage of patients with Alzheimer's disease. Tacrine has been on the market for a longer period of time. It requires close monitoring of liver enzymes and QID dosing. Donepezil requires no laboratory monitoring for adverse effects and is dosed once a day. It must be understood that all patients are not a candidate for these medicines (for example, patients with severe Alzheimer's) and that results will vary.

Clinical trials continue to find medications that retard or even reverse the progression of Alzheimer's disease. Herbs such as gingko biloba and antioxidants such as vitamin E and selegiline may have some modest benefit in slowing the progression. Nonsteroidal anti-inflammatory agents and postmenopausal estrogen replacement may prevent the onset or progression of Alzheimer's disease, but prospective studies have not confirmed these anecdotal findings.

3. What are suggestions the NP could make in terms of family support for ongoing care?
Discuss the availability of support groups and home health care, as well as respite services in the area. Suggest *The 36 Hour Day* as a resource for tips on caring for someone with dementia.

4. What are home safety issues that need to be discussed?
Issues such as cooking safety, firearm safety, environment modification, a fire plan, and how to call for help all should be discussed with Mrs. Emmitt and her family. Suggest telephone reassurances and a life-call program, if available.

5. At what point will Mrs. Emmitt's family know she is unable to care for herself?

It is important to discuss planning for continued care before a patient needs a high level of care that can be provided in the home. Making arrangements for 24-hour in-home care or transfer to some type of institutional living can take time. Waiting for an emergency to begin planning can only lead to frustration.

6. *What are suggestions you can make so Mrs. Emmitt does not feel so lonely?*
Programs such as Meals on Wheels, adult daycare, and supervised senior activities might be helpful in providing companionship and cognitive stimulation for Mrs. Emmitt. Because she previously enjoyed people, she may enjoy getting out of the house.

7. *What are community resources that might be helpful to the NP, Mrs. Emmitt, and her family?*
   • Social workers/elder services: Provide identification of community, financial, and insurance resources, assistance with referral home care agencies, and help in obtaining higher levels of care (nursing home placement) as the need arises.
   • Home health agencies: Provide in-home personal and nursing care, such as bathing assistance, medication setup, BP monitoring, and nursing observations
   • Chaplain/parish nurse: Provide spiritual support for the patient and family. May be aware of volunteers who are able to visit or call.
   • Alzheimer Association and support groups: Provide information and support from those whose families who have similar problems
   • Geriatric evaluation team: Provides comprehensive evaluation of medical problems and mental status. Usually part of a medical school. Aware of new treatments or approaches that may be beneficial.
   • Area Office on Aging: Provides listing of governmental programs for the elderly available in the area.
   • Attorney: Provides assistance in legal matters, such as assigning a power of attorney.
   • Web and organization references:

     Alzheimer's Association
     Chicago, IL
     1-800-272-4380
     http://www.alz.org

     Alzheimer's Disease Education and Referral Center
     Silver Spring, MD
     1-800-438-4380
     http://www.alzheimers.org

     Administration on Aging
     Washington, DC
     206-619-1006
     http://www.aoa.dhhs.gov

Eldercare Locator
Washington, DC
1-800-677-1116
http://www.aoa.dhhs.gov/elderpage/locator.html

American Association of Retired Persons (AARP)
Washington, DC
1-800-424-3410
http://www.aarp.org

Family Caregivers Alliance Website
http://www.caregiver.org

8. *Discuss how the plan of care might need to be readjusted and revised as the dementia progresses.*
This family will need ongoing care and support as they struggle with the demands of deterioration in cognitive abilities. The rate of progression can not be predicted for any individual. Periodic re-evaluation of mental and functional status is needed. Episodic illness may have a prolonged effect; the patient may never quite return to baseline functioning. The needs of Mrs. Emmitt and her family are likely to be dynamic. Families vary in their ability and willingness to care for a loved one with altered mental status. Some graciously accept the challenge, whereas for others it is an overwhelming situation. It is not unusual for one member of the family to be selected by the family to shoulder the greater share of the responsibility. The re-alignment of roles and responsibilities is stressful. The focus of care can shift from the patient to the family, as they are educated and supported during this illness process.

REFERENCES

Agency for Health Care Policy and Research (AHCPR). (1996). *Clinical practice guideline: Recognizing and initial assessment of Alzheimer's and related dementias.* Publication Number 97-0702 (1-800-358-9295).

Brännström, B., Tibblin, Å., & Löwenborg, C. (2000). Counseling groups for spouses of elderly demented patients: A qualitative evaluation study. *International Journal of Nursing Practice, 6*(4), 183–191.

Cohen-Mansfield, J., Golander, H., & Arnhein, G. (2000). Self-identity in older persons suffering from dementia: Preliminary results. *Social Science and Medicine, 51*(3), 381–394.

Geldmacher, D., & Whitehouse, P. (1996). Evaluation of dementia. *New England Journal of Medicine, 335*, 330–336.

Hendryx-Bedalov, P. M. (2000). Alzheimer's dementia: Coping with communication decline. *Journal of Gerontological Nursing, 26*(8), 20–24, 52–53.

Hoffman, S., & Platt, C. (1991). *Comforting the confused.* New York: Springer.

Mace, N., & Rabins, P. (1981). *The 36 hour day.* Baltimore: Johns Hopkins University Press.

Miller, L. L., Nelson, L. L., & Mezey, M. (2000). Comfort and pain relief in dementia: Awakening a new beneficence. *Journal of Gerontological Nursing, 26*(9), 32–40, 55–56.

Reichel, W., & Rabins, P. (1995). Evaluation and management of the confused, disoriented or demented elderly patient. In W. Reichel (Ed.), *Care of the elderly* (pp. 142–154, 4th ed.). Baltimore: Williams and Wilkins.

Richards, S., Emsley, C., Roberts, J., Murray, M., Hall, K., Gao, S., & Henrie, H. (2000). The association between vascular risk factor-mediating medications and cognition and dementia diagnosis in a community-based sample of African-Americans. *Journal of the American Geriatric Society, 48,* 1035–1041.

Schneider, G., Kruse, A., Nehen, H., Serf, W., & Henft, G. (2000). The prevalence and differential diagnosis of subclinical depressive syndromes in inpatients 60 years and older. *Psychotherapy and Psychosomatics, 69*(5), 251–260.

Steele, C. (2000). The genetics of Alzheimer. *Nursing Clinics of North America, 35*(3), 687–694.

Strub, R., & Black, F. (1993). *The mental status examination in neurology.* Philadelphia: F.A. Davis.

Williams, I. (2000). What help do GPs want from specialist services in managing patients with dementia? *International Journal of Geriatric Psychiatry, 15*(8), 758–761.

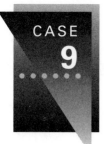

CASE

9

A 36-year-old woman with amenorrhea

Kathleen Andrews presents to the health center with a history of amenorrhea of 2 months' duration. She is married and has no children. She is a partner in an architectural firm, where she works full time.

● TENTATIVE DIAGNOSES

Based on the information presented, what are potential differential diagnoses?

DIAGNOSIS   **RATIONALE**

1.

2.

3.

4.

5.

6.

7.

● HISTORY

What are significant questions in the history for Kathleen? Identify why the information is important to know at this visit.

REQUESTED DATA	DATA ANSWER
Allergies	NKA.
Current medications	Multivitamin daily. Sodium levothyroxine (Synthroid) 0.025 mg daily. No other medications.
Surgery/transfusions	Tonsillectomy, 12 years; appendectomy, 22 years; hemorrhoidectomy, 28 years.
Medical history/ hospitalizations/ fractures/injuries	Chicken pox, mumps, and measles as child. No injuries or fractures.
Immunizations	Believes all vaccinations are up to date. Has had Hepatitis B vaccine series (completed 2 years ago), TB screen 2 years ago. Does not remember date of last tetanus shot.
Adult illness	History of hypothyroidism (since age 22 years).
Ob/Gyn history	Menarche, age 12 years. LNMP: 8 weeks ago, normal flow and duration. Cycles irregular during past 3 years due to Depo-Provera for birth control. Last pelvic: approximately 6 months ago. History of abnormal Pap smear (mild inflammation) 6 months ago. Did not return for second smear. Last injection of Depo-Provera 11 months ago. No birth control method at present, although couple used condoms "sometimes." Possibility of pregnancy is not a problem for her. She and her husband were ready to actively attempt pregnancy. Mammogram: none. BSE: Monthly. Therapeutic abortion, age 18 years.
Appetite/weight change	No changes in appetite. Has lost 2 pounds in the past month; otherwise weight has remained stable over the past years. Attempts to maintain low-fat diet; however she and her husband resort to eating fast food approximately 2 nights per week because of busy work schedules.

(continued)

REQUESTED DATA *DATA ANSWER*

Social history	European American ancestry. Tobacco: never. Alcohol: one 8-ounce glass red wine every evening. Caffeine: 4–5 cups coffee/day. 2–3 colas/day. Drugs: none. Exercise: Works out at gym 4 times per week; weights and treadmill for 1 hour. Has done this for the past 5 years. No history of physical or sexual abuse.
Husband's medical/ surgical/social history	Husband is of Jewish ancestry but raised as a Protestant. Adopted, so he is unsure of his complete medical history. He is in good health. No genetic or familial diseases of which he is aware. His parents are both in good health, as is he. He goes to the gym with her 4 times a week. He does not smoke but does drink occasionally, not to excess. He had a bicycle accident as a child and was hospitalized with a broken leg; otherwise unremarkable history. Enjoys playing golf on the weekend with his father and brother. Ht, 5′ 10″; Wt, 170 lbs; Age, 38 years.
Social organizations	Unity Church, Eastern Star; active in both organizations
Relationship with husband	Husband is active in Masonic Lodge. Both are monogamous. Married 9 years. They have sex about 2 times a week, satisfying. Husband is junior partner in a law firm. They have not been attempting pregnancy, but he agrees with her that if she becomes pregnant, they will both be happy.
Relationship with family	She and her husband value their time together. They have enjoyed traveling together in the United States and abroad. They share numerous activities together, including gardening and gourmet cooking. Close to both her parents and her husband's parents, who live in the same town. Sees brother only occasionally because he lives 1,000 miles away.
Income/insurance/home	She and her husband earn upper-level incomes. Both jobs are secure. Still paying for school loans. Medical and dental insurance through husband's job. They own their home.
Length of symptoms	Amenorrheic for 2 months. Now experiencing nausea and breast tenderness. Her greatest concern is "feeling tired all the time, even though I get 10 hours sleep at night."
How has this affected your ADLs?	The tiredness becomes acute in the afternoon, so she nearly falls asleep at her desk. Has to take a nap when she arrives home after work, sometimes missing going to the gym. Nausea has recently begun, occurs most when she arises in the morning.

(continued

REQUESTED DATA   DATA ANSWER

REQUESTED DATA	DATA ANSWER
How do you manage stress?	Enjoys exercising in the gym and working in the garden. When she and her husband feel stressed, they sometimes have a "getaway" for the weekend. Both have stressful jobs.
Any recent vaginal infections or pelvic pain?	No recent infections. Diagnosed with chlamydia at age 18 years.
Have you traveled recently?	Last traveled to Cancun 2-1/2 months ago. Before that, traveled to Europe 2 years ago. Other traveling inside the United States.
Has she had any recent tattoos or body piercing procedures?	Ears pierced (twice), 3 years ago and 15 years ago. No tattoos.
Any exposure to toxins or chemicals at work or home	She has used some pesticides containing pyrethrums in the garden. No other known exposure.
Regular screenings	Dental every 6 months, last exam 5 months ago; ophthalmologic exam every 2 years, last exam 1 year ago; wears contact lenses. Annual well-woman exam; last exam 6 months ago. PPO pays for dental, Gyn and ophthalmologic exams.

● PHYSICAL ASSESSMENT

What are the significant portions of the physical examination that should be completed for Kathleen?

SYSTEM   RATIONALE   FINDINGS

SYSTEM	RATIONALE	FINDINGS
Vital signs		BP 118/68 mm Hg right arm; HR, 80 bpm; RR, 20; T, 98.6 °F; Ht, 5' 4"; Wt, 128 lbs.
General appearance/skin		Alert, NAD. Skin warm and dry. No lesions noted. No pallor or jaundice.
HEENT		Normocephalic, no sinus tenderness, TMs pearly and WNL. Nose pink and moist with septum midline; oral mucosa moist and pink. Uvula midline. No pharyngeal erythema or oral lesions noted. No LA; supple neck. Thyroid nonpalpable; no masses. No dental caries readily seen.
Lungs		Clear to auscultation

(continued)

SYSTEM	RATIONALE	FINDINGS
Heart		No murmurs noted.
Abdomen		BS present × 4, soft, no splenomegaly. No liver enlargement noted. No tenderness on palpation.
Neurological assessment		Alert and oriented; gait normal. Strength/sensation intact. DTRs 2+. No liver flap.
Pelvic exam		Uterus enlarged to 6 to 8 weeks' size. No tenderness in uterus or adnexal areas on bimanual exam. No lesions; no unusual discharge noted. Pap smear performed. Clear cervical mucus noted. Cervix closed.
Breast exam		Breast tenderness present bilaterally; no masses or LA noted. No discharge noted.
Extremities		Pulses 2+. No edema noted.

● DIFFERENTIAL DIAGNOSES

What are the significant positive and negative findings that support or refute your diagnoses for Kathleen?

DIAGNOSIS	POSITIVE DATA	NEGATIVE DATA
1		
2		
3		
4		
5		
6		
7		

● DIAGNOSTIC TESTS

Based on the history and physical examination, what, if any, diagnostic testing would you obtain? What is your rationale for the testing? What do the test results mean?

DIAGNOSTIC TEST	RATIONALE	RESULTS	INTERPRETATION
Urine HCG		Positive.	
Wet mount of vaginal discharge		No WBCs, clue cells, yeast, or trichomonas seen.	
Rubella titer		Rubella titer, 1:3.	
RH/ABO		AB negative	
Pap smear		Endocervical.	
Thyroid screen		TSH, 4.6 µU/mL.	
CBC		Hgb, 12 g/dL; HCt, 38%.	
HIV		Negative.	
Syphilis serology		Negative.	
Gonorrhea & chlamydia cultures		Negative.	
Vaginal ultrasound		Positive gestational sac; 7-week size.	
Urinalysis		Negative.	

● DIAGNOSES

What diagnoses do you determine as being appropriate after a review of the subjective and objective data?

Data Supporting the Diagnosis

● THERAPEUTIC PLAN

1. How is amenorrhea classified?

2. *What influence does the cause of amenorrhea have on therapeutic treatment plan?*

3. *What will the management of Kathleen's pregnancy consist of?*

4. *When should Kathleen be referred to a specialist and to whom?*

5. *What patient education should you discuss with Kathleen?*

6. *What impact does this pregnancy have in terms of her continuing work?*

7. *What suggestions can you make for Kathleen for her symptoms of early pregnancy?*

8. *When should Kathleen return for her next prenatal visit?*

9. *What are community resources that are available for the NP and Kathleen?*

REFERENCES

Bungum, T., Peaslee, D. Jackson, A., & Perez, M. (2000). Exercise during pregnancy and type of delivery in nulliparae. *JOGNN, 29,* 258–264.

Callister, L. C. (2000). Toward evidence-based practice. Perceived impediments to prenatal care among low-income women. *American Journal of Maternal Child Nursing, 25*(3), 166.

Corbett, J. V. (1996). *Laboratory tests & diagnostic procedures.* Stamford, CT: Appleton & Lange.

Crichton, M. A. (1997). Assessment of needs model in midwifery practice. *British Journal of Midwifery, 5*(6), 330, 332–334.

Dixon, D., Cobb, T. G., & Clarke, R. W. (2000). The first prenatal visit. *Clinician Reviews, 10*(4), 53–66, 71–74, 77–78.

Hauth, J. C., Goldenberg, R. L., Andrews, W. W., DuBard, M. B., & Copper, R. L. (1995). Reduced incidence of preterm delivery with metronidazole and erythromycin in women with bacterial vaginosis. *New England Journal of Medicine, 333,* 1732–1736.

Hillier, S. L., Nugent, R. P., Eschenbach, D. A., et al. (1995). Association between bacterial vaginosis and preterm delivery of a low-birth-weight infant. *New England Journal of Medicine, 333,* 1737–1742.

Hobart, J., & Smucker, D. (2000). The female athlete triad. *American Family Physician, 61,* 3357–3364, 3367.

Johnson, T., Zettelmaier, M., Warner, P., Hayashi, R., Avni, M., & Luke, B. (2000). A competency based approach to comprehensive pregnancy. *Womens Health Issues, 10*(5), 240–247.

Kogan, M. D., Alexander, G. R., Kotelchuck, M., & Nagey, D. A. (1994). Relation of the content of prenatal care to the risk of low birth weight: Maternal reports of health behavior advice and initial prenatal care procedures. *Journal of the American Medical Association, 271,* 1340–1345.

Kogan, M. D., Kotelchuck, M., Alexander, G. R., & Johnson, W. E. (1994). Racial disparities in reported prenatal care advice from health care providers. *American Journal of Public Health, 84,* 82–88.

Kogan, M. D., Martin, J. A., Alexander, G. R., Kotelchuck, M., Ventura, S. J., Frigoletto, F. D. (1998). The changing pattern of prenatal care utilization in the United States, 1981–1995, using different prenatal care indices. *Journal of the American Medical Association, 279,* 1623–1628.

Koniak-Griffin, D., Anderson, N. L. R., Verzemnieks, I., & Brecht, M. (2000). A public health nursing early intervention program for adolescent mothers: Outcomes from pregnancy through 6 weeks postpartum. *Nursing Research, 49*(3), 130–138.

Marantides, D. (1997). Management of polycystic ovary syndrome. *Nurse Practitioner, 22*(12), 34–38.

March of Dimes. (1999). *Folic acid.* Wilkes-Barre, PA: March of Dimes Birth Defects Foundation.

McIver, B., & Romanski, S. (1997). Evaluation and management of amenorrhea. *Mayo Clinic Proceedings, 72,* 1161–1169.

Misra, D. P., & Guyer, B. (1998). Benefits and limitations of prenatal care: From counting visits to measuring content. *Journal of the American Medical Association, 279,* 1661–1662.

Mora, J., & Nestel, P. (2000). Improving prenatal nutrition in developing countries: Strategies, prospects, and challenges. *American Journal of Clinical Nutrition, 71* (5 Suppl), 1353S–1363S.

Newes-Adeyi, G., & Maxwell, J. P. (2000). Preventive care-seeking among inner-city African American pregnant women. *American Journal of Health Behavior, 24*(4), 254–267.

Sanders, J. (2000). Let's start at the very beginning . . . women's comments on early pregnancy care. *MIDIRS Midwifery Digest, 10*(2), 169–173.

Sergent, J. B., Sheahan, S. L., & Latimer, M. (1994). Demographic predictors of smoking at initiation of antenatal care. *Journal of the American Academy of Nurse Practitioners, 6*(12), 573–579.

Weiss, M., & Adams, A. K. (1995). Telephonic nursing: Empowering patients at risk for preterm birth. *Advanced Practice Nursing Quarterly, 1*(3), 58–64.

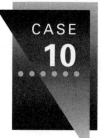

CASE
10

A 48-year-old woman with fatigue and headaches

SCENARIO

Florence McGee is a 48-year-old obese African American woman with fatigue, headaches, decreased libido, and irregular menses. She also has noticed increased skin dryness and sleep disturbances. Occasionally she notices that she shakes in the morning. Florence says she lost her job as a paralegal 3 months ago. Her headaches have worsened since she lost her job. For the headache, she has been taking propranolol, which was prescribed by a physician she saw 6 months ago. Florence says that her last physical was more than 2 years ago. She says she has gained about 15 pounds in the last month.

● TENTATIVE DIAGNOSES

Based on Florence's presentation, what are your tentative differential diagnoses?

● HISTORY

What questions do you want to ask Florence to assist you in developing a diagnosis?

● PHYSICAL ASSESSMENT

Based on the subjective data you have obtained, what parts of the physical examination should be performed and why?

● DIFFERENTIAL DIAGNOSES

Examine all the data obtained. Link the subjective and objective data to the appropriate differential diagnosis. Identify both positive and negative data that support or refute the diagnosis.

● DIAGNOSTIC TESTS

What additional data or diagnostic tests need to be performed to confirm the diagnosis?

● DIAGNOSIS

What is your conclusive diagnosis? What positive and negative data assisted you in your decision?

● THERAPEUTIC PLAN

1. *What are the issues to consider for Florence when deciding on treatment?*
2. *What are the possible treatments?*
3. *What is the efficacy of each treatment?*
4. *What are alternative treatments that might be appropriate for Florence?*
5. *How often and when would you see Florence again?*
6. *Florence has shown little improvement after 6 weeks of treatment. What adjustments would you make in the therapeutic plan?*
7. *Based on the information given about Florence, what impact do think this situation has on Florence's family?*
8. *What would be appropriate interventions for Florence's family?*
9. *Where can a nurse practitioner obtain more information concerning this diagnosis and/or additional resources for the patient and family?*
10. *What community resources can the nurse practitioner refer the client and/or family to?*
11. *What other health care professionals should be involved in a plan of care for Florence? When should Florence be referred for more intensive therapy?*

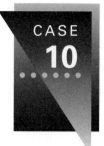

TUTORIAL

A 48-year-old woman with fatigue and headaches

SCENARIO

Florence McGee is a 48-year-old obese African American woman with fatigue, headaches, decreased libido, and irregular menses. She also has noticed increased skin dryness and sleep disturbances. Occasionally she notices that she shakes in the morning. Florence says she lost her job as a paralegal 3 months ago. Her headaches have worsened since she lost her job. For the headaches, she has been taking propranolol, which was prescribed by a physician she saw 6 months ago. Florence says that her last physical was more than 2 years ago. She says she has gained about 15 pounds in the last month.

● TENTATIVE DIAGNOSES

Based on Florence's presentation, what are your tentative differential diagnoses?

DIFFERENTIAL DIAGNOSES	RATIONALE
Brain tumor/primary neurological problem	Florence is presenting with headaches, decreased libido, and irregular menses. These could be caused by a neurological problem.
Depression	Florence is presenting with fatigue, headaches, decreased libido, sleep disturbances, weight gain, and loss of job. These are all symptoms of depression.
Menopause	Florence is c/o irregular menses and decreased libido. Irregular menses may be the first symptom seen in perimenopause.
Hypothyroidism	Florence is c/o fatigue and skin dryness, common symptoms of hypothyroidism.

(continued)

DIFFERENTIAL DIAGNOSES	RATIONALE
Substance abuse	Florence is c/o shakiness in the morning, a sign seen when the body is lacking the abused substance, ie, ETOH.
Anemia	Florence is c/o fatigue and skin dryness, possible indicators of anemia.
Decreased blood sugar	The symptoms of shakiness and fatigue also could lead one to suspect a low blood sugar count.

Note how many of the presenting symptoms overlap and could lead the NP to suspect many different problems.

● HISTORY

What questions do you want to ask Florence to assist you in developing a diagnosis?

REQUESTED DATA	DATA ANSWER
Allergies	NKA.
Medications	Propranolol, 20 mg po BID. Tylenol PRN for H/A. Occasional laxative/antacid. No vitamins.
Childhood diseases	Asthma. Chicken pox.
Immunizations	Unsure about anything except tetanus/TB skin test: done 5 years ago.
Surgery	Tubal ligation 12 years ago: 1983.
Transfusions	None.
Hospitalizations	Vaginal childbirth 2 times: 1978, 1982.
Fractures/injuries, accidents	FX radius at 7 y/o, no problems now. FX two ribs, 1986, slipped on ice.
Adult illness	Pneumonia, 1992. Costochondritis, 1990.

(continued)

REQUESTED DATA   DATA ANSWER

OBG history	LNMP: 7-2-95, periods farther apart. Last pelvic: 2 years ago, WNL. Mammogram: 2 years ago, WNL. BSE: not regularly. G2P2A0.
Last complete PE	In 1982, when pregnant.
Weight changes	Has gained 10–15 pounds in last 2½–3 months.
Appetite	Increased because of "nerves," craves chocolate, eats what she wants, no special diet.
24-Hour diet recall	B: 2 glazed doughnuts, 2 cups coffee. L: peanut butter crackers, apple, soda. D: sphagetti, salad with no-fat ranch dressing, 2 pieces garlic bread, soda.
Sleeping pattern	Problems going to sleep and staying asleep; sleeps about 4 hours per night; naps occasionally during the day.
Family history	Father: died 8 years ago at age of 59 of liver failure (admits father was alcoholic and sexually abusive to her). Mother: living, age 76, mild HTN, nervous breakdown years ago. 2 living brothers: 45, good health; 57, HTN. 1 living sister: 43, good health. 2 children: 16, daughter, good health; 13, son, good health.
Social habits	Smokes ½ pack/day for 25 years; occasional social drinker. Drinks approximately 5 cups of coffee/day plus 3 sodas/day. Denies recreational drug use and does not exercise.
Social organizations	Church women's group; Jaycees; has not been to a meeting in 3 months since losing her job.
Relationship with husband	Feels she and her husband do not talk much anymore. Thinks he is aggravated with her because she is not working. Having intercourse 1 time every other week; little affection exchanged between them.
Relationship with children	Typical teen-agers who know it all and want to do it their way. Has a good relationship with them; they seem concerned about her.
Relationship with mother/siblings	Lives in different town than mother and sibs. Talks to mother 1 time per week, sister 1 time every 2 weeks, brother 1 time every 3–4 weeks. Mother/brothers live in Chicago. Sister lives in Durham, NC.
Income	Husband works as 1st shift supervisor at Lexington computer services. She is drawing unemployment. Things are tight now.

(continued)

REQUESTED DATA   DATA ANSWER

REQUESTED DATA	DATA ANSWER
Insurance	Has medical and dental through husband's work.
Home	Owns their home; live about 3½ miles from health center.
Length of symptoms	Last few months has been sad; really bad in last 6 weeks.
How has this affected your daily activities?	Seems harder to do anything; not as interested in things as I used to be; tired all the time; would rather just sleep. Sometimes I don't even get dressed. I'm also very shaky in the mornings until I really get started.
Losses in your life	Job is probably loss; wasn't really sad when Dad died; have lived away from my family for 15 years. Feels a loss in decrease in communication with husband; her children go their own ways and not needing her as much.
How do you manage stress?	Watch TV; get off by myself; go to room; outside on deck or just driving; have tried praying.
Tell me about your headaches	I had them almost every day. I would get nauseated but did not vomit. They just pulled me down. The doctor put me on this medicine, and it really seemed to decrease how many H/A I get now.
What do you do for your headaches?	Take propranolol every day. Acetaminophen (Tylenol) or ibuprofen as needed. Sometimes have to lie down in quiet room; sometimes in the morning coffee or sodas help.
Do you ever think of hurting yourself, in other words suicide?	No.
On a scale from 1–10, with 1 being terrible and 10 being great, how do you feel?	3.
Have you ever felt this way before?	I've felt sad, but not for this long and this bad.
Are there situations/ instances that make you feel worse?	I feel worse when I think about work or the loss of the closeness to my husband and my weight.
Do you feel bad all the time?	Pretty much. I have a few less sad times, but when I'm sad, I'm sad. I cry some too.
Can you think of anything that would make you feel better?	Not really; not now. Maybe getting a job, getting back to normal, but I don't feel I have enough energy to work.

● PHYSICAL ASSESSMENT

Based on the subjective data you have obtained, what parts of the physical exam should be performed and why?

SYSTEM	RATIONALE	FINDINGS
Vital signs	Provides a baseline assessment.	HR, 72 bpm; RR, 20; BP 116/86 mm Hg; T, 99 °F.
Skin color and character	Provides overall indication of health. Also dry skin is an indicator of hypothyroidism. Pale skin is an indicator of anemia. Spider angiomas may indicate alcohol abuse, as do unexplained cuts and bruises.	Skin brown, mucous membranes and nailbeds are pink. No jaundice, bruises, spider angiomas. Skin dry.
Heart/peripheral pulses	Provides a baseline assessment of cardiovascular status.	S1, S2 without murmur. No venous hum over neck. No carotid bruits. Pulses 2+, no edema.
Lungs	Provides a baseline assessment of respiratory status.	CTA.
Cranial nerves	Needed to rule out neurological dysfunction.	II–XI intact.
Fundoscopic	Can indicate increased intercranial pressure and diabetic retinopathy.	No AV nicking. Disc with clear margins. No disc-to-cup ratio. No hemorrhages, cotton wool spots noted.
Mental status	Important system given her complaints of fatigue, etc. Helps to rule out substance abuse and mental illness.	Mini Mental Status exam performed: score of 30.
Motor function/ muscle strength	Needed to rule out neurological dysfunction.	Gait normal. Negative Romberg. Extremities equal in strength. No tremors noted.
Sensation	Needed to rule out neurological dysfunction.	Pain discrimination intact in all extremities.
Reflexes	Needed to rule out neurological dysfunction and identify baseline.	Biceps, triceps, brachioradialis, patellar, and ankle 2+ bilaterally.

(continued)

SYSTEM	RATIONALE	FINDINGS
Visual acuity	Only needed if complete PE is done, although may be gross screening for diabetic vision loss.	OD, 20/30; OS, 20/20 corrected with glasses.
Confrontation	Gross test for peripheral vision. May indicate neurological dysfunction.	Visual fields intact.
Abdominal	Provides information regarding abdominal function. If concerned about possible substance abuse, may indicate liver enlargement or tender abdomen caused by gastritis	BS present all four quadrants. Abdomen obese and nontender. No splenomegaly or hepatomegaly.
Breasts	Only would be done if time permits and if you are concerned she may not return for annual breast/pelvic exam.	No masses or dimpling noted.
ENT	Looking for indication of substance abuse: nasal lesions; parotid gland enlargement; indications of anemia; pale mucous membranes.	Normocephalic; no sinus tenderness; PERRLA; no pharyngeal erythema or oral lesions noted. Nasal septum midline. TMs gray with light reflex present.
Gynecologic	Would not usually be done; only consider if time permits or you are concerned she may not return for annual exam.	Deferred.

● DIFFERENTIAL DIAGNOSES

Examine all of the available data. Link the subjective and objective data to the appropriate differential diagnosis. Identify both positive and negative data that support/refute the diagnosis.

DIAGNOSIS	POSITIVE DATA	NEGATIVE DATA
Hypothyroidism	Fatigue, weight gain, almost age 50.	No edema, bradycardia, decreased BS, decreased appetite, hyperflexia, hypotension, slurred speech, or hoarseness.
Diabetes	Shakes, fatigue.	No weight loss, visual changes, numbness, tingling of hands/feet; no history of fungal infections, nocturia, polyuria, or thirst.
Brain tumor	Change in personality/ activities, headaches and shakes.	No edema, papilledema, vomiting, change in gait, sensorium, reflexes, cranial nerves.
Substance abuse	Shakes, recent loss, decreased libido, dry skin, sleep abnormality, and fatigue.	No track marks, nasal lesions, GI complaints, vomiting, hepatomegaly, jaundice, palpitations.
Anemia	Shakes, fatigue, irregular menses, and pallor.	No family history; no bruising, hematuria, melena, splenomegaly, hepatomegaly, bone tenderness, murmur, pale mucous membranes.
Depression	Depressed mood, loss of interest or pleasure, weight gain, sleep disturbance, fatigue, feelings of worthlessness and sadness, irregular menses, decreased activity with organizations and parenting of teen-agers. Loss of job and mother's history of "mild" nervous breakdown.	No history of previous depression, suicide attempts, impaired concentration, psychomotor retardation.

● DIAGNOSTIC TESTS

What additional data and/or diagnostic tests need to be performed to confirm the diagnosis?

DIAGNOSTIC TEST	RATIONALE	RESULTS	INTERPRETATION
Self-report depression scales: General Health Questionnaire, Jung Self-Rating Depression Scale, Beck Depression Inventory, Center for Epidemiological Studies Depression Scale	Good choice to help identify depression. Can complete in waiting area. Watch for false positive result, where score indicates depression but patient is not depressed. Do not include questionnaires in chart; validity of test depends on people not having access to test before taking.	Florence scored 55 on the Jung Self-Rating Depression Scale.	This score is equal to 69 on the Jung SDS, indicating depression.
Clinician-completed depression scales: Hamilton Rating Scale for Depression	Good choice. Depends on the amount of time you have to spend with this patient and your familiarity with the tools.	Not completed because the self rating scale was done.	NA.
Clinical interview to assess for DSM IV-R criteria	Good choice. Can be completed as part of the interview or review of systems.	Completed.	Meets DSM criteria for depression.
MRI or CT scan of the head	Very costly and time consuming to get. Wound help only if brain tumor was your primary diagnosis. Even in this case, a neurological consult may be warranted first based on paucity of symptoms.	Not done.	NA.
TSH: Thyroid stimulating hormone T_4	Will help discriminate pituitary and thyroid disorders in combination with T_4. If TSH and T_4 both are low, an anterior	TSH, 2.2 μU/mL.	WNL.

(continued)

DIAGNOSTIC TEST	RATIONALE	RESULTS	INTERPRETATION
	pituitary disorder is suspected. If TSH is high or normal and T_4 is low, a thyroid disorder is suspected. Requires a couple of days to get results. Because Florence is exhibiting nonacute symptoms, refer to endocrinologist first if this is your primary diagnosis. If client were elderly, should get tests.		
Sleep EEG	May help to rule out brain tumor or sleep disorder. Expensive and takes 1–2 hours to perform. Not really warranted in this situation.	Not done.	NA.
Hgb, HCT, CBC	It has been at least 2 years since Florence had this test. Because she is c/o fatigue and irregular menses, you could perform a fingerstick test. If results are abnormal, send for outpatient CBC. Need to think in terms of what do you get from the CBC that you do not get from the Hgb/HCT.	Hgb, 14.8 g/dL.	WNL.
Blood glucose, electrolytes	Could do a fingerstick glucose because patient is c/o shakes in the morning and fatigue. Diabetes runs in her family. Weight gain and stress may	Glucose, 78 mg/dL; Na, 137 mEq/L; K, 3.8 mEq/L; Cl, 101 mEq/L; CO_2, 23 mEq/L; BUN, 11 mg/dL; creatinine 0.8 mg/dL;	WNL.

(continued)

DIAGNOSTIC TEST	RATIONALE	RESULTS	INTERPRETATION
	precipitate diabetes. If glucose is high, arrange to have a glycosolated hemoglobin level drawn. Liver functions tests may provide data supporting substance abuse.	ALT, 20 U/L; AST, 10 U/L; alkaline phosphatase, 41 U/L; bilirubin, 1.0 mg/dL.	
Mammogram/ Papanicolaou smear	Florence is due for one. However, if you are busy today, you may have to arrange for these and a complete physical at another date. Find out how far Florence lives from the facility. If it is far, you may wish to complete all health maintenance activities at this time. An issue of concern: will Florence return for health maintenance activities since it has been > 2 years since her last full exam.	Not done.	Appointment made for 2 weeks.
CAGE, SMASK	Screening questionnaires for alcohol dependence. Good choice. Can be integrated into interview.	Denies feeling angry because people criticize her drinking; has not ever felt guilty about drinking or felt the need to cut down on drinking. Denies drinking first thing in morning as an eye opener to steady nerves.	Negative CAGE.

(continued)

DIAGNOSTIC TEST	RATIONALE	RESULTS	INTERPRETATION
U/A, drug Screen	U/A may be appropriate if done as part of a routine yearly exam. If not, consider what data it will contribute to diagnosis. Drug screen probably not indicated because it was not supported by data in history.	Not done.	NA.

● DIAGNOSES

What is your conclusive diagnosis? What positive and negative data assisted you in your decision?

Depression, nonsuicidal
    Rationale:
    According to DSM IV criteria, 5 of following are present at the same time: One of the following two must be present:

- Depressed mood most of day or every day;
- Markedly diminished interest or pleasure in almost all activities.

Plus

- Significant weight gain or loss;
- Insomnia/hypersomnia.

    Psychomotor agitation/retardation

- Fatigue;
- Feelings of worthlessness;
- Impaired concentration;
- Recurrent thoughts of death or suicide.

Six of these criteria are applicable for Florence, thus meeting DSM IV criteria for depression.

● THERAPEUTIC PLAN

1. *What are the issues to consider for Florence when deciding on treatment?*
    Some issues to consider when deciding on the treatment are

    - the need to educate about the illness, its prognosis, and a treatment plan;
    - the ultimate selection of first treatment is a collaborative process between patient and caregiver;

- visits should be frequent enough to optimize adherence; and
- outcomes must be carefully assessed by interviews and self-rating scales.

2. *What are the possible treatments?*
   Effectiveness depends on cooperative effort to empower the patient, which helps increase compliance/adherence and helps the patient learn health maintenance strategies and gain coping skills. Choices for treatments include medications, psychotherapy, combined medications and psychotherapy, and electroconvulsive therapy.

3. *What is the efficacy of each treatment?*
   I. *Medication*
      Consider

      - side effect profiles
      - history of prior response
      - family history of response
      - type of depression
      - concurrent general medical or psychological illness
      - other medications
      - cost
      - length of treatment: short vs long term.

      Consider when

      - moderate to severe depression
      - psychotic, melancholic or atypical
      - patient requests
      - psychotherapy not available
      - prior positive response to medication
      - maintenance is planned.

      1st and 2nd line choices:
      A. Secondary amine tricyclics (nortriptyline [Pamelor]; desipramine [Norpramin] 25 to 50 mg/day) (a 2nd line choice)
      B. Bupropion (Wellbutrin) (Heterocyclic)
      C. Fluoxetine (Prozac) (SSRIs) 20 mg/day
      D. Paroxetine (Paxil) (SSRI) 20 mg/day
      E. Sertraline (Zoloft) (SSRI) 20 mg/day
      F. Trazodone (Desyrel) (Heterocyclic) (a 2nd line choice)
         Side effects are most likely to occur at initiation or when medications are increased; adaptation occurs with time.
         Once-daily dosing at bedtime minimizes side effects and does not diminish efficacy, because the half-life is 24 hours. The full therapeutic dosage is maintained until the patient has either had a response or clearly failed to have a response (evaluate at 6 weeks and 12 weeks).
   II. *Psychotherapy*
      Few clinical trials are available demonstrating efficacy.
      Consider:

      - useful for depression is of the mild to moderate type;
      - when patient requests.

III. *Medication and psychotherapy*
Consider when:

- Either treatment alone only has partial response or poor interepisode recovery;
- Most patients do best when combined therapy is used.

IV. *Electroconvulsive therapy*
Consider when:

- More severe or psychotic forms are present
- Other therapies have failed
- Medication conditions preclude the use of medications
- There is need for a rapid response.

5. *How often and when would you see Florence again?*
Providing patient support and education optimizes adherence, facilitates dosage adjustment, minimizes side effects, and allows monitoring of clinical response. AHCPR (1993) recommends seeing more severely depressed patients weekly for the first 6 to 8 weeks. Less severely depressed patients may be seen every 10 to 14 days.

6. *Florence has shown minimal improvement after 6 weeks of therapy with fluoxetine (Prozac) 20 mg/day. What adjustments would you make in the therapeutic plan?*
Failure to have a response necessitates two steps:

a. *Reassessment of the adequacy of the diagnosis;*

b. *Reassessment of the adequacy of treatment.*
Ongoing, undisclosed substance abuse or an underlying general medical condition are two common pitfalls.

Medication underdosing is common. Increasing doses of medications should be given in the first few weeks for most antidepressants.

Medication is recommended for 4 to 9 months after an acute episode. Recurrences require longer treatment with medications. Patient with more than three recurrences may need to continue medications for life.

7. *Based on the information given about Florence, what impact do you think this situation has had on Florence's family?*
Although Florence has been depressed for an extended period of time, if the depression continues or becomes more severe, the impact will likely become more serious. Families with a member with depression frequently report feelings of:

- Grief over the loss of the person they once knew;
- Guilt that perhaps they are to blame for the illness;
- Anger directed toward the depressed person and other feelings directed at other family members as a release of frustrations;
- Powerlessness with the thought that the depression can not be "cured" or that it may become a chronic condition; and
- Fear of the unknown and future and even of the depressed person.

In addition, in Florence's case and similar ones, depression alters the emotional and functional equilibrium of the family by creating:

- Marital strain and stress;
- Altered communication/interaction patterns;
- Worry and concern by family members regarding the patient's lack of interest in personal hygiene, ADLs, usual activities and interests, altered social interactions, and feelings of hopelessness;
- Altered roles and responsibilities;
- Psychosocial impairment of spouse and increased risk of the children developing a psychiatric disorder; and
- Fatigue and the potential for "burn out" of caregivers.

8. *What would be appropriate interventions for Florence's family?*
   Appropriate interventions for Florence's family could include:

- Education for the family concerning depression;
- Family/marital counseling (individual and/or group);
- Attending a community support group;
- Encouragement of continuation of normal activities/routines as much as possible;
- Family meetings to negotiate needed changes in shifting of responsibilities;
- "Time out" breaks as needed to maintain balance;
- Use of existing social support networks and development of new ones with help;
- Make sure "crisis hot line" phone numbers and other needed phone numbers are near at hand for emergency use.

9. *Where can a nurse practitioner obtain more information concerning depression or additional resources for assisting depressed clients?*

Phone Book: Look for numbers of

- local crisis/hot lines
- social support groups/hospitals with psychiatric units

Other:

National Alliance for the Mentally Ill (NAMI)
Arlington, VA
703-524-7600
www.nami.org

National Depressive & Manic Association (NDMDA)
Chicago, IL
312-642-0049
www.ndmda.org

National Foundation for Depressive Illness
1-800-248-4344

National Mental Health Association Information Center
1021 Prince Street
Alexandria, VA 22314
1-800-969-6642
http://depression-screening.org/nmha/nmha.htm

Information Referral and Crisis Hotline
1-800-233-4357

American Psychological Association
1-202-336-6062
www.apa.org

National Institute of Mental Health
http://www.nimh.nih.gov

Information about DSM IV:
http://www.a-silver-lining.org/BPNDepth/dsmiv.html

Information about suicide/crisis intervention:
http://www.mhsanctuary.com/suicide/index.html

10. *To what community resources can the nurse practitioner refer the depressed client or family?*
The NP should have learned and identified the resources in his/her community that serve the needs of the depressed client and family. This will be different in each community and will require research on the practitioner in advance of the need.

11. *What other health care providers/professional disciplines could/should be included in a therapeutic plan of care for Florence? When should Florence be referred for more intensive therapy?*
- Physician/psychiatrist for consultation and referral;
- Psychologist for referral for counseling/consultation; and
- Licensed clinical social worker or psychiatric nurse/specialist for consultation and referral.

Florence should be referred to a specialist if her depression is severe, she exhibits suicidal ideation, she requires multiple medications for control or improvement, or if you determine she has bipolar depression.

REFERENCES

Agency for Health Care Policy Research (AHCPR) Depression Guideline Panel. (1993, April). *Depression in primary care: Volume 1. Detection and diagnosis.* Clinical practice guideline, Number 5. Rockville, MD: US Department of Heath and Human Services, Public Health Service, Agency for Health Care Policy Research. AHCPR Publication No. 93-0550.
Agency for Health Care Policy Research (AHCPR) Depression Guideline Panel. (1993,

April). *Depression in primary care: Volume II. Treatment.* Clinical practice guideline, Number 5. Rockville, MD: US Department of Heath and Human Services, Public Health Service, Agency for Health Care Policy Research. AHCPR Publication No. 93-0550.

American Psychiatric Association. (1994). *Diagnosis and statistical manual of mental disorders.* Washington, DC: American Psychiatric Association.

Betrus, P. A., Elmore, S. K., Woods, N. F., & Hamilton, P. (1995). Women and depression. *Health Care for Women International, 16,* 243–252.

Bierut, L. J., Heath, A. C., Bucholz, K., Dinwiddie, S., Madden , P., Statham, D., Dunne, M., & Martin, N. (1999). Major depressive disorder in a community-based twin sample: Are there different genetic and environmental contributions for men and women? *Archives in General Psychiatry, 56,* 557–563.

Burkhart, K. S. (2000). Diagnosis of depression in the elderly patient. *Lippincott's Primary Care Practice, 4*(2), 149–162.

Davis, K., & Mathew, E. (1998). Pharmacologic management of depression in the elderly. *Nurse Practitioner: American Journal of Primary Health Care, 23*(6), 16, 18, 26.

Hassell, J. S. (1996). Improved management of depression through nursing model application and critical thinking. *Journal of the American Academy of Nurse Practitioners, 8,* 161–166.

D'Epiro, N. W. (2000). Chronic depression: Now, a treatable condition. *Patient Care Nurse Practitioner, 3*(1), 54–56, 59, 62.

D'Epiro, N. W., & Cirigliano, M. (1999). CAM spotlight. St. John's wort and depression. *Patient Care Nurse Practitioner, 2*(8), 50–52.

Floyd, B. J. (1997). Problems in accurate medical diagnosis of depression in female patients. *Social Science Medicine, 44,* 403–412.

Garcia, G., & Ghani, S. (2000). Newer medications and indications used in psychiatry. *Lippincott's Primary Care Practic, 4,* 207–208.

Horsfall, J. (1997). Women's depression: Nursing theory and practice. *Contemporary Nurse, 6*(34), 129–135.

Kasper, S., Praschak-Rieder, N., Tauscher, J., & Wolf, R. (1997). A risk-benefit assessment of mirtazapine in the treatment of depression. *Drug Safety, 17*(40), 251–264.

Kessler, R. C., McGonagle, K. A., Zhao, S., Alelson, C., Hughes, M., Eghleman, S., Wittchen, H., & Kendler, K. (1994). Lifetime and 12-month prevalence of DSM-III-R psychiatric disorders in the United States. *Archives in General Psychiatry, 51,* 8–19.

Kupecz, D. (1995). New antidepressants. *Nurse Practitioner, 20*(5), 64, 66, 67.

Lucas, B. (1999). Coping with psychiatric emergencies in the office. *Patient Care Nurse Practitioner, 2*(2), 25–26, 29–38, 41–42.

Martin, A. (2000). Major depressive illness in women: Assessment and treatment in the primary care setting. *Nurse Practitioner Forum, 11*(3), 179–186.

McCabe, S., & Grover, S. (1999). Psychiatric nurse practitioner versus clinical nurse specialist: Moving from debate to action on the future of advanced psychiatric nursing. *Archives Psychiatric Nursing, 13*(3), 111–116.

Nemeroff, C. B. (1994). Evolutionary trends in the pharmacotherapeutic management of depression. *Journal of Clinical Psychiatry, 55,* 3–15.

Pinkowish, M. D. (1999). Clinical clips. Identifying premenopausal women at risk of depression. *Patient Care Nurse Practitioner, 2*(8), 54–55.

Preskorn, S. H. (1993). Pharmacokinetics of antidepressants: Why and how they are relevant to treatment. *Journal of Clinical Psychiatry, 54*(Suppl. 9), 14–34.

Rickert, V. I., Wiemann, C. M., & Berenson, A. B. (2000). Ethnic differences in depressive symptomatology among young women. *Obstetrics and Gynecology, 95,* 55–60.

Roberts, S. B., & Kendler, K. S. (1999). Neuroticism and self-esteem as indices of the vulnerability to major depression in women. *Psychological Medicine, 29,* 1101–1109.

Skaer, T., Sclar, D., Robison, L., & Galin, R. (2000). Trend in the use of antidepressant pharmacotherapy and diagnosis of depression in the US: An assessment of office-based visits 1990 to 1998. *CNS Drugs, 14*(6), 473–481.

West, M., Rose, S. M., Spreng, S., Verhoef, M., & Bergman, J. (1999). Anxious attachment and severity of depressive symptomatology in women. *Women's Health, 29,* 47–56.

Woods, N. F., & Mitchell, E. S. (1997). Pathways to depressed mood for midlife women: Observations from the Seattle midlife women's health study. *Research in Nursing and Health, 20,* 119–129.

Yonkers, K. A., & Austin, L. S. (1996). Mood disorders: Women and affective disorders. *Primary Psychiatry, 3,* 27–28.

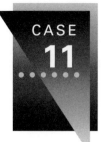

CASE

11

An 8-month-old boy with diaper rash

SCENARIO

Gloria brought her 8-month-old son (Stefan) in because he has had diarrhea for the last 2 days. Now he has a diaper rash, and he cries whenever he urinates.

● TENTATIVE DIAGNOSES

*Based on the information provided, what are potential differential diagnoses? What are **red flag** diagnoses that you cannot miss?*

DIAGNOSES   *RATIONALE*

1

2

● HISTORY

What are significant questions in the history for Stefan?

REQUESTED DATA   *DATA ANSWER*

Health history   Normally healthy. Has had "colds" but has not been hospitalized or had any surgery

(continued)

REQUESTED DATA   *DATA ANSWER*

REQUESTED DATA	DATA ANSWER
Childhood illnesses	None.
Birth history	Prenatal: unplanned pregnancy, mother is only 17. Had prenatal care; took prenatal vitamins. L & D: full term; 18-hour labor; vaginal delivery with epidural. Wt, 8 lbs, 11 oz. Length, 20.5″. APGAR: unknown but states infant cried vigorously at birth. Postnatal: some jaundice, did not require phototherapy. Formula fed, tolerated well. Went home with mother after 48 hours.
Allergies	NKA.
Medications	Uses acetaminophen (Infant Tylenol) as needed for fever.
Immunizations	2 months: Hepatitis B vaccination, DTAP, *Haemophilus influenza*, IPV, Prevnar. 4 months: Hepatitis B vaccination, DTAP, *Haemophilus influenza*, IPV, Prevnar. 6 months: DTAP, IPV, *Haemophilus influenza*.
Developmental history	Growth: 18 lbs, 27 inches currently. Milestones: rolled over at 4 months; sat alone at 6 months. Eats finger foods, drinks from sippy cup. Verbalizes sounds; responsive smile; laughs.
Habits	Uses pacifer much of time.
Sleep	Sleeps from 9 pm to 7 am; seldom awakens. Has cried a few times during the night last night. Usually naps 1–2 hours in afternoon. Has his own bedroom.
Temperament	Generally in happy mood. Fussy if tired.
Diet history	Uses Enfamil with iron; drinks about 4 bottles and uses sippy cup. Eats baby food.
24-hour intake	B: ½ cup cereal + ½ cup formula. S: ½ banana and formula from cup. L: ½ jar meat, ½ jar vegetable, ½ jar fruit + formula. S: ½ banana. D: same as lunch. S: ½ piece toast.
Family health history	Mother: 17, in good health, lives with her mother. Father: nonparticipative in care. MGM: 40, in good health.
Social history	Mother smokes 1 pack a day and is working on her GED.
Environmental history	Lives in housing project with about 300 families; area somewhat "rough."

What are the key points to cover on the review of systems?

SYSTEM	DATA ANSWER
General	Healthy, awake, and happy.
HEENT	No URI.
CV	No history of heart murmur.
Lungs	No problems with breathing.
GI	Diarrhea started 2 days ago. Mom was sick with diarrhea and vomiting before Stefan. Taking fluids but not eating as much as normal. Has had BMs 6 times in last day. All liquid.
GU	Urinating a little less than normal.
Musculoskeletal	No problems.
Skin	Has bright red rash on buttocks that started last night. Cries when diaper gets wet. Mom usually uses emollient (A & D Ointment) and disposable wipes. She has stopped using the wipes because they make him cry.

● PHYSICAL ASSESSMENT

What are the significant portions of the physical examination that should be completed for Stefan?
What is your rationale behind doing each part of the exam?

SYSTEM	RATIONALE	FINDINGS
Vital signs		T, 99.8°F; P, 128; RR, 30; Wt, 17 lbs, 10 oz.
General appearance		Mom holding him. Sitting quietly.
HEENT		Normocephalic. TM: gray and pearly with good movement. Nose: no drainage. Pharynx: no erythema or exudate. Mouth with moist mucus membranes. Neck: no LA.
Lungs		CTA.
CV		Sinus tachycardia; no murmurs noted.

(continued)

SYSTEM	RATIONALE	FINDINGS
Abdomen		BS hyperactive; no tenderness noted; no HSM; no rebound tenderness.
Genitalia		Intensely red rash on perineum; skin folds spared. Satellite lesions around the main area of rash. Penis and scrotum involved. See Figure 11–1.

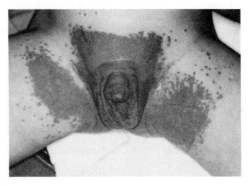

Figure 11–1. From Sauer, p. 358.

● DIFFERENTIAL DIAGNOSIS

What are the significant positive and negative findings that support or refute your tentative diagnoses for Stefan?

DIAGNOSES	POSITIVE DATA	NEGATIVE DATA
1		
2		
3		
4		

● DIAGNOSTIC TESTS

Based on the history and physical examination, what, if any, diagnostic testing will you obtain? What is your rationale for doing the tests, and what is your interpretation of the results obtained?

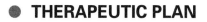

TEST	RATIONALE	RESULTS	INTERPRETATION
KOH slide		+ hyphae.	
Fungal culture		Not done.	

● DIAGNOSIS

What diagnosis(es) do you determine are appropriate for Stefan?

● DATA SUPPORTING THE DIAGNOSIS

Identify the data that support your final diagnosis(es).

Pathophysiology

Explain the pathophysiology for Stefan's condition.

● THERAPEUTIC PLAN

1. What is the treatment for Stefan's diaper rash?

2. How can Gloria prevent his rash from worsening?

3. What other teaching would you do for Gloria related to Stefan's rash?

4. You determine that Stefan is behind in one set of immunizations. Is this an appropriate time to give them to him?

5. How would you instruct Gloria concerning Stefan's diarrhea?

6. What teaching would you do concerning the issue of dehydration?

REFERENCES

Arad, A., Mimouni, D., Ben-Amitai, D., Zeharia, D., & Mimouni, M. (1999). Efficacy of topical application of eosin compared with zinc oxide paste and corticosteroid cream for diaper dermatitis. *Dermatology, 199*(4), 319–322.

Arnsmeier, S. L., & Paller, A. S. (1998). Getting to the bottom of diaper. *Contemporary Pediatrics, 14*(11), 115–116, 118, 120.

Berg, R. W., Milligan, M. C., & Sarbaugh, F. C. (1994). Association of skin wetness and pH with diaper dermatitis. *Pediatric Dermatology, 11*(1), 18–20.

Boiko, S. (1999). Treatment of diaper dermatitis. *Dermatology Clinics, 17*(1), 235–240.

Fleischer, A., & Feldman, S. (1999). Prescription of high-potency corticosteroid agents and clotrimazole-betamethasone dipropionate by pediatricians. *Clinical Therapeutics, 21,* 1725–1731.

Gregory, T. (1998). Getting to the bottom of diaper dermatitis. *Patient Care, 32*(17), 85–86, 91–92, 95–96.

Hoppe, J. (1997). Treatment of oropharyngeal candidiasis and candidal diaper dermatitis in neonates and infants: Review and reappraisal. *Pediatric Infectious Disease Journal, 16*(9), 885–894.

Lund, C. (1999). Prevention and management of infant skin breakdown. *Nursing Clinics of North America, 34*(4), 907–920.

Lund, C., Kuller, J., Lane, A., Lott, J. W., & Raines, D. A. (1999). Neonatal skin care: The scientific basis for practice. *Neonatal Network, 28,* 241–254.

Odio, M., O'Connor, R., Sarbaugh, F., & Baldwin, S. (2000). Continuous topical administration of a petrolatum formulation by a novel disposable diaper: Effect on skin condition. *Dermatology, 200*(3), 238–243.

Ryan-Wenger, N. A., & Lee, J. E. M. (1997). The clinical reasoning case study: A powerful teaching tool . . . two sample case studies are provided: 'A child with a heart murmur' and 'An infant with diaper rash.' *Nurse Practitioner: American Journal of Primary Health Care, 22*(5), 66–67, 70, 76–79.

Sauer, G., & Hall, J. (1996). *Manual of skin diseases* (7th ed.). Philadelphia: Lippincott-Raven.

Ward, D., Fleischer, A., Feldman, S., & Krowchuk, D. (2000). Characterization of diaper dermatitis in the United States. *Archives in Pediatric Adolescent Medicine, 154*(9), 943–946.

Wisscher, M., Chatterjee, R., Munson, K., Bare, D., & Hoath, S. (2000). Development of diaper rash in the newborn. *Pediatric Dermatology, 17*(1), 52–57.

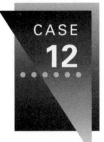

A 28-year-old woman with abdominal pain

SCENARIO

Misty Harbor presents to the health center for an evaluation of abdominal pain experienced during the past 10 months. She has recently separated from her husband of 5 years. They have twin boys, who are 2 years old. She works full time as a legal assistant.

● TENTATIVE DIAGNOSES

*What are the potential diagnoses you have identified based on this scenario? What are the **red flag** diagnoses that you cannot miss?*

DIAGNOSIS	SUPPORTING DATA
1	
2	
3	
4	
5	
6	
7	
8	
9	
10	

● HISTORY

Which of the following questions are significant ones in the history for Misty based on the tentative diagnoses? Identify which of the following data can be delayed until the next visit. Also identify if there is any important information missing.

REQUESTED DATA   DATA ANSWER

REQUESTED DATA	DATA ANSWER
History of current illness	Misty Harbor reports abdominal pain that started approximately 10 months ago. She reports at that time the pain was intermittent, occurring approximately once a month. In the past 3 months, she has noticed a significant increase in abdominal pain, occurring at least once a week. She describes her pain as dull, with occasional crampy feelings. The pain lasts as long as 3–4 hours and as short as 5–15 minutes. She points to her lower abdomen, below the umbilicus, and the left lower quad as the prominent areas of her pain. She states that greasy/spicy foods make the pain worse and make her nauseated. She has a lot of bloating and gas daily.
	She reports she has been having alterations in her bowel pattern. She reports intermittent diarrhea and constipation, occurring once a week. She will go 3 days without a bowel movement. At that point she has more abdominal pain and difficulty moving her bowels. She states she does a lot of straining. After a constipated day, the next day begins with soft, brown stool, leading to four to five bowel movements, ending with watery diarrhea. She denies any blood, melena, or mucus in the stool. She says defecation relieves her pain for a short while. She had a normal bowel pattern of every other day, brown in color, soft in consistency, prior to 10 months ago. She denies any tenesmus, anal itching, or loss of control. She admits to occasional urgency. She also notes a pattern of needing to defecate approximately 1 hour after eating. She states her pain and urgency are worse when eating out. She denies any vomiting, recent infections, travel, fevers, or chills. She denies any alteration in her ADLs because of the bowel pattern alteration or pain. She denies any change in appetite or weight
Past medical history	This includes hypothyroidism, anxiety disorder (panic attacks), depression (diagnosed 2 months ago), childhood chicken pox.
OB/GYN history	OB/GYN: G1P2. LNMP: currently. She states she has a normal flow, regular pattern and duration of 4–5 days, every 30 days. Her children were delivered vaginally. She obtains yearly Pap and pelvic exams.

(continued)

REQUESTED DATA   *DATA ANSWER*

Allergies	Sulfa, reaction of hives.
Medications	Levothyroxine sodium (Synthroid), 50 μg QD; citalopram hydrobromide (Celexa), 20 mg QD; alprazolam (Xanax), 0.25 mg Q12 PRN; aspirin and caffeine (Excedrin), PRN (up to 5–6 times a week). Sees psychiatrist for counseling and meds.
Family history	Father: expired age 60, MI. Mother: age 59, cholecystectomy for cholelithiasis at age 32; otherwise healthy. Maternal grandmother: diagnosed with colon cancer at age 45. Sister: expired at age 16, related to MVA. Brother: age 30, diagnosed with Crohn's disease at age 22.
Social history	Misty denies any ETOH, smoking, or recreational drug use. She drinks 2–3 12-oz cans of cola a day. She works full time as a legal assistant. She received her education at a 2-year college. She does not exercise routinely. She participates in church activities.
Stress management/coping	While talking with Misty, she volunteers that she and her husband have recently separated after a 5-year marriage. She states they are going to marriage counseling. She states she is under a lot of stress with this separation, as well as trying to take care of her twin boys (age 2) and continue working full time. She reports having a difficult time dealing with her father's death. He apparently died of a heart attack about 1 year ago. It was unexpected.
Spirituality	Attends church on a weekly basis; Catholic.
Recent travel	No recent travel. Has never been outside the USA.
Illness in family	No recent sickness in family.

● PHYSICAL ASSESSMENT

What are the significant portions of the physical examination that should be completed for Misty based on the history and chief complaint?

SYSTEM   *RATIONALE*   *FINDINGS*

Vital signs		BP, 120/80 mm Hg; HR, 88; RR, 18; T, 98.7 °F; Ht, 5'5"; Wt, 145 lb

(continued)

SYSTEM   RATIONALE   FINDINGS
....

System	Rationale	Findings
General appearance		Misty Harbor is a pleasant 28-year-old white woman, who presents in NAD. She is alert and oriented, well nourished, and nicely dressed. Her gait is steady. Sclerae nonicteric. Skin pink, dry, warm; good turgor; mucous membranes moist.
Neurological assessment		DTRs, 2+; alert and oriented; speech appropriate; PERRLA; neck supple; CN II–XII intact; no motor or sensory deficits; normal gait.
Lungs		Chest clear to auscultation.
Cardiac		Heart with a normal S1, S2; no murmurs or gallops; RRR.
Abdomen		Abdomen soft, mild LLQ tenderness; BS × 4 present; no masses; no organomegaly; no guarding.
Rectal		No tenderness; no masses; negative hemoccult; external hemorrhoids mildly inflamed. She exhibits a normal Wink reflex.
Lymphatics		No LA noted.
Extremities		No edema, erythema, ecchymosis; pulses palpable.
HEENT		Conjunctiva WNL. Ears: TM pearly, no erythema. Nose: slight erythema. Mouth: no erythema or exudate. Neck supple; no LA; thyroid nonpalpable.

● DIFFERENTIAL DIAGNOSES

What are the significant positive and negative findings that support or refute your diagnoses for Misty?

DIAGNOSIS   POSITIVE DATA   NEGATIVE DATA
....

Diagnosis	Positive Data	Negative Data
1		
2		
3		
4		
5		
6		

(continued)

DIAGNOSIS	POSITIVE DATA	NEGATIVE DATA
7		
8		
9		
10		

● DIAGNOSTIC TESTS

Based on the history and physical examination, what are the tests that should be done? Indicate which tests should be done first and which ones might be done at a later time. Interpret the results. What do they indicate?

DIAGNOSTIC TEST	RATIONALE	RESULTS	INTERPRETATION
GB ultrasound		No evidence of gallstones or inflammation.	
Flat and upright of the abdomen		No abnormalities; normal gas pattern. No free air.	
Flexible sigmoidoscopy		Mildly inflamed external hemorrhoids.	
Barium enema		The X ray was unable to differentiate an area in the ascending colon as stool or a possible mass. It could not entirely rule out inflammatory disease.	
Colonoscopy		The biopsies were negative for any inflammatory disease; no masses or strictures were noted. One polyp was removed at the descending colon, which was hyperplastic.	

(continued)

DIAGNOSTIC TEST	RATIONALE	RESULTS	INTERPRETATION
CBC		Hgb, 13.5 g/dL (normal 11.9–15.7 g/dL); HCT, 39.8% (normal, 35–45.9%); RBC, 4.53 million/mm³ (normal 4.0–5.13); WBC, 10.3 1000/mm³ (normal, 4.0–11.0).	
TSH		TSH, 2.5.	
CMP (comprehensive metabolic panel)		Na, 140 mEq/L; K, 3.7 mEq/L; BUN, 22 mg/dL; Glucose, 118 mg/dL; Cl, 101 mEq/L; Bicarbonate, 25 Creatinine 1.4 mg/dL.	
Hemoccult		No blood present.	
ESR		20 mm/h.	
Small bowel series		Normal.	
Lactose hydrogen breath test		Trace amount hydrogen in the expired air.	

● DIAGNOSIS

What diagnoses do you determine as being appropriate after a review of the subjective and objective data?

1.

2.

3.

4.

5.

● DISCUSSION

Discuss why the diagnoses you identified are pertinent in this case. Include some information related to demographics and how the diagnosis is commonly made.

● THERAPEUTIC PLAN

1. *What medicine is appropriate for Misty?*
2. *What type of foods may aggravate Misty's condition?*
3. *What is the holistic management plan for Misty?*
4. *What should Misty know about her diagnoses?*
5. *When should Misty return for a follow-up visit?*

RESOURCES

What are organizations that will help provide information for Misty and the NP?

REFERENCES

American Gastroenterological Association. (1997). American Gastroenterological Association Medical position statement: Irritable bowel syndrome. *Gastroenterology, 112,* 2118–2119.

Blackington, E. (2000). Irritable bowel syndrome: An update on treatment options. *Advance for Nurse Practitioners, 8*(10), 32–40.

Bueno, L., Fioramonti, J., Delvaux, M., & Frexinos, J. (1997). Mediators and pharmacology of visceral sensitivity: From basic to clinical investigations. *Gastroenterology, 112,* 1714–1743.

Camilleri, M., Lee, J., Viramonte, B., Bharucha, A., & Tangalos, E. (2000). Insights into the pathophysiology and mechanisms of constipation, irritable bowel syndrome, and diverticulosis in older people. *Journal of American Geriatric Society, 48,* 1142–1150

Carlson, E. (1998). Irritable bowel syndrome. *Nurse Practitioner, 23,* 82–91.

Drossman, D., Leserman, J., Nachman, G., Li, Z., Gluck, H., Toomey, T., & Mitchell, C. (1990). Sexual and physical abuse in women with functional or organic gastrointestinal disorders. *Annals of Internal Medicine, 113,* 828–833.

Drossman, D., Patrick, D., Whitehead, W., Toner, B., Diamant, N., Hu, Y., Jia, H., & Bangdiwala, S. (2000). Further validation of the IBS-QOL: A disease-specific quality-of-life. *American Journal of Gastroenterology, 95,* 999–1007.

Gralnek, I., Hays, R., Kilbourne, A., Naliboff, B., & Mayer, E. (2000). The impact of irritable bowel syndrome on health related quality of life. *American Journal of Gastroenterology, 119,* 654–660.

Heymann-Myonnikes, I., Arnold, R., Florin, I., Herda, C., Melfsen, S., & Myonnikes, H. (2000). The combination of medical treatment plus multicomponent behavioral therapy is superior to medical treatment alone in the therapy of irritable bowel syndrome. *American Journal of Gastroenterology, 95,* 981–994.

Houghton, L., Jackson, N., Whorwell, P., & Morris, J. (2000). Do male sex hormones protect from irritable bowel syndrome? *American Journal of Gastroenterology, 95,* 2296–2300.

Jailwala, J., Imperiale, T. F., & Kroenke, K. (2000). Pharmacologic treatment of the irritable bowel syndrome: A systematic review of randomized, controlled trials. *Annals of Internal Medicine, 133,* 136–147.

Janssen, H., Borghouts, J., Muris, J., Metsemakers, J., Koes, B., & Knottnerus, J. (2000).

Health status and management of chronic non-specific abdominal complaints in general. *British Journal of General Practice, 50*(454), 375–379.

Licht, H. M. (2000). Irritable bowel syndrome: Definitive diagnostic criteria help focus symptomatic treatment. *Postgraduate Medicine, 107*(3), 203–207, 277.

Locke, G., Zinsmeister, A., Talley, N., Fett, S., & Melton, L. (2000). Familial association in adults with functional gastrointestinal problems. *Mayo Clinic Proceedings, 75*, 907–912.

Sperber, A., Carmel, S., Atzmon, Y., Weisberg, I., Shalit, Y., Neumann, L., Fich, A., Friger, M., & Buskila, D. (2000). Use of the Functional Bowel Disorder Severity Index (FBDSI) in a study of patients with the irritable bowel syndrome and fibromyalgia. *American Journal of Gastroenterology, 95*, 995–998.

Thompson, W., Longstreth, G., Drossman, D., Heaton, K., Irvine, E., & Miller-Lissnor, S. (1999). Functional bowel disorders and functional abdominal pain. *Gut, 45*(Suppl 2), 1143–1147.

Wootton, J. (2000). How effective are antidepressant medications in the treatment of irritable bowel syndrome and nonulcer dyspepsia? *Journal of Family Practice, 49*(5), 396.

A 15-year-old girl with abnormal menstrual bleeding

SCENARIO

Samantha Blank presents to the health center with a history of abnormal menstrual bleeding for 3 weeks. She is a freshman in high school.

● TENTATIVE DIAGNOSES

*What are the potential diagnoses you have identified based on this scenario? Make sure you include any vital **red flag** diagnoses that cannot be missed.*

DIAGNOSIS	RATIONALE
1	
2	
3	
4	
5	
6	

● HISTORY

What are significant questions in the history for Samantha?

REQUESTED DATA	DATA ANSWER
Allergies	NKA.
Medications	None.
Surgery/Transfusion	None.
Medical history and hospitalizations/ injuries/accidents	Chicken pox.
Family history	Father, age 45; good health. Mother, age 43; good health. Sister, age 12; good health. Denies any history of bleeding or endocrine disorders.
Social history	Tobacco: never. Alcohol: never. Caffeine: none. Drugs: none. Exercise: cheerleader, aerobics 3 times/week.
GYN history	Menarche at age 13; has cycles every 28 days, usually bleeds for 7 days, with heavy flow on the first day of cycles, and has dysmenorrhea on day 1 of cycles. LNMP 5 weeks ago; bled for 7 days but 1 week later began having menstrual bleeding every day for the last 3 weeks. No dysmenorrhea in the past 3 weeks. Has been using one pad a day for the last 3 weeks. Blood is dark red with no clots. Contraceptive and sexual history—denies vaginal discharge, sexually transmitted diseases, or pelvic pain. Became sexually active 4 months ago with one partner, uses condoms. First pelvic exam three months ago, Pap smear was normal.
Have you noticed any symptoms of pregnancy?	No nausea, vomiting, breast tenderness, weight gain, fatigue.
Have you noticed any symptoms of thyroid disease?	No weakness, fatigue, hair loss, sleep problems, weight changes, cold intolerance, constipation. Has been attending school normally.
Have you noticed any bruising or nosebleeds?	Denies any bruising or nosebleeds.

● PHYSICAL ASSESSMENT

What are the significant portions of the physical examination that should be completed for Samantha?

SYSTEM	RATIONALE	FINDINGS
Vital signs		BP, 110/70 mm Hg right arm; HR, 72 bpm; RR, 18; T, 98.6 °F; Ht, 5′ 4″; Wt, 120 lbs
General appearance/skin		Alert; NAD; skin warm and dry, no pallor. No acne, hirsutism, petechiae, or eccyhmosis.
HEENT		Normocephalic; no pallor of conjunctiva; no epistaxis; thyroid nonpalpable, no masses.
Lungs		CTA.
Heart		S1, S2 normal; no MRG.
Breasts		Tanner IV; no galactorrhea.
Pelvic		No cervical lesions; no foreign objects; no Hegar's sign; no Chadwick's sign; no discharge. Small amount of blood noted in vaginal vault. No adnexal tenderness or uterine enlargement. Tanner IV.
Neurological assessment		Alert and oriented; gait steady; DTRs 2+.

● DIFFERENTIAL DIAGNOSES

What are the significant positive and negative findings that support or refute your diagnoses for Samantha?

DIAGNOSIS	POSITIVE DATA	NEGATIVE DATA
1		
2		
3		
4		
5		
6		

● DIAGNOSTIC TESTS

DIAGNOSTIC TEST RATIONALE	RESULTS/INTERPRETATION
CBC with differential	Hgb, 15 g/dl; HCT, 43.1%; MCV, 85; Platelets, 200,000; PT—12 seconds/PTT—35 seconds; WBC, 7.0 1000/mm³.
Thyroid studies	TSH, 4.6
FSH/LH, prolactin level	Not done because this was the first episode of bleeding.
Pregnancy test	HCG, negative.
Vaginal wet prep	

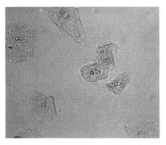

Figure 13–1. *Vagina wet mount (400X).*

Gen Probe	No chlamydia or gonorrhea.
Pelvic ultrasound	Not done

● DIAGNOSES

What diagnoses do you determine as being appropriate after a review of the subjective and objective data? Indicate what data support your diagnosis.

● THERAPEUTIC PLAN

1. How is dysfunctional uterine bleeding classified?

2. What influence does the classification have on the therapeutic treatment plan?

3. *Describe the management plan for Samantha's dysfunctional uterine bleeding.*

4. *When should Samantha be referred to a specialist?*

5. *What patient education should you discuss with Samantha?*

6. *What impact does this problem have in terms of lifestyle?*

7. *When should Samantha return for follow-up?*

8. *What resources are available for Samantha and the NP?*

REFERENCES

Bayer, S. R., & DeCherney, A. H. (1993). Clinical manifestations and treatment of dysfunctional uterine bleeding. *Journal of the American Medical Association, 269,* 1823–1828.

Bhattacharjee, B., Ghosh, A., Murray, A., & Murray, A. (2000). A study on the possible association of dysfunctional uterine bleeding with bacterial vaginosis, mycoplasma, ureaplasma, and Gardnerella vaginalis. *Sexually Transmitted Infections, 76,* 407.

Baughan, D. M. (1993). Challenges in the management of the patient with dysfunctional uterine bleeding. *Family Practice Recertification, 15,* 68–78.

Bravender, T., & Emans, S. (1999). Menstrual disorders. Dysfunctional uterine bleeding. *Pediatric Clinics of North America, 46*(3), 545–553.

Chen, B., & Giudice, L. (1998). Dysfunctional uterine bleeding. *Western Journal of Medicine, 169*(5), 280–284.

Dealy, M. F. (1998). Dysfunctional uterine bleeding in adolescents. *The Nurse Practitioner, 23*(5), 12–23.

Langer, R. D., Pierce, J. J., O'Hanlan, K. A., Johnson, S. R., Espeland, M. A., Trabal, J. F., Barnabei, V., Merino, M., & Scully, R. (1997). Transvaginal ultrasonography compared with endometrial biopsy for the detection of endometrial disease. *New England Journal of Medicine, 337,* 1792–1798.

Munro, M. (2000). Medical management of abnormal uterine bleeding. *Obstetrics and Gynecology Clinics of North America. 27*(2), 287–304.

Oriel, K., & Schrager, S. (1999). Abnormal uterine bleeding. *American Family Physician, 60*(5), 1371–1380.

Smith-Bindman, R., Kerlikowske, K., Feldstein, V. A., Subak, L., Scheidler, J., Segal, M., Brand, R., & Grady, P. (1998). Endovaginal ultrasound to exclude endometrial cancer and other endometrial abnormalities. *Journal of American Medical Association, 280,* 1510–1517.

Spencer, C. P., Cooper, A. J., & Whitehead, M. I. (1997). Management of abnormal bleeding in women receiving hormone replacement therapy. *British Medical Journal, 315,* 37–42.

Uphold, C. R., & Graham, M. V. (1998). *Clinical guidelines in family practice* (3rd ed.). Gainesville, FL: Barmarrae.

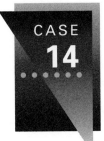

A 51-year-old woman with fatigue, irregular menstrual cycles, and night sweats

SCENARIO

Barbra Hudson presents to the women's health center with a history of night sweats, irregular menstrual bleeding, and labile emotions for the past 6 months. She is married and works as an RN in the emergency department at the local hospital.

● TENTATIVE DIAGNOSES

Based on the this scenario, what are the potential diagnoses for Barbra?

DIAGNOSIS	RATIONALE
1	
2	
3	
4	
5	
6	
7	

● HISTORY

What are significant questions in the history for Barbra?

REQUESTED DATA   DATA ANSWER

Allergies	NKA.
Medication	OTC medication for colds and headaches. Vitamins/iron.
Surgery/transfusion	Tonsillectomy (1960). Blood transfusion (1983). Exploratory laparotomy (1983).
Medical history/hospitalizations	Spontaneous vaginal delivery (1970). MVA (1983).
Fractures/injuries/accidents	MVA 1983: fracture right femur, internal bleeding.
OB/GYN history	LNMP, 6 months prior. Light to heavy flow. History of shortened intervals between cycles, varies 15–18 days for the 6 months prior to cessation of cycle. Last pelvic exam 1 year ago. Pap cytology has been within normal limits for the past 10 years. Previous abnormal Pap with appropriate follow-up. No sequelae. SBE: admits to intermittent exam every 3–4 months. Mammogram every 2 years for the past 10 years. G1P1A0L1.
Appetite/weight changes	No changes in weight or appetite. Stable weight for 5 years.
Social history	Tobacco: never. Alcohol: socially; 1–2 glasses wine per week. Caffeine: 2–3 cups of coffee/day and 2–3 colas/day. Illicit drug use: denies. OTC: acetaminophen (Tylenol), ibuprofen (Motrin), various cold remedies. Prescription drugs: none.
Exercise	Aerobics 2–3 times a week.
Family history	Father: deceased at age 33. Mother: 78, good health. Brothers: none. Sisters: 1, age 54, good health. Spouse: 59, good health. Children: 1 son, 30, good health.
Social organizations	Jewish synagogue.
Relationship with husband	Both are in monogamous relationship. Married 2 years ago. Engage in intercourse 1–2 times a week, and both report satisfaction. Husband a retired physician.

(continued)

REQUESTED DATA   DATA ANSWER

REQUESTED DATA	DATA ANSWER
Relationship with children	Reports good relationship with son. Engages in social activities with son and phones him 1–2 times a week. Son lives in another city. Vacations with son in California every year.
Income/insurance/home	Husband has healthy retirement income based on investments and stock market earnings. Has health insurance provided through employment. They own their own home.
Sexual history	Denies history of sexually transmitted diseases. Reports 5 partners since divorce 10 years ago. Admits to only occasional condom use. Reports decrease in desire for intimacy.
History of current symptoms	Reports fatigue for 6 months and shortening of intervals between menstrual cycles. Has noted cycles may be heavy one month and then light the next month. She wakes up 4–5 nights per week "drenched in sweat." Husband has noticed irritability and mood swings in association with night sweats. Both report satisfaction with sexual intercourse, but frequency has decreased.
How has this affected your ADLs?	Inability to determine next date of cycle, which disrupts day-to-day events. The night sweats disrupt sleep cycle, leading to irritability and sleep deprivation. Currently no loss of work has been reported.
How do you manage stress?	Aerobic exercise 2–3 times per week. Walks in park. Swims when not on menstrual cycle.
Any evidence of blood loss?	On last physical exam, stools were hemoccult negative. Approximately 9 months ago, menstrual cycle heavy and irregular. No menstrual loss in the past 6 months.
Any recent needlesticks/tattoos?	Denies.
Any known exposure to tuberculosis or HIV?	Denies.
Any travel recently?	Denies recent travel. Last trip 1 year ago to San Diego, California.
Has anyone in family been sick?	Denies.
Any change in energy level?	Only when sleep deprived.

● PHYSICAL ASSESSMENT

What are the significant portions of the physical assessment that should be completed for Barbra?

SYSTEM	RATIONALE	FINDINGS
Vital signs		BP 126/80 mm Hg right arm; HR, 76 bpm; RR, 18; T, 98.7 °F; Wt, 156 lbs; Ht 5'8"
General appearance/ skin		Alert, warm, and dry; color natural with varying degrees of pigmentation; no petechia. No pallor or jaundice; skin turgor elastic.
HEENT		Normocephalic; thyroid nonpalpable, no LA; PERRLA. TMs gray, without erythema or bulging. No oral lesions; uvula midline; teeth in fair repair.
Lungs		CTA.
Heart		S1, S2 WNL.
Abdomen		BS+; no organomegaly; no pain/tenderness; no LA.
Neurological assessment		Alert and oriented; DTRs, 2+.
Rectal		No masses noted; brown stool noted.
Extremities		ROM intact upper and lower extremities; pulses 2+; no edema; small varicosities noted on backs of thighs.
Pelvic		Thinning of labial tissue and vaginal rugae. Cervix pink. No abnormal discharge noted. No cervical motion tenderness. No masses palpated.

● DIFFERENTIAL DIAGNOSES

What are the significant positive and negative findings that support or refute your diagnoses for Barbra?

DIAGNOSIS	POSITIVE DATA	NEGATIVE DATA
1		
2		
3		
4		
5		
6		
7		

● DIAGNOSTIC TESTS

Based on the history and physical examination, what, if any, diagnostic testing would you obtain?

DIAGNOSTIC TEST	RATIONALE	RESULTS	INTERPRE-TATION
Hemoccult testing		Negative ×3.	
PPD		0 mm.	
CXR		Normal.	
TSH		TSH, 4.1 mU/mL.	
FSH		72 mLU/mL.	
Gen probe		Negative for chlamydia and gonorrhea.	
CBC		Hgb, 13.2 g/dL; HCt, 38.4%; WBC, 4 1000/mm³.	
Pap smear		Hormonally equated with menopause.	
Endometrial biopsy		(To be completed later.)	

● DIAGNOSES

What diagnoses do you determine as being appropriate after a review of the subjective and objective data?

Data Supporting the Diagnosis

● THERAPEUTIC PLAN

1. *How will the nurse practitioner manage the diagnosis?*
2. *When should Barbra be referred to a specialist and to whom?*
3. *What patient education should you discuss with Barbra?*
4. *What impact does this illness have on the family and work environment?*
5. *What suggestions can you make for Barbra and her family to control symptoms while her condition stabilizes?*
6. *When should Barbra return for follow-up?*
7. *What community resources are available for the NP and Barbra?*

REFERENCES

Abraham, D., & Carpenter, P. C. (1997). Issues concerning androgen replacement therapy in postmenopausal women. *Mayo Clinic Proceedings, 72,* 1051–1055.

Andrews, W. (1995). Continuous combined estrogen/progestin hormone replacement therapy. *Nurse Practitioner: American Journal of Primary Health Care, 20*(11 part 2), 1–11.

Barbach, L. (1996). Sexuality through menopause and beyond. *Menopause Management, 5*(6), 18–21.

Barrett-Connor, E., Timmons, C., Young, R., Wiita, B., & the Estratest Working Group. (1996). Interim safety analysis of a two-year study comparing oral estrogen-androgen and conjugated estrogens in surgically menopausal women. *Journal of Women's Health, 5,* 593–602.

Carlson, E., & Li, S. (1998). Androgen therapy for menopausal women. *Clinical Excellence for Nurse Practitioners, 2*(6), 324–328.

Coope, J. (1996). Hormonal and non-hormonal interventions for menopausal symptoms. *Maturitas, 23,* 159–168.

Lichtman, R. (1996). Perimenopausal and postmenopausal hormone replacement therapy. *Journal of Nurse- Midwifery, 41,* 3–28.

Mansfield, P. K., & Voda, A. M. (1997). Woman-centered information on menopause for health care providers: Findings from the midlife women's health survey. *Health Care for Women International, 18,* 55–72.

Mansfield, P. K., Voda, A. M., & Koch, P. (1995). Predictors of sexual response changes in heterosexual midlife women. *Health Values, 19,* 10–20.

Marten, S. (1993). Complications of menopause and the risks and benefits of estrogen replacement therapy. *Journal of American Academy of Nurse Practitioners, 5*(2), 55–61.

Masten, Y., & Gary, A. (1999). Is anyone listening? Does anyone care? Menopausal and postmenopausal health risks, outcomes, and care. *Nurse Practitioner Forum, 10*(4), 195–200.

Moore, A. A., & Noonan, M. D. (1999). A nurse's guide to hormone replacement therapy. *Journal of Obstetric, Gynecologic and Neonatal Nursing, 28*(Suppl 1), 13–20.

Myers, L. S. (1995). Methodological review and meta-analysis of sexuality and menopause research. *Neuroscience and Biobehavioral Reviews, 19,* 331–341.

Palacios, S., Menendez, C., Jurado, A. R., Castano, R., & Vargas, J. C. (1995). Changes in sex behavior after menopause. *Maturitas, 22,* 155–161.

Peterson, C. M. (1995). The rational use of androgens in hormone replacement therapy. *Clinical Obstetrics and Gynecology, 38,* 915–920.

Rako, S. (1996). Testosterone deficiency and supplementation for women: What do we need to know? *Menopause Management, 5*(5), 10–15.

Rousseau, M. (1998). Hormone replacement therapy. *Nurse Practitioner Forum, 9*(3), 147–153.

Sands, R., & Studd, J. (1995). Exogenous androgens in postmenopausal women. *American Journal of Medicine, 98,* 76.

Taylor, D. (1995). Perimenopausal symptoms and hormone therapy. In W. L. Star, L. L. Lommel, & M. T. Shannon (Eds.), *Women's primary health care: Protocols for practice* (pp. 12–140). Washington, DC: American Nurses Publishing.

Thyland, S., & Scharbo-DeHaan, M. (1995). Endometriosis may develop after menopause . . . possible risk/rewards of hormone replacement therapy. *Nurse Practitioner: American Journal of Primary Health Care, 20*(4), 15–16.

Voda, A. M. (1997). Menopause, me and you. Binghampton, NY: The Haworth Press.

Watts, N. B., Notelovitz, M., Timmons, M. C., Addison, W. A., Wiita, B., & Downey, L. J. (1995). Comparison of oral estrogens and estrogens plus androgen on bone mineral density, menopausal symptoms, and lipid-lipoprotein profiles in surgical menopause. *Obstetrics and Gynecology, 85,* 529–537.

Wetzel, W. (1998). Human identical hormones: Real people, real problems, real solutions. *Nurse Practitioner Forum, 9*(4), 227–234.

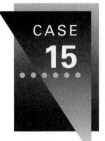

A 6-year-old boy with a red, itchy eye

SCENARIO

Mary Jennings has brought her 6-year-old son Joe to the office. He presents with the complaint of an itchy, red eye. Mary states that it was crusted with dry yellow drainage from his eye several times this morning. Joe has complained to Mary frequently about pain in his eye.

● TENTATIVE DIAGNOSES

At this point, what tentative diagnoses can you identify based on Joe's presentation and Mary's brief history?

● HISTORY

What questions would you ask Mary and Joe that would facilitate you in developing a diagnosis?

● PHYSICAL ASSESSMENT

Is a complete physical exam necessary? What parts of the exam would you include and why? How did your interpretation of the subjective data direct your physical examination?

● DIFFERENTIAL DIAGNOSES

List and prioritize your four most probable differential diagnoses. With each diagnosis, list the positive and negative data that validate or refute the diagnoses.

● DIAGNOSTIC TESTS

What, if any, additional data should be obtained? Would any diagnostic tests be appropriate in this case? Include your rationale for the testing.

● DIAGNOSIS

What is your conclusive diagnosis? What positive and negative data assisted you in arriving at your decision?

● THERAPEUTIC PLAN

1. *What therapeutic agent would you use in planning care for Joe?*
2. *What is your rationale for choosing this particular agent?*
3. *What are some alternatives to this treatment?*
4. *What education does Mary need to provide relief for Joe and decrease the risk of reinfection?*
5. *What follow-up care will Joe need?*

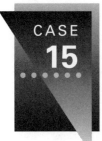

TUTORIAL

A 6-year-old boy with a red, itchy eye

SCENARIO

Mary Jennings has brought her 6-year-old son Joe to the office. He presents with the complaint of a red, itchy eye. Mary states that it was crusted with dry yellow drainage from his eye several times this morning. Joe has complained to Mary frequently about pain in his eye.

● TENTATIVE DIAGNOSES

What are the potential diagnoses you have identified based on this scenario?

DIFFERENTIAL DIAGNOSES	RATIONAL

1. Conjunctivitis
  a. Allergic
  b. Bacterial
  c. Chemical
  d. Viral
	Joe presents with itching, erythema, and pain in his OD. Mary has described a mucopurulent drainage from his OD. All of these symptoms are associated with conjunctivitis. Bacterial (gonococcal) conjunctivitis is **red flag.**

2. Corneal abrasion/eye trauma	Joe complains of erythema and pain in his OD. These symptoms and the unilateral involvement are associated with corneal abrasion and eye trauma. Hyphema is a **red flag.**
3. Herpes simplex blepharitis	Joe's complaints of itching, erythema, and pain are associated with herpes simplex blepharitis. With this diagnosis there is usually unilateral involvement. Herpes zoster is **red flag.**
4. Iritis	Joe's complaints of erythema, eye pain, and eye drainage are associated with iritis.
5. Glaucoma	Joe's complaints of pain and erythema of the eye are symptoms of glaucoma. Acute angle glaucoma is **red flag.**

● HISTORY

What questions would you ask Mary and Joe that would facilitate you in developing a diagnosis?

REQUESTED DATA	DATA ANSWER
Allergies	NKA.
Medication	None.
Recent changes in health	No problems until present complaint. Last check up 3 months ago.
Chief complaint: onset, location, quality, aggravating/alleviating factors	Joe describes burning, itching, and pain in OD. States that pain is not "too bad." Mary describes a thick yellow drainage. States it looks like pus. Joe's eyelids got stuck together by drainage. Joe denies a change in vision and blurred vision. Pain is bad when he looks at bright lights. Mary states warm wet washcloths have helped relieve burning.
Associated manifestations	No history of recent or concurrent respiratory infection.
Associated symptoms	Denies history of throat pain, ear pain, rhinorrhea.
History of exposure to conjunctivitis	None.
History of swimming in chlorinated or contaminated water	Swam two times in the past week in nonchlorinated pool.
History of trauma to eye	None.
History of exposure to chemicals	None.
Recent cold sores or exposure to herpes lesions	None.
Recent history of impetigo	None, but his younger brother was started on cephalexin (Keflex) 3 days ago for impetigo on his face.
Family members with eye problems	Joe has two younger siblings who do not have any eye symptoms.
Past medical history	Normally healthy. No hospitalizations or surgeries.

● PHYSICAL ASSESSMENT

What parts of the physical exam would you perform? Is a complete physical exam necessary? What parts of the exam would you include and why?

SYSTEM	RATIONALE	FINDINGS
Vital signs	Gives an indication of possible infection.	T (oral) 98 °C; HR, 84 bpm; RR, 22; BP 88/56 mm Hg.
Skin	Overall quick assessment of visible skin should be performed. Particular attention should be given to the face.	Skin is pink and supple, no lesions noted.
Ear, nose, throat	Gives an indication of possible infection.	TMs pearl gray bilaterally. Nares patent and free of drainage. No pharyngeal erythema or edema. No oral lesions.
Eyes	Need to evaluate eyes thoroughly to identify possible diagnoses. Visual acuity should be completed for all patients with eye problems. It is vital for patients with decreased vision. This testing may be painful if the child has photophobia.	OS sclera white, without infection, erythema, or edema. OD edema of eyelids present. Crusted yellow drainage on lashes. Conjunctiva markedly inflamed. Cornea and eyelid margins without ulceration. PERRLA with positive red reflex bilaterally. Visual acuity reveals OD 20/20, OS 20/20.
Fundoscopic	Provides a quick indication of eye healthiness. This testing may be difficult because of photophobia and constriction of pupils.	Discs well marginated. No AV nicking.
Heart sound	Provides baseline information.	S1 and S2 normal, without murmur
Breath sounds	Allows the NP to determine if there has been respiratory involvement.	CTA.
Lymphatics	Palpation of lymph nodes can provide an indication of infection.	No palpable lymph nodes in the head or neck.

● DIFFERENTIAL DIAGNOSIS

What are the significant positive and negative findings that support or refute your diagnoses for Joe?

DIAGNOSIS	POSITIVE AND NEGATIVE DATA
Allergic conjunctivitis	Conjunctiva inflamed. Itching and burning present. Cornea, pupil and vision normal. No watery discharge, profuse tearing, LA, bilateral involvement.
Bacterial conjunctivitis	Edema of eyelids, conjunctiva inflamed; itching, burning and pain present. Mucopurulent discharge, photophobia, cornea, pupil, vision normal. Unilateral involvement; history of recent impetigo in family. No eyelid margin ulceration.
Chemical conjunctivitis	Burning, itching, and pain present. Photophobia and unilateral involvement. Denies history of exposure to chemicals. No excessive tearing or thin water discharge.
Viral conjunctivitis	Edema of eyelids with burning and itching. Conjunctiva inflamed. Cornea, vision, and pupil normal. Denies history of recent or concurrent URI or viral illness. No bilateral involvement. Profuse watery discharge not evident. No preauricular LA. No hypertrophy of lymphoid follicles of lower palpebral conjunctiva.
Corneal abrasion/eye trauma	Conjunctiva inflamed with itching, burning, and photophobia present. Unilateral involvement. No history of trauma, cornea, vision, and pupil normal. No thin watery discharge.
Herpes simplex blepharitis	Conjunctiva inflamed with itching, burning, and photophobia. Unilateral involvement. No history of herpes or herpes involvement. No thin watery discharge or corneal or lid ulcerations. No corneal or eye lid ulcerations, severe pain or LA.
Iritis	Conjunctiva erythremic, with unilateral involvement. Complaining of mild to moderate pain. No decreased vision, severe pain, or decreased pupil sign with poor pupil reaction.
Glaucoma	Conjunctiva erythremic with mild to moderate pain. No severe pain. Eye pressure normal. No cornea cloudiness or marked decrease in vision. Pupil is not fixed or dilated.

● DIAGNOSTIC TESTS

Would any diagnostic tests be appropriate in this case? What is your rationale for the tests?

DIAGNOSTIC TEST	RATIONALE	RESULTS
Eye culture and gram stain	Would probably not be necessary for Joe at this point. If his infection is resistant or recurring, this might be considered. Eye cultures should always be done on children younger than 1 month of age. Cultures of the eye and nasopharynx should be done concurrently for gonococcal, chlamydial, and bacterial infections (Baker, 1999).	Test not done.

● DIAGNOSES

What diagnoses do you determine as being appropriate after a review of the subjective and objective data?

DIAGNOSIS	RATIONALE
Conjunctivitis: bacterial	Positive history of exposure to causative bacteria. All of the symptoms Joe is experiencing can be the effect of bacterial conjuctivitis. The negative finding of eyelid margin ulceration is not a consistent finding in patients with bacterial conjunctivitis and does not eliminate this diagnosis.

● THERAPEUTIC PLAN

1. *What therapeutic agent would you use in planning your care for Joe?*
   Because most causes of bacterial conjunctivitis are due to *Haemophilus influenza* or *Streptococcus pneumoniae*, it would be important to treat with the most effective medication. Ciprofloxacin (Ciloxan) 1 to 2 gtts while awake for 2 days, then 1 to 2 gtts every 4 hours while awake.

2. *What is your rationale for choosing this particular agent?*
   Ciprofloxacin, ofloxacin, and tetracycline are the most active agents against pediatric conjunctivitis. Gentamicin, tobramycin, and polymyxin

B-trimethoprim are intermediately active. Sulfamethoxazole possesses no activity against either *S. pneumoniae* or *H. influenza* (Block et al., 2000).

3. *What are some alternatives to this treatment?*
   Tobramycin ointment or polymixin B trimethoprim solution would be an alternative treatment for Joe. Gentamicin and neomycin are options for use but have a higher incidence of allergic reactions (Merenstein, Kaplan, & Rosenberg, 1994).

4. *What education does Mary need to provide relief for Joe and decrease the risk of reinfection?*

Medication Administration

- Clean the eye before medication administration. Wipe eye with a wet cotton ball, from the inner to outer canthus. Throw away cotton ball.
- To apply or instill: Gently separate eyelids, pull down inner canthus or lower lid toward center of the eye. Place the drops or thin line of ointment in the pocket that is formed (Boynton, Donn, & Stephens, 1998).
- Infection should respond to treatment in 2 to 3 days.

Comfort Measures

- Wet compresses, cool or warm per child's preference. Use cotton balls.
- Joe may need distraction to keep him from rubbing or scratching his eye.

Infection Control

- Good handwashing by entire family.
- Have Joe keep his hands away from his face and eye.
- Keep Joe's face cloths and towels separate from those of other family members. Use these linens one time only.
- Monitor Joe's siblings for symptoms.

5. *What follow-up care will Joe need?*
   Joe should stay home from school until inflammation and discharge are gone. Instruct Mary to call in 2 to 3 days if no improvement is seen. Instruct Mary to call if symptoms worsen or vision decreases. No follow-up visit is necessary if Joe has a response to the medication. The infection should be resolved in 1 week.

REFERENCES

Alessandrini, E. (2000). The case of the red eye. *Pediatric Annals, 29* (2), 112–116.
Baker, L., Burton, J. & Steve, P. (1999). Principles of ambulatory medicine (5th ed.). Philadelphia: Lippincott Williams & Wilkins.
Block, S., Hedrick, J., Tyler, R., Smith, A., Findlay, R., Keegan, E., & Stroman, D. (2000).

Increasing bacterial resistance in pediatric acute conjunctivitis (1997–1998). *Antimicrobial Agents Chemotherapeutics, 44,* 1650–1654.

Boynton, R., Dunn, E., & Stephens, G. (1998). *Manual of ambulatory pediatrics* (4th ed.). Philadelphia: Lippincott Williams & Wilkins.

Coston, C. C., & Craven, R. A. (1994). Reading the red eye: Conjunctivitis and its mimics. *Emergency Medicine, 26*(11), 15–20, 23–26, 29.

Lee, A. G., Beaver, H. A., & Hamill, M. B. (1998). What's causing that red eye? Clues to the underlying source. *Hospital Medicine, 34*(12), 30–32, 35–38, 57–58.

Leibountz, H. (2000). The red eye. *New England Journal of Medicine, 343,* 345–351.

Marsden, J. (1998). Identifying and managing non-traumatic red eye in A&E. *Emergency Nurse, 5*(9), 34–40.

Merenstein, G., Kaplan, D., & Rosenberg, A. (1994). *Handbook of pediatrics.* Norwalk, CT: Appleton and Lange.

Ruppert, S. D. (1996). Differential diagnosis of pediatric conjunctivitis (red eye). *Nurse Practitioner: American Journal of Primary Health Care, 21*(7), 12, 15–16, 18.

Small, R. G. (1995). Ophthalmology in primary care: Office workup for red eye. *Consultant, 35,* 321–324, 327.

Trobe, J. D. (1994). Red eye: Spotting the seven dangerous causes. *Consultant, 34,* 1657–1660, 1662.

Weber, C. M., & Eichenbaum, J. W. (1997). Acute red eye: Differentiating viral conjunctivitis from other, less common causes. *Postgraduate Medicine, 101*(5), 185–186, 189–192, 195–196.

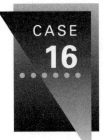

A 54-year-old man with blurred vision, polyuria, and fatigue

SCENARIO

Joe Hobbs is a 54-year-old obese white man who presents to your clinic. Joe has not seen a health care provider in 6 years. He states that until 3 months ago he was feeling fine. Joe has slowly experienced a blurring of his vision. He also relates that he has been having polyuria, polydipsia, and fatigue. He currently takes no medications.

● TENTATIVE DIAGNOSES

*Based on the information provided, what are the potential differential diagnoses? What are **red flag** diagnoses that cannot be missed?*

DIAGNOSIS	RATIONALE
1	
2	
3	
4	
5	

● HISTORY

What are significant questions in the history for Joe? What are the key points to cover on the review of systems?

REQUESTED DATA   DATA ANSWER

REQUESTED DATA	DATA ANSWER
Allergies	NKDA.
Current medications	None.
Surgery/transfusions	Tonsillectomy at age 10.
Medical history/ hospitalizations/ fractures/injuries/ accidents	Unremarkable (should ask about prior or current infections of the skin, feet, gums, teeth, and GU system).
Sleeping pattern	Getting up recently to urinate 3–4 times a night.
Appetite/weight change	Has gained approximately 20 lbs in past year but has lost 5 lbs in past 2 weeks without really trying. Has noticed that his thirst is tremendous, and he is unable to quench his thirst, even with his usual soft drink.
24-hour diet recall	B: sausage biscuit with gravy, coffee, and orange juice. L: hamburger, french fries, soda. D: meat, potato, gravy, vegetable, and salad. S: potato chips or ice cream.
Social history	Tobacco: none. Alcohol: none. Drugs: denies. Caffeine: 2 cups coffee/day. Exercise: none.
Family history	Father: died at age 55, HTN, DM. Mother: age 74, breast cancer. PGF: deceased 49, MI. MGM: deceased 65, CVA.
Employment	New job in past year as salesperson, does a lot of traveling.

SYSTEM REVIEWED   DATA ANSWER

SYSTEM REVIEWED	DATA ANSWER
General	Feels fatigued after lunch. At times he does not feel he has enough energy to do his usual activities.
Skin	Dry, but no problems. Denies problems with healing.
HEENT	Vision change recently. He noticed his vision is blurry and has difficulty with reading. He does not wear corrective lenses. Denies loss of peripheral vision or difficulty with glare.

(continued)

SYSTEM REVIEWED   DATA ANSWER

SYSTEM REVIEWED	DATA ANSWER
Lungs	Denies problems breathing or SOB.
Cardiac	Denies chest pain or palpitations.
GI/GU	Denies dysuria, frequency or urgency, hesitancy in starting stream, no dribbling, retention (should also ask about sexual function).

● PHYSICAL ASSESSMENT

What are the significant portions of the physical examination that should be completed for Joe?

SYSTEM	RATIONALE	FINDINGS
Vital signs	Provides baseline data.	BP, 130/86 mm Hg; HR, 78 bpm; RR, 22; T, 98.2 °F.
General appearance/skin	General overall picture of patient's status.	Alert; NAD.
Eyes	Look for changes in blood vessels of retina.	Optic disc margins well defined. No nicking or hemorrhages.
Neck	Check vascular status/thyroid.	Supple; no thyromegaly or bruits.
Lungs	Provides baseline data.	CTA.
Heart	Provides baseline data. Important to evaluate because he has a + FH.	RRR; no MRG.
Abdomen	Baseline data, able to check vascular status.	BS+, soft; no masses, tenderness, HSM, or bruits.
Extremities/feet	Assessment of peripheral vascular system. A monofilament test for sensation is quick and should be done on a yearly basis to identify if his feet are at high risk for vascular problems.	Pulses 2+; skin warm and pink; no edema. Sensation intact. Able to detect the monofilament in all areas. Feet dry, no callus, no open lesions.

(continued)

SYSTEM	RATIONALE	FINDINGS
Rectal	Assessment of prostate, check for blood loss.	Anal sphincter WNL; prostate firm, nonenlarged; no nodules; brown soft stool.

● DIFFERENTIAL DIAGNOSES

What are the significant positive and negative data that support or refute your diagnoses for Joe?

DIAGNOSIS	POSITIVE DATA	NEGATIVE DATA
1		
2		
3		
4		
5		
6		

● DIAGNOSTIC TESTS

Based on the history and physical assessment, what, if any, diagnostic testing would you do. Include your rationale for the testing.

DIAGNOSTIC TEST	RATIONALE	RESULTS	INTERPRETATION
CBC	Provide baseline information, rule out anemia	WBC, $5.9 \times 10^3/\mu L$; RBC, $5.03 \times 10^6/\mu L$; Hgb, 15.8 g/dL; HCT, 46.8%; MCV, 92.1; MCH, 31.5; RDW, 11.8%; platelet, 236.	WNL.

(continued)

DIAGNOSTIC TEST	RATIONALE	RESULTS	INTERPRETATION
Lipid profile	Provide baseline information, particularly since patient has a + FH.	Cholesterol, 260 mg/dL; LDL, 188 mg/dL; HDL, 47 mg/dL; triglycerides, 330 mg/dL.	Elevated cholesterol, LDL, and triglycerides.
Chemistry	Provide baseline information.	FBS, 350 mg/dL; BUN, 17 mg/dL; creatinine 1.4 mg/dL; Na, 143 mEq/L; K, 4.4 mEq/L; CO_2, 27 mEq/L; calcium, 10.1 mg/dL; albumin, 4.7 g/dL; bilirubin, 1.3 mg/dL; alkaline phosphatase, 89 U/L; AST, 41 U/L; ALT, 47 U/L.	Elevated glucose, all others WNL.
Thyroid profile	Rule out thyroid dysfunction, given the high prevalence with other autoimmune diseases.	TSH, 1.2; T_4 7.0 μg/dL.	WNL.
Hgb A1C	Provides indication of glucose levels for past 10–12 weeks. Not generally used for diagnostic purposes.	12%.	Out-of-control diabetes.
U/A	Rule out UTI, check for ketones, microalbuminuria, and glucose.	3+ glucose; ketones, negative; protein, negative; SG, 1.018; pH, 6.0; blood, negative; nitrite, negative; leukocytes, negative; microalbumin, negative	WNL.

(continued)

DIAGNOSTIC TEST	RATIONALE	RESULTS	INTERPRETATION
Electrocardiogram	Document cardiac functions. Provide a baseline for future comparisons.	Rate, 86; PR, 0.16; QRS, 0.08; QT, 0.36; No ST depression or elevation.	Normal sinus rhythm, normal electro-cardiogram results.

● DIAGNOSIS

What diagnoses do you determine as being appropriate for Joe?

● THERAPEUTIC PLAN

1. *Identify the risk factors that contributed to Joe's disease.*
2. *Why did Joe exhibit the symptoms of polyuria, polydipsia, fatigue, and blurred vision?*
3. *What are the short-term management goals for Joe?*
4. *What patient education should Joe receive related to his medications and management of his disease when ill?*
5. *What type of surveillance needs to be done to monitor the existence of chronic complications from his disease?*
6. *When should Joe return for follow-up?*
7. *What are support systems that are available to assist the NP, Joe, and his wife in the management of his disease?*

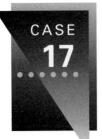

A 20-year-old woman with vaginal itching and malodorous discharge

SCENARIO

Kate Warren presents to the Student Health Clinic stating, "I think I have a yeast infection." She reports a 4-day history of vaginal discharge, itching, and foul odor. She attends college full time and shares an apartment with three other students.

● TENTATIVE DIAGNOSES

What potential diagnoses have you identified based on the scenario presented? Identify any red flag conditions that you cannot miss.

DIAGNOSIS	RATIONALE
1	
2	
3	
4	
5	
6	
7	
8	

● HISTORY

What are significant questions in the history for Kate?

REQUESTED DATA   DATA ANSWER

REQUESTED DATA	DATA ANSWER
Allergies	NKA.
Medications	No prescription medications. Occasional OTC pain reliever for minor aches and pains.
Previous vaginal infections and treatment	Self-diagnosed "yeast" infection about 1 year ago. Had severe itching, a very thick, white discharge but does not remember having an odor. Successfully self-treated with OTC vaginal cream for yeast.
OB/GYN history	Menarche, age 14. Periods regular; moderate flow; occur about every 30 days; last 4–5 days. Uses unscented tampons. LNMP, 2 weeks ago; usual flow and duration. Birth control: Condoms. G0P0A0 Last pelvic exam: age 18 with normal Papanicolaou smear results. Mammogram: none. BSE: no. Use of vaginal sprays, powders, douching: none. Showers daily, "never" takes tub baths, has used same antibacterial soap for bathing past 4–5 years.
Sexual history	Sporadic heterosexual intercourse since age 17. Has had current sexual partner for 2 years. She is monogamous and believes him to be as well. Sexual intercourse about 2 times a week in past month. Uses condoms every time with no known breaks. Used same brand condoms for 2 years. Last sexual intercourse 5 days ago with no discomfort. Partner has not shared history of any symptoms. Both tested negative for HIV 1 year ago.
Onset of symptoms	Noticed vaginal itching, discharge, and odor about 4 days ago. Itching not intense but is noticeable. Vaginal discharge thin, gray-white, and has a "fishy," unpleasant odor.
Other significant past medical history	Tonsillectomy and adenoidectomy age 8. Mumps, measles, and chicken pox as child. Mononucleosis, age 16 with no sequelae. Considers self "healthy," no recent illnesses.
Social history	Tobacco: none. Alcohol: 2–3 alcoholic drinks 1 night a week. Occasionally has 2–3 alcoholic drinks on weekends. No DUIs or other legal infractions.

(continued)

REQUESTED DATA   DATA ANSWER

	Caffeine: 2 cups coffee most mornings: 2–3 sodas a day.
	Recreational drugs: none.
	Drinks 2–3 8-ounce bottles of water a day.
	Attends classes at the university daily. Studies 3–4 hours a day after classes.
	Exercise: aerobic 3 times a week.
	Stress: relieves with exercise and occasional "flag" football.
Income/insurance	Parents are paying tuition and expenses. Has a "drug card" for buying prescription medications.

What are the key points to cover in the review of systems?

SYSTEM   DATA RECEIVED

SYSTEM	DATA RECEIVED
General	Denies chills, fever, loss of appetite, or weight changes
HEENT	Denies URI, sore throat, or congested nose.
Chest	Denies palpitations, chest pain, or SOB.
Gastrointestinal GI	Denies abdominal pain, nausea, or vomiting
GU	Denies frequency, urgency, or dysuria. Denies pelvic pain, pressure, or genital lesions.
Lymphatics	Has noticed no enlarged lymph nodes in groin or other part of body.
Skin	Denies rashes or lesions.

● PHYSICAL ASSESSMENT

What are the significant portions of the physical examination that should be completed for Kate? What is your rationale for including the system identified?

SYSTEM   RATIONALE   FINDINGS

SYSTEM	RATIONALE	FINDINGS
Vital signs		T, 97.7 °F; P, 76; RR, 16; BP 104/62 mm Hg; Ht, 5′5″; Wt, 123 lbs.
General appearance		Alert, friendly, NAD. Skin warm and dry.

(continued)

SYSTEM	RATIONALE	FINDINGS
Heart		Regular rate and rhythm. No murmurs.
Lungs		CTA.
Abdomen		BS+ all four quadrants; soft, nontender. No organomegaly; no LA; no CVAT.
Pelvic		External genitalia: no swelling, redness, ulceration, lesions or infestation; no LA.
		Vagina: pink with prominent rugae; adherent gray-white homogenous discharge; fishy odor prominent.
		Cervix: pink, nulliparous os, no discharge. Nonfriable.
		Bimanual exam: uterus small, firm, mobile, nontender, anteverted. No adnexal masses or tenderness; ovaries not palpable. No CMT.

● DIFFERENTIAL DIAGNOSES

What are the significant positive and negative findings that support or refute your diagnoses for Kate?

DIAGNOSIS	POSITIVE AND NEGATIVE DATA
1	
2	
3	
4	
5	
6	
7	

● DIAGNOSTIC TESTS

Based on the history and physical examination, the following tests were done. What is the significance of these findings?

DIAGNOSTIC TEST	RATIONALE	RESULT	INTERPRETATION/ SIGNIFICANCE
Wet mount (saline)		See Figure 17-1.	

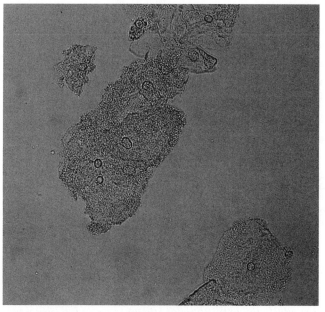

Figure 17–1. (400×). From Robinson & McKenzie, p. 343.

Wet mount (KOH)		No budding yeast or pseudohyphae.	
Whiff test		+ whiff test.	
Vaginal pH		4.7.	
U/A		Negative for bacteria and leukocytes.	
Urine HCG		Negative urine HCG.	

Other diagnostic tests to consider, depending on the patient's history, symptoms, and clinical findings are:

DIAGNOSTIC TEST	RATIONALE	RESULTS	INTERPRETATION
Cultures of cervical discharge		Clear cervical discharge.	
Culture of genital lesions		No lesions present.	
Veneral Disease Research Laboratory Test (VDRL) or rapid plasma reagin test (RPR)		Nonreactive.	
White count with differential		Not done.	
Fasting blood sugar		Glucose, 116 mg/dL.	

● DIAGNOSIS

Based on a review of the subjective and objective data, what is the appropriate diagnosis? What is the pathophysiology of the condition?

How is vaginitis classified?

Identify and compare the most common causes of vulvovaginitis:

COMPARISON OF COMMON CAUSES OF VULVOVAGINITIS

Predisposing factors

Clinical findings

Lab findings

Complications if misdiagnosed or untreated

● TREATMENT PLAN

	BACTERIAL VAGINOSIS	VULVOVAGINAL CANDIDIASIS	TRICHOMONIASIS
Acute treatment			
Alternative treatment			
Treatment during pregnancy			

1. What are the warnings for each of the treatments listed?

2. How does the classification of vaginitis affect the treatment plan?

3. What will be the management plan for Kate?

4. What patient education should be discussed with Kate?

5. When should Kate be referred to a specialist and to whom?

6. What other sources of information might be beneficial to Kate?

REFERENCES

(2000). Updates. Diagnosing vaginal trichomoniasis. *Contemporary OB/GYN, 45*(8), 114, 117.

Abbott, J. (1995). Clinical and microscopic diagnosis of vaginal yeast infection: A prospective analysis. *Annals of Emergency Medicine, 25,* 587–591.

Amankawa, L., & Frank, D. (1991). Vulvovaginal conditions: A study of immediate vs. delayed treatment on patient comfort. *Nurse Practitioner, 16*(6), 23–27.

Antonelli, N, Diehl, S., & Wright, J. (2000). A randomized trial of intravaginal nonoxynol 9 versus oral metronidazole in the treatment of vaginal trichomoniasis. *American Journal of Obstetrics and Gynecology, 182,* 1008–1010.

Association of Professors of Gynecology and Obstetrics. (1996). *Diagnosis of vaginitis.* St. Paul: 3M Pharmaceuticals, 1–9.

Buttaro, T. M., Trybulski, J., Bailey, P. P., & Sandberg-Cook, J. (1999). *Primary care: A collaborative practice.* St: Louis: Mosby, 699–704.

Centers for Disease Control and Prevention. (1998). 1998 Sexually transmitted disease guidelines. *MMWR, 47,* 1–111.

Coco, A. S., & Vandenbosche, M. (2000). Infectious vaginitis: An accurate diagnosis is essential and attainable. *Postgraduate Medicine, 107*(4), 63–66, 69–74

Cleveland, A. (2000). Vaginitis: Finding the cause prevents treatment failure. *Cleveland Clinic Journal of Medicine, 67*(9), 634, 637–642, 645–646.

Cullins, V. E., Dominquez, L., Guberski, T., Secor, R. M., & Wysoki, S. J. (1999). Treating vaginitis. *The Nurse Practitioner, 24,* 10, 46–65.

Eckert, L. O., Hawes, S. E., Stevens, C. E., Koutsky, L. A., Eschenbach, D. A., Holmes, K. K. (1998). Vulvovaginal candidiasis: Clinical manifestations, risk factors, management algorithm. *Gynecology, 92,* 757–765.

Egan, M. E., & Lipsky, M. S. (2000). Diagnosis of vaginitis. *American Family Physician; 62,* 1095–1104.

Lipsky, M., Waters, T., & Sharp, L. (2000). Impact of vaginal antifungal products on utilization of health care services: Evidence from physician visits. *Journal of American Board of Family Practice, 13*(3), 178–182.

Lowe, N., & Ryan-Wenger, N. (2000). A clinical test of women's self-diagnosis of genitourinary infections. *Clinical Nursing Research, 9*(2), 144–160

Mead, P. B., Eschenbach, D. A., & Sobel, J. D. (1999). Update on management of vaginitis. *Contemporary OB/GYN, 44*(11), 26–28, 31–32, 34.

Rex, J., Walsh, T., Sobel, J., Filler, S., Pappas, P., Dismukes, W., & Edwards, J. (2000). Practice guidelines for the treatment of candidiasis. Infectious Diseases Society of America. *Clinical Infectious Diseases, 30*(4), 662–678.

Robinson, D., Kidd, P., & Rogers, K. M. (2000). *Primary care across the lifespan.* St. Louis: Mosby.

Robinson, D., & McKenzie, C. (2000). *Procedures for primary care providers.* Philadelphia: Lippincott Williams & Wilkins.

Sweet, R. (2000). *The vaginitis report.* St. Paul: 3M National Vaginitis Association, Spring, 1–4.

Witkin, S. S., & Giraldo, P. C. (2000). The quandary of recurrent vaginal candidiasis. *Patient Care, 34*(2), 123–126, 129.

Woodward, C., & Fisher, M. A. (1999). Drug treatment of common STDs: Part II. Vaginal infections, pelvic inflammatory disease and genital warts. *American Family Physician, 60,* 1716–1722.

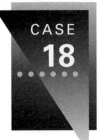

A 68-year-old woman with severe dizziness

SCENARIO

Grace Brown is a 68-year-old, slender African-American woman who presents with complaints of severe dizziness, nausea, and vomiting. She states she has had bouts of dizziness over a 3-day period, and the nausea had increased to the point that she has had four violent vomiting episodes since awakening early this morning. She complains of weakness.

● TENTATIVE DIAGNOSES

Based on Grace's presentation, what are the tentative differential diagnoses?

● HISTORY

What questions do you want to ask Grace to assist you in developing a diagnosis?

● PHYSICAL ASSESSMENT

What parts of the physical examination are needed? Are there any special maneuvers that need to be included in the exam?

● DIFFERENTIAL DIAGNOSES

What are the significant positive or negative data that support or refute the differential diagnoses for Grace?

● DIAGNOSTIC TESTS

What additional data or diagnostics are needed to confirm the priority diagnosis? Include your rationale for testing.

● DIAGNOSIS

After combining subjective and objective data with test findings, what is the diagnosis? Identify data that support this diagnosis. Include information about the pathophysiology for this condition.

● THERAPEUTIC PLAN

1. *What is the basic teaching you will do for Grace about this condition?*
2. *What self-care measures would be helpful for Grace in terms of exercise, diet, and monitoring?*
3. *What referrals would be appropriate for Grace?*
4. *What medications might be appropriate for Grace based on the severity of her symptoms?*
5. *What follow-up should be planned for Grace?*
6. *What impact might this condition have on her family? Identify needed education for the family.*
7. *What resources are available for Grace and her family?*

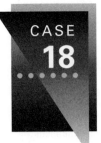

TUTORIAL

A 68-year-old woman with severe dizziness

SCENARIO

Grace Brown is a 68-year-old, slender African-American woman who presents with complaints of severe dizziness, nausea, and vomiting. She states she has had bouts of dizziness over a 3-day period, and the nausea has increased to the point that she has had four violent vomiting episodes since awakening early this morning. She complains of weakness.

● TENTATIVE DIAGNOSES

Based on Grace's presentation, what are the tentative differential diagnoses?

DIFFERENTIAL DIAGNOSIS	RATIONALE
1. Peripheral vertigo	Peripheral vestibular disorder, trauma, or age-related changes of the inner ear can cause the sensation of spinning or motion.
a. Benign paroxysmal positional vertigo	Accumulation of organic debris in postsemicircular canal. Patient c/o a spinning sensation with position change. All of these symptoms are associated with BPPV.
b. Peripheral vestibulopathy	A spinning sensation of dizziness with nausea is an indicator of vestibulopathy. A primary cause of vestibulopathy is tertiary syphilis or labrynthitis.
c. Meniere's disease	Patient c/o dizziness: a symptom of Meniere's disease.
d. Post-traumatic vertigo	Dizziness can be caused by trauma. Until recent trauma is ruled out, this diagnosis needs to be considered.
e. Ototoxic drugs	Various drugs can cause the adverse effect of dizziness and nausea. Drugs such as aspirin and aminoglycosides should be considered potential causes of dizziness.

(continued)

DIFFERENTIAL DIAGNOSIS	RATIONALE
2. Central vertigo	Neoplastic and vascular disorder of the lower brainstem and cerebellum can cause unsteadiness, imbalance, and a feeling that a fall is imminent.
a. Acoustic neurinoma	Patient c/o hearing loss and vertigo. Symptoms of acoustic neurinoma include a slowly progressing unilateral hearing loss and dizziness.
b. Vertibrobasilar arterial disease	Hearing loss and vertigo are symptoms of inadequate bloodflow to the brain. **Red flag.**
3. Syncope/near syncope	These conditions are caused by cardiovascular, cerbrovascular, or psychogenesis, with feelings of lightheadedness, fainting, or impending loss of consciousness.
a. Hypotension, from vasodilating-dilating drugs and decreased blood volume	Dizziness and nausea are indicators of hypotension. Until blood loss from recent trauma is ruled out, it must be considered a potential diagnosis. **Red flag.**
b. Cardiac disease, such as aortic stenosis, arrhythmia, carotid sinus hypersensitivity, and diminished vascular reflexes of the elderly	Patient's report of dizziness supports the possible diagnosis of cardiac disease. In addition, given her age, cardiac causes need to be considered a possibility of etiology.
c. Metabolic conditions, such as hypo- or hyperglycemia, hypothyroidism and anemia	Dizziness is a possible symptom for increased glucose or decreased glucose or thyroid function. Elderly women are at risk for hyperglycemia and hypothyroidism. In addition, anemia with its resultant lowered hemoglobin could cause dizziness and must be considered.
d. Intracranial conditions, such as seizure disorder, migraine, and increased intracranial pressure	Patient's c/o dizziness and nausea can be the primary symptoms noted for an intercranial lesion. **Red flag.**
e. Psychiatric disorders, such as anxiety, depression, psychosis	Because you do not know patient's living situation, coping abilities, or social situation, dizziness and nausea should be considered symptoms of psychiatric disorders. A vague history along with stress can indicate psychogenic disorders.

● HISTORY

What questions do you want to ask Grace to assist you in developing a diagnosis?

QUESTION	ANSWER
Allergies?	NKA.
Current medications?	Prescribed: Atenolol (Tenormin), 50 mg po QD. HCTZ, 25 mg po QD. OTC: Acetaminophen (Tylenol Extra Strength) prn for pain (approximately 2 times month.)
When did the symptoms start?	About 3 days ago.
How long does the dizziness last?	Not long—a few seconds, then it stops. Then I feel sick to my stomach.
Do you have a sensation of spinning or the room moving around you?	Mostly spinning, like the room is moving. Then I feel a little off balance.
Does any certain movement precipitate the dizziness?	It seems to start first thing in the morning when I roll over to get out of bed. And then, when I try to lay down on the couch because I'm sick at my stomach, it starts over again.
Do you have any changes in vision with the dizziness?	No.
Have you had any other illness in the past 3 months?	No.
Do you have any pain with the dizziness?	No.
Do you have any loss of balance with the dizziness or any loss of consciousness?	No.
Have you noticed any hearing loss or ringing in your ears?	My daughter says I'm getting hard of hearing, but I haven't noticed it getting worse. No ringing of the ears.
Difficulty walking or weakness?	I feel weak today because I can't keep anything down. I've thrown up four times today. It is difficult to walk when you are so dizzy and sick.
Any history of seizures or convulsions?	No.
Have you hit your head lately or been in any kind of accident where you might have hit your head?	No.

(continued)

QUESTION	ANSWER
Do you feel like you're going to pass out or faint?	No.
Any history of heart disease for you or your family?	No.
Have you ever had this type of dizziness before?	No.
Describe what you were doing before the dizziness occurred and what position you were in. Did you have any chest pain or palpitations before the dizziness?	The dizziness occurred after I got out of bed. No chest pain or palpitations.
Describe your diet for the past 24 hours	Breakfast: 1 piece toast, cup of hot tea. Lunch: sliced tomato and tuna with crackers, glass of milk. Dinner: chicken and rice frozen dinner, tea.
Have you been able to maintain your normal activities since you have been sick?	Can't do my volunteer job at the library. I've had to call in sick the last 3 days. When I bend over to clean up at the bathroom sink, I feel like the dizziness is going to start again, and I just can't get any of my housework or yardwork done. My neighbor and I take a walk every night after dinner, and I haven't felt like doing that.
Do you live alone?	Yes, my husband passed on 8 years ago. I stay busy with my friends and children, and I do volunteer at the local library a few hours in the morning. I love books and I love to read. I am able to drive but today felt too sick to drive.
Have you had a recent weight gain or loss?	No.
Do you have any problems sleeping?	I usually get 7–8 hours a night. Haven't had any problems with sleeping, but in the last couple of days, I have this dizziness in bed sometimes, especially when I roll over to look at the clock. It makes getting to sleep hard.
Social habits: Tobacco	No.
ETOH	Occasionally have a cocktail when out to dinner with friends 1–2 times a month.

It is important to determine if syncope actually occurred. This information needs to be collected from family if possible. The presyncopal period probably is the most important period upon which to focus. In addition, ask about premonitory symptoms and their duration. Nausea and vomiting are nonspecific; symptoms such as chest pain or palpitations imply cardiac disease, whereas vertigo, diplopia, dysarthria, hemiparesis, or aura shift the focus to the nervous system. Little or no warning suggests an arrhythmia or seizure.

Questions Useful in the Differential Diagnosis of Vertigo

QUESTION	BPPV	H/A	EH	LABYR	CVA	TIA	FISTULA	AN	MVC
Sudden onset	+++		a	++	+++	+++	+++	May occur	+++
Gradual onset		+++	++	May occur				May occur	
Constant		b	+++	c	c	+++	+++	May occur	
Episodic	+++	+++	+++			+++	+++	May occur	+++
Duration	< 1 min	30 min–days	30 min–hours	Days	Days	2–5 min	Seconds	Seconds	Second–minutes
Caused by head movement with respect to gravity	+++							May occur	++
Caused by valsalva, cough, laugh, straining, air travel	d	May occur					+++		May occur
Tinnitus or ear pressure associated with vertigo			+++				May occur	May occur	May occur
A single or very few major episodes				+++	+++				
Multiple episodes	+++	++	++			e	+++	May occur	+++

BPPV = benign paroxysmal positional vertigo; H/A = migraine; EH = endolymphatic hydrops (Meniere's); Labyr = labyrinthitis/vestibular neuritis; CVA = stroke; TIA = transient ischemic attack; AN = acoustic neuroma; MVC = microvascular compression.

++ common
+++ less common
a = A form of Meniere's disease, otolithic crisis of Tumarkin, has extremely sudden onset.
b = Vestibular migraine can present as a constant vague dizziness as well as an episodic vertigo.
c = A stroke and labyrinthitis usually produce a constant vertigo that improves over days to weeks.
d = Only if caused by a corresponding head movement.
e = A very large number of TIAs without a complete stroke is unlikely.
From: Barker, L., Burton, J., & Zieve, P. (1999). *Principles of ambulatory medicine* (5th ed., p 1254). Baltimore: Williams & Wilkins.

● PHYSICAL ASSESSMENT

What parts of the physical examination are needed? Are there any special maneuvers that need to be included in the exam?

EXAMINATION	RATIONALE	FINDINGS
Vital signs, orthostatics	Baseline information. Orthostatics indicated for possible hypovolemia.	Supine BP, 136/88 mm Hg right arm and 138/88 mm Hg left arm; HR, 76 bpm; Standing BP, 134/86 mm Hg right arm and 136/86 mm Hg left arm; HR, 78 bpm; RR, 20; T, 97.4 °F oral.
Skin mucous membranes	Check for hydration status.	Pale, dry, turgor fair. Mucus membranes and nailbeds pink. No jaundice, bruising, spider angiomas noted.
Eye	Indicated to check for visual changes as well as spontaneous nystagmus in both peripheral and central vestibular dysfunction. Also important to evaluate secondary to HTN (Williams, Schneiderman, & Algranati, 1994).	No AV nicking. No exudate or hemorrhage noted. Disk well marginated. Visual acuity OD 20/40, OS 20/30 corrected with glasses.
Ear	Indicated for evaluation of hearing loss, a symptom of Meniere's syndrome.	Denies tenderness of external ear. TMs gray; light reflex present. Rinne/Weber WNL. Hearing handicap inventory for the elderly score of 6; a score of 8 shows probable screening vision hearing loss.
Neck	Indicated to check for bruit, which may be manifestation of blockage of vessels and a cause of dizziness.	S1, S2, regular rhythm without murmur. No venous hum over neck vessels; no carotid bruits heard.
Chest	Baseline data.	CTA.

(continued)

EXAMINATION	RATIONALE	FINDINGS
Heart	Baseline data. Allows for evaluation of irregular heart rhythm that may have impact on dizziness, as well as CHF resulting from HTN.	S_1 and S_2 WNL. No murmur or extra heart sounds auscultated.
Abdomen	Important to evaluate because of nausea and vomiting.	Soft, nontender BS + in all quads. No HSM or splenomegaly.
Neurological assessment	Important data related to chief complaint.	Alert and oriented × 3. CN I-VII, IX-XII intact, VIII diminished bilaterally to whisper test. No spontaneous nystagmus. Motor function/muscle strength. gait normal. Romberg test negative. Heel/toe walking normal, slow on turn. Extremities equal in strength. Sensory function; intact pain discrimination in all extremities.

Special maneuvers that need to be included in the exam.

SPECIAL MANUEVER	RESULTS	RATIONALE
Barany maneuver	Nystagmus elicited in 10 seconds with head turned 45° to the right. Nystagmus movement: upward fashion toward the right ear.	Allows for observation of nystagmus, dizziness, and vertigo when head is rotated into a horizontal position with the affected posterior semicircular canal 30–45° below the horizontal plane. Direction of nystagmus helps to distinguish BPPV from other types of positional vertigo. Nystagmus goes counterclockwise when the right ear canal is abnormal and clockwise when the left ear is abnormal.

● DIFFERENTIAL DIAGNOSES

What are the significant positive or negative data that support or refute the differential diagnoses for Grace?

DIFFERENTIAL DIAGNOSES	POSITIVE DATA	NEGATIVE DATA
Benign positional vertigo	Spinning sensation of dizziness with positional change. Nausea. Positive nystagmus elicited with Barany maneuver.	Hearing deficit.
Peripheral vestibulopathy	Spinning sensation of dizziness with nausea.	TMs gray, with light reflex present. No erythema or exudate of oropharynx. Nasal passages normal. Breath sounds clear. Abdomen soft, nontender. No hearing deficit. No spontaneous nystagmus.
Meniere's disease	Vertigo.	Tinnitus, ear discomfort, tandem gait normal. No hearing deficit.
Post-traumatic vertigo		No history of recent trauma to head, fall, or whiplash type injury. No Battle's sign.
Ototoxic drugs	Atenolol and HTCZ both have the possible adverse effects of dizziness and N/V.	No history of taking aminoglycosides, salicylates, ethacrynic acid, or furosemide. No tinnitus; Rinne and Weber tests normal.
Acoustic neuroma	Vertigo.	No unsteadiness or loss of balance when upright; no unilateral hearing loss; tinnitus; V and VII cranial nerves intact.
Vertibrobasilar arterial disease	Weakness, vertigo, nausea and vomiting.	No visual changes, perioral numbness, clumsiness, ataxia, unilateral hearing loss.
Volume depletion/anemia	Nutritional intake history, vertigo, weakness, nausea and vomiting, diuretic: HTCZ.	Fair skin turgor, BP and P within normal range; no significant orthostasis; mucus membranes and nailbeds pink.
Cardiac disease, hypotension, arrhythmia, syncope		Vital signs stable; no significant orthostasis; HR regular; S1S2 without murmur; denies fainting feeling or LOC.

(continued)

DIFFERENTIAL DIAGNOSES	POSITIVE DATA	NEGATIVE DATA
Cerebellar disease	Vertigo. Nausea and vomiting.	No truncal ataxia.
Hypothryoidism	Vertigo, weakness	No weight gain, hoarseness, depression, bradycardia, thickened skin, hypersomnia.
Psychiatric illness	At risk since living alone; loss of spouse; advanced age.	No history of recent stress; no vague history; denies depressed mood, weight gain or loss, sleep disturbances, impaired concentration, or substance abuse.

● DIAGNOSTIC TESTS

What additional data or diagnostics are needed to confirm the priority diagnosis? Include your rationale for testing. Interpret the test results that are available.

TEST	RATIONALE	RESULTS	INTERPRETATION
TSH	Vertigo and decreased hearing may be symptoms of hypothyroidism. If elevated, suspect hypothyroidism.	3.2 μU/mL.	WNL.
Hgb/HCT	To check for anemia as possible cause of vertigo. Further testing with CBC is warranted if any abnormalities are found.	Hgb, 12.5 g/dL; HCT, 38%.	WNL.
Fasting blood sugar	Initial screening for diabetes mellitus.	95 mg/dL.	WNL.
Electrolytes, renal, and liver function tests	Basic screening tests.	Na, 147 mEq/L; K, 4.2 mEq/L; Cl, 100 mEq/L; CO_2, 100 mEq/L; calcium, 10.0 mg/dL; alkaline phosphatase, 85 U/L;	WNL.

(continued)

TEST	RATIONALE	RESULTS	INTERPRETATION
		ALT, 38 U/L; AST, 30 U/L; BUN, 14 mg/dL; creatinine, 0.9 mg/dL.	
ECG/Holter monitor	Allows for identification of cardiac arrhythmias.	NSR.	WNL EKG.
Antinuclear antibody	Check for the presence of autoimmune diseases.	Negative at 1:20 dilution.	No autoimmune diseases.
FTA-ABS	Inflammatory labryinthitis may be caused by syphilis, and nontreponemal tests may be negative in tertiary syphilis. Patients with symptoms of peripheral vertigo should be screened for syphilis.	Nonreactive.	Normal.
ESR	Screen for vasculitis.	30 mm/hr.	No vasculitis.

What other testing may be done at a later time, typically by a consulting otolaryngologist.

DIAGNOSTIC TEST	RATIONALE	RESULTS	INTERPRETATION
Vestibulo-Occular Reflex Evaluation (VOR)	Blurring occurs, as well as image movement with head movement. With loss of VOR function, visual acuity decreases by more than one line on the Snellen chart during passive horizontal and vertical head oscillations. VOR	Not done.	NA.

(continued)

DIAGNOSTIC TEST	RATIONALE	RESULTS	INTERPRETATION
	deficits are due to bilateral labrynthine damage, usually the result of ototoxic drugs.		
Caloric test	Normal response with use of warm water is nystagmus toward warm irrigation. Normal response with use of cold water is nystagmus away from cold irrigation. This test causes profound discomfort and nausea.	Nystagmus toward stimulated ear (with warm water).	WNL.
Electronystagmography	Useful in Meniere's disease and persistent BPPV to determine the degree and progression of vestibular deficit, side affected, and surgical intervention, if needed. Done by audiologist on referral. Also provides objective data for cases with clients with psychogenic vertigo who need reassurance that no organic diseases are present. Picks up subtle nystagmus and differentiates central from peripheral nystagmus.	WNL.	WNL.

(continued)

DIAGNOSTIC TEST	RATIONALE	RESULTS	INTERPRETATION
MRI	Very expensive. Indicated if diagnosis of central vertigo is suspected. Small lesions can cause significant symptoms. Bone structures can cause artifact with CT scans, and enhanced resolution makes MRI preferable to CT.	No lesions seen.	WNL.
Audiometry with speech discrimination	Provides screening for acoustic neuroma hearing loss of Meniere's disease. Usually includes pure tone audiometry, speech audiometry, tone decay testing, and acoustic reflex testing.	No audiometric abnormality.	WNL.

● DIAGNOSIS

After combining subjective and objective data with test findings, what is the diagnosis? Identify data that support this diagnosis.

DIAGNOSES	SUPPORTING DATA
Benign paroxysmal positional vertigo (BPPV)	Hallpike-Dix/Barany maneuver is positive for latent nystagmus elicited with upward movement and torsionally counterclockwise toward the right ear. Episodes of dizziness do not last more than 1 minute individually, although the episodes have occurred in clusters in the past 3 days.

Pathophysiology

BPPV is the most common cause of vertigo in the adult. It occurs at most ages but is most common after the age of 40 years and in those with recent head trauma.

It results from pathology in the posterior semicircular canal approximately 95% of the time but can occur in any canal. It usually is caused by inappropriate activation of the canal by calcium carbonate particles, which normally are found in the macula of the utricle and saccule (Barker, Burton, & Zieve, 1999). Vertigo usually is noted when the patient lies down, gets up from a recumbent position, rolls over in bed, looks up while standing, or bends forward. Each episode is short, lasting less than 1 minute. Each episode is stimulated by head position change relative to gravity. Usually the patient does not complain of tinnitus or hearing loss. Nausea and vomiting may occur with the vertigo. BPPV usually is limited to 2 weeks' duration but may persist for months or years in approximately 20% of patients.

● THERAPEUTIC PLAN

1. *What is the basic teaching you will do for Grace about BPPV?*
   - Most cases of BPPV are self-limiting and end within weeks to months.
   - Some people with BPPV have a course of remissions and reoccurrence for months to years.
   - Some people have permanent symptoms, and they may be candidates for surgery.
   - Follow-up visits may be necessary if the current symptoms do not subside and will be extremely important if other accompanying symptoms should occur. Atypical results of follow-up assessment may indicate the need for a referral.
   - Periods of dizziness and associated nausea from BPPV usually are very brief and intense, and the use of sedating medications can cause impaired mental alertness and clarity, with a resulting change in lifestyle for this active woman.

2. *What self-care measures would be helpful for Grace in terms of exercise, diet, and monitoring?*
   Positional exercises (Brandt's-Darroff exercises) should be taught to the patient, and prescribed to be done every 3 hours or 3 times a day until the patient is symptom free for 2 consecutive days. This exercise often leads to a remission of BPPV within 2 weeks. The patient should sit on the edge of a bed and then to lie down quickly on one side with the symptomatic ear down. After the vertigo resolves the patient should sit up.
   Exercises that can be performed by an otolaryngologist or a neurologist are the liberatory maneuver of Siment and the Canolith repositioning procedure. These exercises are done in an effort to move free-floating deposits out of the semicircular canal.
   Diet: A diet low in Na+ and MSG may benefit Grace. Salt and MSG may lead to fluid retention and increase the production and retention of endolymph, which deflates the cupula of the semicircular canal.
   Monitoring: Teach Grace to keep a log of activities and symptoms, so she can learn which movements should be adjusted.

3. *What referrals would be appropriate for Grace?*
Refer Grace to an audiologist for hearing loss determination.

4. *What medications might be appropriate for Grace based on the severity of her symptoms?*
Treatment with an antivertigo medication may provide relief of symptoms, although the use of such medications remains a matter of controversy because of the side effects, especially in the elderly.

First and second line drug choices are:

- Meclizine (Antivert) 25 to 100 mg/day in divided doses, antihistamine, antiemetic
- Dimenhydrinate (Dramamine) 50 to 100 mg po, antiemetic
- Diphenidol (Vontrol) 25 to 50 mg p, antiemetic
- Diazepam (Valium), CNS depressant
- Scopolamine, anticholinergic

These medications have adverse effects of dizziness, drowsiness, ataxia, sedation, and scopolamine may cause depressed respirations.

5. *What follow-up should be planned for Grace?*
Test results of TSH, HCT, blood glucose, and FTA-ABS per telephone call if normal as soon as results are available. Follow up in 2 to 4 weeks after prescribing at-home Brandt's exercises and diet changes for reevaluation, looking for evidence of other causes of vertigo.

Serial follow-up visits to reevaluate, looking for evidence of other possible causes of dizziness. If at-home exercises and diet changes have not alleviated the symptoms, you may refer Grace to an audiologist, otolaryngologist, or neurologist for additional testing/treatment.

Surgical follow-up for clients whose dizziness and accompanying symptoms are chronic may include:

- Posterior semicircular canal occlusion
- Laser partitioning of the labyrinth to create semicircular occlusion

6. *What impact might BPPV have on her family? Identify needed education for the family.*

- Teach family about the nature of BPPV and exercises that may relieve the vertigo.
- Follow-up should occur earlier than the 2- to 4-week appointment if symptoms worsen, continue for a prolonged period, or if other symptoms appear.
- If medication is prescribed, family should be educated on possible side effects, especially of sedation and possible respiratory depression. Family may need to stay with Grace when medicated to monitor ambulation because she would be at high risk for falls.
- Family/friends may be needed to do grocery shopping and essential errands until the episodes have been abolished. For safety reasons, she should not drive at this time or while taking antivertigo medication.

- Teach about prognosis and alternatives to care.
- Teach family to be supportive of Grace continuing her present active independent lifestyle as much as possible.

7. *What resources are available for Grace and her family?*

Vestibular Disorders Association
PO Box 4467
Portland, OR 97208-4467
503-229-7705
http://www.teleport.com/~veda/
Multiple links to various vestibular disorder groups:
http://www.teleport.com/~veda/links.html.

REFERENCES

(2000). Vertigo: Taking the spin out of life. *Mayo Clinic Health Letter, 18*(7), 1–3.

Ahmad, A., Cooley, R., & Akhtar, M. (2000). Evaluation and management of patients with unexplained syncope. *Home Health Care Consultant, 7*(7), 11–15.

Barker, L., Burton, J., & Zieve, P. (1999). Principles of ambulatory medicine (5th ed., p. 1254). Baltimore: Williams & Wilkins.

Burke, M. (1995). Dizziness in the elderly: Etiology and treatment. *Nurse Practitioner: American Journal of Primary Health Care, 20*(12), 28, 31–32, 34.

Clark, M. R. (1994). Chronic dizziness: An integrated approach. *Hospital Practice, 29,* 57–64.

Cox, M. M., & Kaplan, D. (Eds.). (2000). Uncovering the cause of syncope. *Patient Care, 34*(10), 39–42, 45–46, 48.

Drozd, C. E. (1999). Short communications. Acute vertigo: Peripheral versus central etiology. *Nurse Practitioner: American Journal of Primary Health Care, 24*(4), 147–148.

Grimm, R. J. (1996). Dizziness. *Nurse Practitioner Forum, 7*(4), 160–166.

Maurer, M., Karmall, W., Rivadineira, H., Pardis, M., & Bloomfield, D. (2000). Upright posture and postprandial hypotension in elderly persons. *Annals of Internal Medicine, 133*(7), 533–536.

McGee, S. R. (1995). Dizzy patients: Diagnosis and treatment. *Western Journal of Medicine, 162,* 37–42.

McNaboe, E., & Kerr, A. (2000). Why history is the key in the diagnosis of vertigo. *Practitioner, 244*(1612), 648–653.

Neatherlin, J. S., & Egan, J. (1994). Benign paroxysmal positional vertigo. *Journal of Neuroscience Nursing, 26,* 330–335.

Ojala, M., & Palo, J. (1991). The aetiology of dizziness and how to examine a dizzy patient. *Annals of Medicine, 23,* 225–230.

Olshansky, B. (2000). Syncope: Step by step through the workup. *Consultant, 40,* 702–704, 706–711.

Paluso, K. A. (2000). The fainting patient: First and foremost, a meticulous evaluation. *Journal of the American Academy of Physician Assistants, 13*(8), 40–42, 48–49, 53–54.

Porterfield, J. G., Porterfield, L. M., & Khattak, T. A. (2000). Case & comment. A syncopal episode. *Patient Care, 34*(6), 137–139.

Ruchenstein, M. J. (1995). A practical approach to dizziness. Questions to bring vertigo and other causes into focus. *Postgraduate Medicine, 97,* 70–81.

Sisson, S., & Kramer, P. (1999). Dizziness, vertigo, motion sickness, syncope and near syncope and disequilibrium. In L. Barker, J. Burton, P. Zieve (Eds), *Principles of ambulatory medicine* (5th ed., pp. 1252–1273). Baltimore: Williams & Wilkins.

Weinstein, B. E., & Devons, C. (1995). The dizzy patient: Stepwise workup of a common complaint. *Geriatrics, 50,* 42–50.

Wlliams, J. L., Schneiderman, H., & Algranati, P. S. (1994). *Physical diagnoses: Bedside evaluation of diagnosis and function.* Baltimore: Williams & Wilkins.

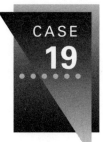

A 26-year-old woman requesting a postpartum follow-up 6 weeks after childbirth

SCENARIO

Anne Luckhurst, a married 26-year-old woman, underwent a vacuum-assisted vaginal delivery of her first child, a daughter, 6 weeks ago. She presents for a postpartum follow-up visit.

● HISTORY

What are the significant questions from Anne's history/prenatal record? What are key points from the labor and delivery record? What is the significant information from the postpartum hospital record? What information do you need from the interval history (the time between hospital discharge and this visit) to assist in making a diagnosis?

● PHYSICAL ASSESSMENT

What are the significant portions of the physical examination that should be completed?

● DIFFERENTIAL DIAGNOSES

What are the significant positive and negative data that support or refute your diagnoses?

● DIAGNOSTIC TESTS

Based on the history and physical assessment, what, if any, diagnostic testing would you do? Include your rationale for the testing.

● DIAGNOSIS

What diagnoses are appropriate for Anne?

● THERAPEUTIC PLAN

1. *How will you manage Anne's anemia?*
2. *How will you manage Anne's hypoestrogenized vagina/dyspareunia?*
3. *How will you manage Anne's lack of immunity to rubella?*
4. *What anticipatory guidance will you give Anne related to resumption of sexual relations?*
5. *What other teaching will you do at this visit?*
6. *When should Anne return for follow-up?*
7. *What community resources are available to the NP and Anne?*

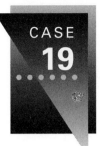

TUTORIAL

A 26-year-old woman requesting a postpartum follow-up 6 weeks after childbirth

SCENARIO

Anne Luckhurst, a married 26-year-old woman, underwent a vacuum-assisted vaginal delivery of her first child, a daughter, 6 weeks ago. She presents for a postpartum follow-up visit.

● TENTATIVE DIAGNOSIS

What are the tentative diagnoses that you would identify at this point based on the scenario presented?

DIAGNOSIS	RATIONALE
6 weeks postpartum	By history.

● HISTORY

What are the significant questions from Anne's history/prenatal record?

REQUESTED DATA	DATA ANSWER
Allergies	NKA.
Current medications	Prenatal vitamin daily. Occasionally acetaminophen (Tylenol) for H/A.

(continued)

REQUESTED DATA   DATA ANSWER
· ·

Medical history	Chickenpox, mumps, and measles in childhood. Has not had rubella; prenatal rubella titer, 1:6 (nonimmune). No prior hospitalizations or transfusions. Had fractured arm at age 15 from basketball injury; no sequela. No serious adult illnesses.
Ob/Gyn	G1P0 on prenatal admission. Menarche at age 13. LNMP prior to pregnancy. Menses usually every 30 days for 4 days; normal flow, no cramping or PMS. BSE monthly since college. Last pelvic, pregnancy related. Used progestin-only OCPs before pregnancy.
Social history	Tobacco: never. Alcohol: never. Caffeine: 1–2 cups coffee and 1–2 diet colas daily before pregnancy; none during pregnancy or breastfeeding. Drugs: never. Exercise: walked at least 2 miles daily before and during pregnancy. Minimal exercise since delivery. Married 3 years to (Steve) a 27 y/o seminary student with part-time job as youth minister in local church. Both active in First Baptist Church Comanages "The Stitcher's Dream," a cross-stitch shop and framery; works 3–5 days in shop and does "display" projects at home.
Family history	Father: 54 y/o, good health. Mother: 52 y/o, good health. Brother: 20 y/o, paraplegia from MVA. Spouse: 27 y/o, good health. Newborn: 6 weeks 1 day old, good health.
Income/ insurance	Minimal income and insurance; husband in Baptist seminary completing Master of Divinity degree; will have 6 months until graduation when baby is born. Insurance pays for 48-hour childbirth stay. Patient's income essentially part-time wages. Resides in graduate student housing on university campus.

● SUMMARY OF SIGNIFICANT POINTS FROM PRENATAL COURSE

Initial prenatal visit at 7 weeks' gestation after positive home pregnancy test. Pregnancy $2°$ contraceptive failure; wants a child but had hoped to see husband graduated first.

Prenatal course essentially normal with exceptions as follows: Treated for tonsilitis/bronchitis at 26 weeks with erythromycin. Prescribed bedrest for several days at 35 weeks $2°$ mild PIH.

Lab results: A+ blood type with negative antibody screen.
AFP at 15 weeks, negative (8 ng/mL).
Beta strep, negative.
HIV, HbsAg, RPR, GC, chlamydia, HSV, negative.
Hgb/HCT at 38 weeks, 10.2 g/dL and 31%.
PAP, negative.
Diabetes screen at 24 weeks, negative.

What are key points from the labor and delivery record?

REQUESTED DATA   DATA ANSWER

Weeks' gestation	40.4
Duration of labor	1st stage: 12 hours 8 minutes. 2nd stage: 1 hour 10 minutes. 3rd stage: 17 minutes. Total: 13 hours 35 minutes.
Type delivery	Vacuum-assisted vaginal delivery.
Episiotomy	Midline with 2nd degree extension.
Anesthesia	Epidural.
Medication administered	Oxytocin (Pitocin IV) augmentation of labor according to ACOG protocol. Oxytocin (Pitocin) in IV fluids after delivery of placenta. Promethazine (Phenergan) 25 mg IM × 2 for nausea/vomiting.

Gender/Apgar score/
  Wt/Length of Infant
Resuscitation of
Infant/Infant
Complications
	Female; 9/9; 7 lb 3 oz; 20 inches.
	  Bulb syringe and blow-by oxygen only.
	  Normal female at term.

(continued)

REQUESTED DATA   DATA ANSWER
....

Maternal complications	Episode of uterine atony 2 hours after delivery; responded to fundal massage and additional oxytocin (Pitocin) 10 units added to 1000 mL Lactated Ringers for 8 hours. Estimated total blood loss, 750 mL.

What is the significant information from the postpartum hospital record?

Significant Information on Anne's In-Patient Postpartum Course at Time of Hospital Discharge

Stable vital signs; T< 100.4 °F on 2nd postpartum day.

Able to ambulate without difficulty.

No undue pain. Discharged with Rx for ibuprofen (Motrin) 600 mg Q 6 hours × 20 and × 6.

Docusate sodium and casanthranol (Peri-Colace) daily until BM.

Breasts soft, nontender with intact nipples. Breastfeeding well on demand.

Fundus firm at U/2.

Voiding without difficulty.

Intact perineum; well-approximated midline episiotomy with 2nd degree extension; no undue redness, edema, ecchymosis, or discharge.

Lochia rubra, moderate amount at discharge.

Hemoglobin 9 g/dL (to continue prenatal vitamins/iron).

Homan's negative bilaterally.

Postpartum medications, prenatal vitamin daily; laxative (Peri-Colace) at HS daily; ibuprofen (Motrin) 600 mg Q 6 hr × 2 days.

What information do you need from the interval history (the time between hospital discharge and this visit) to assist in making a diagnosis?

REQUESTED DATA   DATA ANSWER

REQUESTED DATA	DATA ANSWER
Readmissions/ER visits/ visits to health care providers since discharge from postpartum unit	Has done well since discharge; has not seen health care provider except for pediatrician 2 weeks ago at baby's first follow-up visit. Did call lactation consultant for advice about sore nipples day after discharge. Used air drying, Masse cream, and position changes during nursing, as advised to resolve problem.
Problems with pain, bowel or bladder elimination, vaginal bleeding, healing of episiotomy	No significant pain. Denies fever. Has not needed ibuprofen (Motrin) since 2 days after discharge. Taking occasional acetaminophen (Tylenol) for headache. Has resumed normal bowel pattern. Voiding without difficulty. Episiotomy "seems to be healed."
Progression of lochia/ resumption of menses	Lochia ceased about 2 weeks ago. Has not resumed period.
Resumption of sexual relations	She and husband decided to wait until after today's exam to make sure everything checks out first.
Family support	Both mother and mother-in-law live nearby and spent the first 2 weeks at home alternating in helping out. Husband helps with baby and housework when possible but is very busy between school and part-time job.
Family-infant bonding	"The baby [Morgan] is wonderful! We are crazy about her and are now glad we didn't wait until after graduation to have her. Of course her crying and not sleeping through the night interrupt Steve's study time, and we are both really tired."
Infant feeding	Breastfeeding on demand. No problems. Plans to breastfeed at least 6 months.
General adaptation	Exhausted. No getting much sleep. Not getting much exercise. Back at work 3 days/week with baby in portable crib in shop. With husband's part-time job in youth ministry comes expectation of her involvement in church activities several times a week. Getting out for private time with spouse every other week, even if for walk in park or hamburger and movie; one of baby's grandmothers baby-sits. Appetite good. Has to remind self to drink extra fluids.
Follow-up with pediatrician/concerns about infant	Saw pediatrician 2 weeks ago. Baby is gaining weight and doing well. No concerns; infant care is going well.
Plans for contraception	Plans to use condoms and spermicide until stops breastfeeding at 6 months. Will likely start OCPs again; wants information about new combined pills with low estrogen.

● PHYSICAL ASSESSMENT

What are the significant portions of the physical examination that should be completed?

SYSTEM	RATIONALE	FINDINGS
Vital signs	Baseline data. Allows comparison with prenatal and in-patient vital signs.	T, 97.8 °F; P, 118; RR, 18; BP, 112/76 mm Hg.
Height/weight	Determines weight loss since delivery. Women tend to retain 60% of weight > 24 lb gain.	5′5″, 122 lb. Weighted 112 at 1st prenatal visit and 140 at last prenatal visit
General appearance	Provides general indication of overall status.	Alert. No distress. Positive affect. Extremely pale skin with pale conjunctiva and mucous membranes.
Heart	Screening data appropriate in all physical exams.	S1, S2 WNL. No murmurs.
Lungs	Quick screen to rule out respiratory problems.	CTA.
Breast	Evaluation of lactation status and integrity of nipples.	Full, lactating breasts, nontender, without undue warmth. Nipples, no cracks or fissures. No axillary or supraclavicular nodes palpable. Wearing supportive nursing bra.
Thyroid	6% postpartum patients have transient thyroid problems.	Normal contour. No nodules, no enlargement.
Abdomen	Evaluate for diastasis recti, subinvolution.	BS + × 4; abdomen soft, nontender; no organomegaly; no diastasis recti; fundus nonpalpable.
Back	Helps to rule out UTI and tenderness or problems related to epidural anesthesia.	No CVAT; no tenderness along paraspinous muscles.
Lower extremities	Rules out postpartum thrombophlebitis and varicosities.	No edema or varicosities. Negative Homan's bilaterally. No redness or calf tenderness or warmth. No inquinal nodes

(continued)

SYSTEM	RATIONALE	FINDINGS
Pelvic	Assess process of involution, healing of episiotomy, pelvic muscle integrity.	BUS normal. Midline episiotomy well healed. Vaginal mucosa sl.pale, thin, dry, consistent with low estrogen of lactation; normal rugae. Good muscle tone. Posterior vaginal septum intact without tenderness. Cervical os closed. No lesions on cervix or vaginal walls. No cervical discharge or CMT. Uterus nonpregnant size with smooth contour. Adnexa negative. Rectum: normal spincter tone; rectovaginal septum at episiotomy site WNL. No masses or fistulas noted. Small clustered external hemorrhoids noted.

● TENTATIVE DIAGNOSIS

- Normal involution at 6 weeks' postpartum exam, with lactation progressing well and episiotomy well healed.
- Rubella nonimmune.
- Rule out anemia.

● DIFFERENTIAL DIAGNOSES

What are the significant positive and negative data that support or refute your diagnoses?

DIAGNOSIS	POSITIVE	NEGATIVE DATA
Normal involution at 6-week postpartum exam with lactation progressing well and episiotomy well healed	Lochia ceased 2 weeks ago. Uterus nonpregnant size. Reports breastfeeding success; breasts full but without signs of mastitis or cracked nipples; episiotomy site intact, without signs of infection or tenderness.	None.

(continued)

DIAGNOSIS	POSITIVE	NEGATIVE DATA
Rubella nonimmune	Prenatal rubella titer < 1:10.	None.
Possible anemia	Episode of uterine postpartum uterine atony; EBL = 750 mL; Hgb at time of postpartum discharge, 9 g/dL; generalized pallor, tachycardia, fatigue.	Has continued prenatal vitamins with iron since discharge; eating high-iron diet. Taking prenatal vitamins with tea.

● DIAGNOSTIC TESTS

Based on the history and physical assessment, what, if any, diagnostic testing would you do? Include your rationale for the testing.

DIAGNOSTIC TEST	RATIONALE	RESULTS	INTERPRETATION
Hgb/HCT	History of postpartum blood loss; signs of anemia	Hgb, 8.8 g/dL; Hct, 25%.	Iron deficiency anemia.
Urinalysis	Routinely screened at 6 weeks' postpartum; UTI common.	Negative protein, glucose, nitrites, leukocytes, or blood.	WNL.

● DIAGNOSIS

What diagnoses are appropriate for Anne?
- Normal involution at 6-week postpartum exam.
- Rubella nonimmune.
- Iron-deficiency anemia.

● THERAPEUTIC PLAN

1. How will you manage Anne's anemia?
- Prescribe high-iron diet.
- Prescribe ferrous sulfate (Feosol) 65 mg po TID.
- Instruct to take between meals if possible or with meals if causes GI problems. Advise to maximize effect by taking with citrus juice. Advise that taking

BRIEF PATHOPHYSIOLOGY IN THE CASE

Normal involution is an expectation at 6 weeks' postpartum. The placental site at delivery is raw and oozing. The uterine musculature helps maintain pressure against the site by firm contraction, and blood loss gradually decreases. Immediately after childbirth, the fundus is located in the midline of the abdomen and is firmly contracted, positioned halfway between the symphysis pubis and umbilicus. Within the first 12 hours, the fundus rises to the level of the umbilicus and then descends into the pelvis at the rate of 1 cm per day. By day 10, it should no longer be palpable abdominally. At the postpartum follow-up visit at 6 weeks, the uterus should be normal, nonpregnant size. Lochia, the shed intrauterine contents, gradually decreases in amount and changes in color as follows: bright red (lochia rubra), days 1–3; pink or brown (lochia serosa), days 3–10; and creamy (lochia alba), days 10–35.

Immunity to rubella is conferred in seronegative women with vaccine. The rubella immunization consists of a live virus that is contraindicated in pregnancy. Because the rubella virus is teratogenic, it is important that women be immunized either before pregnancy or after delivery, and in the latter case, to avoid a subsequent pregnancy for 3 months. Breastfeeding is not a contraindication to the vaccine.

In general, the woman who undergoes vaginal delivery loses about 500 mL of blood during childbirth and the postpartum period; those experiencing Cesarean childbirth lose as much as 1000 mL. Uterine atony is the primary cause of postpartum hemorrhage. A postpartum hemoglobin of < 9 grams is considered treatable anemia.

drug with tea, milk, or antacid will make it ineffective. Caution that stools will be dark. Advise that may cause constipation or diarrhea and to report problems.

2. *How will you manage Anne's lack of immunity to rubella?*
   - Assure that vaccine is not contraindicated by assessing the following before administration: allergy to neomycin or duck eggs; blood transfusion within last 3 months; immunosuppression of patient or person in home.
   - Administer rubella vaccine (Meruvax 2) 1 vial (0.5 mL) SC at this visit.
   - Advise of potential side effects: brief soreness at injection site; slight fever or aching responsive to acetaminophen or ibuprofen; rash, malaise, sore throat, headache in 2 to 4 weeks.
   - Caution patient that this live-virus vaccine is unsafe in pregnancy; thus, pregnancy must be avoided for at least 3 months after the injection. Conscientious contraception is imperative.

3. *What anticipatory guidance will you give Anne related to resumption of sexual relations?*

- Advise that vaginal and perineal tissues are well healed, and resumption of sexual intercourse is safe.
- Suggest a water-soluble lubricant, such as K-Y jelly or Astroglide, until the vaginal mucosa has responded to exogenous estrogen. Spermicide, which she plans to use with condoms for contraception, may provide adequate lubrication.
- Suggest breastfeeding baby before lovemaking to eliminate interruption and to prevent leakage of milk during foreplay or orgasm.
- Suggest gentle intercourse, with time and attention given to arousal. Advise that the woman-dominant position may place less pressure against the site of the episiotomy.
- Advise Kegel's exercises several times daily to strengthen the pelvic musculature. Provide detailed explanation.

4. *What other teaching will you do at this visit?*
   - Teach foods on high-iron diet.
   - Advise to rest or sleep when infant does and to continue to assert her need for help at home or to be excluded from some church activities.
   - Encourage resumption of routine pattern of exercise.
   - Provide verbal and written information related to OCPs with low estrogen, as requested by patient.

5. *When should Anne return for follow-up?*
   Anne will need her annual exam and Papanicolaou smear in 4 to 5 months. At that time, her desires for contraception can be re-evaluated. A repeat hemoglobin and hematocrit at that visit can be used to evaluate response to iron therapy. She should be encouraged to come to the clinic PRN or to call with questions or concerns in the meantime.

6. *What community resources are available to the NP and Anne?*

   LaLeche League International
   9616 Minneapolis Avenue.
   Box 1209
   Franklin Park, IL 60131-8209
   708-455-7730

   Postpartum Support International
   927 North Kellogg Avenue.
   Santa Barbara, CA 93111
   206-881-6580

REFERENCES

Akridge, K. M. (1998). Postpartum and lactation. In E. Q. Youngkin & M. S. Davis (Eds.), *Women's health: A primary care clinical guide* (2nd ed., pp. 639–701). Stamford, CT: Appleton & Lange.

Alteneder, R. R., & Hartzell, D. (1997). Addressing couples' sexuality concerns during the childbearing period: Use of the PLISSIT model. *JOGNN, 26,* 651–658.

AWHONN. (1998). Guidelines for planning family centered care to meet the needs of mother and baby. In *Standards and guidelines for professional nursing practice in the care of women and newborns* (5th ed.). Washington, DC: Author.

Beck, C. T. (1998). A checklist to identify women at risk for developing postpartum depression. *JOGNN, 27,* 39–46.

Berger, D., & Cook, D. L. (1998). Postpartum teaching priorities: The viewpoints of nurses and mothers. *JOGNN, 27,* 161–168.

Birk, D. (1996). Postpartum education: Teaching priorities for primipara. *Journal of Perinatal Education, 5*(2), 7–12.

Brown, K. M. (2000). *Management guidelines for women's health nurse practitioners.* Philadelphia: F.A. Davis.

Chute, G. (1992). Promoting breastfeeding success: An overview of basic management. *NAACOG's Clinical Issues in Perinatal and Women's Health Nursing, 3*(4), 570–572.

Fishbein, E. G., & Burggraf, E. (1998). Early postpartum discharge: How are mothers managing? *JOGNN, 27,* 142–148.

Grace, J. (1993). Mothers' self-reports of parenthood across first 6 months postpartum. *Research in Nursing and Health, 16*(6), 431–439.

Hills-Bonezyk, S. G. (1993). Women's experiences with combining breastfeeding and employment. *Journal of Nurse Midwifery, 38*(5), 257–266.

Johnson & Johnson Consumer Products, Inc. (1996). *Compendium of postpartum care.* Skillman, NJ: Author.

Kish, C. P. (2000). The postpartum family at risk. In S. B. Olds, M. L. London, & P. A. W. Ladewig (Eds.), *Maternal-newborn nursing: A family and community-based approach* (6th ed., pp. 979–1008). Upper Saddle River, NJ: Prentice Hall.

Kish, C. P. (1993). Postpartum home care. In I. Bobak (Eds.), *Maternity and gynecologic care* (5th ed., pp. 735–766). St. Louis: CV Mosby.

Milligan, R., Lenz, E. R., Parks, P. L., Pugh, L. C., & Kitzman, H. (1996). Postpartum fatigue: Clarifying the concept. *Scholarly Inquiry for Nursing Practice, 10*(3), 279–291.

Moran, C. F., Holt, V. L., & Martin, D. P. (1997). What do women want to know after childbirth? *Birth, 24,* 27–34.

Price, W. R. (1993). Strictly for parents: Making love after birth. *The Journal of Perinatal Education, 2*(2), 7–8.

Rarick, T., & Tchabo, J. (1994). Timing of the postpartum Papanicolaou smear. *Obstetrics and Gynecology, 83*(5), 761–764.

Ruchala, P., & Halstead, L. (1994). The postpartum experience of low risk women: A time of adjustment and change. *Maternal-Child Nursing Journal, 22*(3), 83–89.

Sammons, L. N. (1990). Postpartum visit. In W. L. Star, M. T. Shannon, L. N. Shannon, L. L. Lommel, & Y. Gutierrez (Eds.), *Ambulatory obstetrics: Protocols for nurse practitioner/nurse midwives* (pp. 12–17). San Francisco: The Regents University of California at San Francisco.

Sampselle, C. M., Seng, J., Yeo, S., Killion, C., & Oakley, D. (1999). Physical activity and postpartum well-being. *JOGNN, 28,* 41–49.

Sheil, E.P., Bull, M.J., Moxon, B.E., Muehl, P.A., Koening, K.L., Peterson, C., Palmberg, G., & Kelber, S. (1995). Concerns of childbearing women: A maternal concerns questionnaire as an assessment tool. *JOGNN, 24,* 149–155.

Smith-Hanrahan, C., & Deblois, D. (1995). Postpartum early discharge: Impact on maternal fatigue and functional ability. *Clinical Nursing Research, 4*(1), 50–66.

Stover, A. M., & Marnejon, J. G. (1995). Postpartum care. *American Family Physician, 52*(5), 1465–1472.

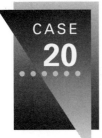

A 33-year-old woman with left lower extremity pain and swelling

SCENARIO

Sue Howard presents to the health center with a 4-day history of left lower extremity tenderness and swelling. She is married, the mother of three, and works part time in a garden supply store.

● TENTATIVE DIAGNOSES

*What are the potential diagnoses you have identified based on this scenario? Make sure you include any vital **red flag** diagnoses that cannot be missed.*

DIAGNOSIS   **RATIONALE**

1

2

3

4

5

6

7

● HISTORY

Here are elements of the history that pertain to Sue. Which of these are the most relevant to this case?

REQUESTED DATA	DATA ANSWER
Allergies	NKDA.
Medications	Oral contraceptives; no OTC medications.
Surgery/transfusion	Appendectomy, age 12; no transfusions.
Medical history/hospitalizations/ fractures/injuries	Chicken pox, measles, and mumps in childhood; no fractures or injuries; hospitalization for appendectomy.
Adult illnesses	None.
OB/GYN history	LNMP: 1 week ago, normal flow and duration. Last pelvic exam: approx. 3 months ago. Mammogram: none. SBE: monthly for past 5 years. G3P3A0.
Appetite/weight change	Stable weight and appetite.
Social history	Tobacco: 1½ packs per day for 10 years. Caffeine: 2–3 colas per day. Recreational drugs: none. Exercise: rare.
Family history, specifically focus on a history of thrombosis, hereditary thrombotic disorders, myeloproliferative disorders, hemolytic anemia, connective tissue diseases or inflammatory disorders	Father: age 58, alive and healthy. Mother: age 56, HTN. Brother: age 28, alive and healthy. Spouse: age 40, alive and healthy. Children: daughters 11, 9, 8, alive and healthy.
Onset and duration of symptoms	Nagging pain and full feeling in left calf for 6 days; edema and frank pain for 4 days. No memory of injury to left calf region.
How have symptoms affected ADLs?	Pain intensified with weight bearing. Spent most of past 2 days on the couch with left leg elevated on a pillow. Children fixed supper last evening.
Any recent conditions that predisposed to immobility?	No recent travel, surgeries, or illnesses requiring prolonged sitting or bed rest. No recent pelvic, orthopedic, or abdominal surgeries.
Any recent trauma?	None known.

● PHYSICAL ASSESSMENT

What are the significant portions of the physical examination that should be completed for Sue?

SYSTEM	RATIONALE	FINDINGS
Vital signs		BP, 122/84 mm Hg right arm; HR, 92 bpm; RR, 20: T, 99.4 °F; Ht, 5'2"; Wt, 141 lbs.
General appearance/skin		Well-developed, well-nourished woman in no acute distress. No pallor noted. Mucous membranes moist; sclera nonicteric.
Lungs		CTA.
Heart		RRR; S1, S2, no MGR.
Abdomen		Soft, nontender, negative organomegaly. BS active; no guarding, rebound tenderness, or distention.
Lower extremities		Left calf tender along the great saphenous vein. Edema 1+ in left ankle. Right calf circumference, 14"; left calf circumference, 16". No Baker's cyst appreciated; no pain with knee flexion. Pulses 2+ where tested. Homan's sign negative.

● DIFFERENTIAL DIAGNOSES

What are the significant positive and negative findings that support or refute your diagnoses for Sue?

DIAGNOSIS	POSITIVE DATA	NEGATIVE DATA
1		
2		
3		
4		
5		
6		
7		

● DIAGNOSTIC TESTS

Here are the tests that were performed. What do the test results indicate? What impact do the lab results have on Sue's condition?

DIAGNOSTIC TESTS	RATIONALE	RESULTS	INTERPRETATION
Duplex Doppler ultrasonography of left lower extremity		Incompressibility and abnormal Doppler flow signals of the great saphenous vein.	
CBC and blood smear		Hgb, 13.8 g/dL. HCt, 42%. RBC, 4.8 million/mm^3. WBC, 7.5 1000/mm^3. Platelets, 280,000.	
PTT		28 seconds.	
Factor V Leiden		Factor V Leiden absent; no evidence of mutation of Factor V.	
CXR		No evidence of acute changes.	
Electrolytes, renal panel, and liver function studies			

Other Diagnostic Tests That Can Be Ordered if Indicated

DIAGNOSTIC TESTS	RATIONALE	EXPLANATION
D-dimer assays		
Ventilation-perfusion scan		
Contrast venography		

(continued)

DIAGNOSTIC TESTS	RATIONALE	EXPLANATION
Initial testing before initiation of heparin therapy if indicated: fibrinogen; thrombin time; lupus anticoagulant assay (RVVT); ELSA for anticardiolipin antibodies; prothrombin 20210 mutation; fasting homocysteine level; Factor VIII level; Antithrombin III activity; protein C, free protein S		

● DIAGNOSES

What diagnoses do you determine as being appropriate after a review of the subjective and objective data?
Discuss the incidence, risk factors, and pathogenesis of this condition

Data Supporting the Diagnosis

● THERAPEUTIC PLAN

1. *How is this condition classified?*

2. *What influence does the classification have on the therapeutic treatment plan?*

3. *What will the management of Sue's condition consist of?*

4. *Should Sue be referred to a specialist and to whom?*

5. *What impact does this illness have on Sue's lifestyle and activities?*

6. *What special diet, if any, should Sue follow?*

7. *What patient education should you discuss with Sue?*

8. *What is the family impact of this diagnosis?*

9. *When should Sue return for follow-up?*

10. *What community resources are available for the NP and Sue?*

REFERENCES

Becker, R., & Ansell, J. (1995). Antithrombotic therapy: An abbreviated reference for clinicians. *Archives of Internal Medicine, 155,* 149–161.

Brigden, M. (1996). Oral anticoagulant therapy: practical aspects of management. *Postgraduate Medicine, 99,* 81–102.

Creager, M. A., & Dzau, V. J. (1994). Vascular diseases of the extremities. In K. J. Isselbacher, et al. (Eds.), *Harrison's principles of internal medicine* (13th ed.) New York: McGraw-Hill.

Eftychiou, V. (1996). Clinical diagnosis and management of the patient with deep venous thromboembolism and acute pulmonary embolism. *Nurse Practitioner, 21*(3), 50–62.

Hathaway, W., & Goodnight, S. (1993). *Disorders of hemostasis and thrombosis: A clinical guide.* New York: McGraw-Hill.

Hirsh, J., Dalen, J., Deykin, D., Poller, L., & Bussey, H. (1995). Oral anticoagulants: Mechanism of action, clinical effectiveness and optimal therapeutic range. *Chest, 108,* 231S–246S.

Kearon, C., Julian, J. A., Newman, T. E., et al. (1998). Noninvasive diagnosis of deep venous thrombosis. *Annals of Internal Medicine, 28,* 663–667.

Komblit, P., Senderoff, J., Davis Ericksen, M., & Zenk, J. (1990). Anticoagulation therapy: Patient management and evaluation of an outpatient clinic. *Nurse Practitioner, 15,* 21–32.

Rubins, J., & Rice, K. (2000). Diagnoses of venous thromboembolism. *Postgraduate Medicine, 108,* 175–180.

Stone, A. (2000). Anticoagulation therapy. In D. Robinson, P. Kidd, & K. Rogers (Eds.), *Primary care across the lifespan* (pp. 69–74). St. Louis: Mosby.

Stone, A. (2000). Thrombophlebitis. In D. Robinson, P. Kidd, & K. Rogers (Eds.), *Primary care across the lifespan* (pp. 1085–1089). St. Louis: Mosby.

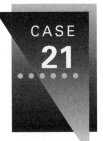

An 8-year-old boy with sore throat and fever

SCENARIO

Sam presents to the family practice office with a 2-day history of sore throat and fever. He has a history of recurrent sore throats, both streptococcal and viral.

● TENTATIVE DIAGNOSIS

*What are the potential diagnoses you have identified based on this scenario? Make sure you include any vital **red flag** diagnoses that cannot be missed?*

DIAGNOSIS	RATIONALE
1	
2	
3	
4	
5	
6	

● HISTORY

What are significant questions in the history for Sam? Are there any other questions that need to be asked in this situation?

REQUESTED DATA   DATA ANSWER

Allergies	PCN and amoxicillin.
Medications	None.
Treatment prior to arrival	Ibuprofen (Advil) 1 hr ago for a temperature of 101.4 °F.
Childhood illnesses	Chicken pox.
Immunizations	Up to date.
Surgery	None.
Medical history/ hospitalizations	Frequent episodes of sore throats, both strep positive and negative, during last 4 years.
Appetite	Not eating well yesterday or today but drinking plenty of fluids because it feels good on his throat.
Exposure to anyone with strep throat/illness	Other children at school have strep throat. No one at home is ill.
Family history	Father: 29, healthy. Mother: 27, healthy. Sister: 5, healthy.

SYSTEM REVIEWED   DATA ANSWER

General	Patient states just doesn't feel good, and his throat hurts.
Skin	No problems.
HEENT	Slight clear runny nose. No ear pain or discharge. C/o difficulty swallowing because throat hurts.
Lungs	Slight nonproductive cough. No wheezing or SOB.
Cardiac	No problems.
GI/GU	Vomited small amount of emesis in AM. No nausea at this time. No diarrhea or abdominal pain.
Neurological assessment	C/o headache for last couple days.

● PHYSICAL ASSESSMENT

What are the significant portions of the physical examination that should be completed for Sam?

SYSTEM	RATIONALE	FINDINGS
Vital signs		BP, 102/60 mm Hg; HR, 92 bpm; RR, 20; T, 98.8 °F; Wt, 41 lbs.
General appearance/skin		Alert, sitting on exam table. Cheeks flushed.
HEENT		Normocephalic; no sinus tenderness. Ear: TMs normal bilaterally. Nares: normal bilaterally. Pharynx: soft palate petechiae; tonsils edematous; erythema with moderate amount of white exudate noted. No difficulty swallowing saliva. Neck: supple; tender and enlarged tonsillar and anterior cervical lymph nodes. Negative Kernig and Brudzinkski signs.
Lungs		CTA bilaterally.
Heart		RRR; no MRG.
GI		BS+; no tenderness; no guarding; no rebound tenderness.

● DIFFERENTIAL DIAGNOSES

What are the significant positive and negative findings that support or refute your diagnosis for Sam?

DIAGNOSIS	POSITIVE DATA	NEGATIVE DATA
1		
2		
3		
4		

(continued)

DIAGNOSIS	POSITIVE DATA	NEGATIVE DATA
5		
6		

● DIAGNOSTIC TESTS

Based on the history and physical assessment, what, if any, diagnostic testing would you do? Include your rationale for the testing and interpret the test results.

DIAGNOSTIC TEST	RATIONALE	RESULTS	INTERPRETATION
Rapid strep screen		Positive.	
CBC		Not done.	
Mono spot		Negative.	

● DIAGNOSIS

What diagnoses do you determine as being appropriate for Sam?

Data Supporting the Diagnosis

Discuss pathophysiology of condition.

● THERAPEUTIC PLAN

1. *Based on your diagnosis, how will you treat Sam?*
2. *What are nonpharmacological therapies you would recommend to Sam's mom?*
3. *When can Sam return to school?*
4. *What information needs to be given to Sam's mom regarding the illness and the likelihood of others in the house contracting the disease?*
5. *What warning signs should be discussed with Sam's mom?*
6. *When should Sam return for follow-up?*

REFERENCES

Bass, J., Person, D., & Chan, D. (2000). Culture confirmation of negative rapid strep test results. *Journal of Family Practice, 49,* 371–372.

Cecchini, J. A. (1996). Streptococcus 'A' screens. *Nurse Practitioner, 21,* 152–153.

Demarest, P. L. (2000). Review: Antibiotics for sore throat reduce symptoms at day 3 and the incidence of rheumatic fever and otitis media. (Commentary on Del Mar, C. B., Glasziou, P. P., & Spinks, A. B. Antibiotics for sore throat. *Cochrane Review,* latest version 2000, issue 1.) *Evidence-Based Nursing, 3*(3), 78.

DiMatteo, L. (1999). Pearls for practice. Managing streptococcal pharyngitis: A review of clinical decision- managing strategies, diagnostic evaluation, and treatment. *Journal of the American Academy of Nurse Practitioners, 11*(2), 57–62.

Fries, S. M. (1995). Diagnosis of group A streptococcal pharyngitis in a private clinic: Comparative evaluation of an optical immunoassay method and culture. *The Journal of Pediatrics, 126,* 933–936.

Gerber, Tanz, R., Kabat, W., Beer, G., Siddiqui, P., Lever, T., et al. (1999). Potential mechanisms for failure to eradicate group A streptococci from the pharynx. *Pediatrics, 104*(4 PT 1), 911–917.

Gerber, M. A., Tanz, R. R., Kabat, W., Dennis, E., Bell, G. L., Kaplan, E. L., & Schulman, S. (1997). Optical immunoassay test for group A beta hemolytic streptococcal pharyngitis: An office based, multicenter investigation. *Journal of the American Medical Association, 277,* 899–903.

Graham, A., & Fahey, T. (1999). Evidence based case report. Sore throat: Diagnostic and therapeutic dilemmas. *British Medical Journal,* 319(7203), 173–174.

McIsaac, W., Goel, V., To, T., & Low, D. (2000). The validity of a sore throat score in family practice. *Canadian Medical Association Journal, 163,* 811–815.

Perkins, A. (1997). An approach to diagnosing the acute sore throat. *American Family Physician, 55*(1)131–138.

Pichichero, M. E. (2000). Pharyngitis: When to culture. *Consultant, 40,* 1663–1664, 1666, 1668.

Pichichero, M. E. (2000). Pharyngitis: When to treat. *Consultant, 40,* 1669–1674.

Pribyl, S., & Force, F. (1999). Cost-effectiveness analysis of management of sore throats in children. *Journal of Family Practice, 48,* 913–914.

Robinson, D. L, Kidd, P., & Rogers, K. (2000). *Primary care across the lifespan.* St. Louis: Mosby.

Sheer, B. (2000). Case study. Young boy presenting with swollen glands and sore throat. *Lippincott's Primary Care Practice, 4,* 524–528.

Stephenson, K. N. (2000). Differential diagnosis. Acute and chronic pharyngitis across the lifespan. *Lippincott's Primary Care Practice, 4,* 471–489.

Stewart, M. H., Siff, J. E., & Cydulka, R. K. (1999). Evaluation of the patient with sore throat, earache, and sinusitis: An evidence based approach. *Emergency Medicine Clinics of North America, 17*(1), 153–187.

Tsevat, J., & Kotagall, U. (1999). Management of sore throats in children: A cost-effectiveness analysis. *Archives in Pediatric Adolescent Medicine, 153*(7), 681–688.

Webb, K., Needham, C., & Kurtz, S. (2000). Use of a high-sensitivity rapid strep test without culture confirmation of negative results: 2 years' experience. *Journal of Family Practice, 49*(1), 34–38.

Zwart, S., Sachs, A., Ruijs, A., Gubbels, J., Hoes, A., & de Melker, R. (2000). Penicillin for acute sore throat: Randomized double blind trial of seven days versus three days treatment or placebo in adults. *British Medical Journal, 320*(7228), 150–154.

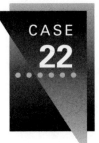

A 72-year-old woman with productive cough, nausea, and itching

SCENARIO

Elizabeth is a 72-year-old woman who presents with a productive cough, nausea, and itching over her entire body. She has had the cough for about 1 month. The nausea and pruritus are acute onset. She is accompanied by her daughter, who lives next door to her.

● TENTATIVE DIAGNOSES

*Based on the information presented, what are potential differential diagnoses? What are the **red flag** diagnoses that you cannot miss?*

DIAGNOSIS	RATIONALE
1	
2	
3	
4	
5	
6	
7	
8	
9	

● HISTORY

What are significant questions to ask Elizabeth? What are the key points to cover on the ROS? Are any data missing that are important for you to know?

REQUESTED DATA   DATA ANSWERS

REQUESTED DATA	DATA ANSWERS
Current illness	Elizabeth's main complaint is pruritis. She describes it as itching all over for the last 2 weeks. The itching is not associated with a rash. She denies any change in soaps, detergents, linens, food, or medications. She has tried OTC creams (such as Cortaid and Panalog) without relief. She denies ever having a visible rash. She has had nausea for several days, with one episode of vomiting. The nausea and vomiting are not related to meals. She denies any abdominal pain, anorexia, or epigastric pain. She started to have clay colored stools and dark urine 2 days ago. She has not had diarrhea or constipation. Elizabeth denies any change in weight. She has had fatigue, but she associates that with recovery from gallbladder surgery 1 month ago. Elizabeth also came in because she is having a productive cough of yellow sputum. She states her sore throat is better since taking the antibiotic. She denies nasal congestion, fullness in the ears, SOB, wheezing. She has had diaphoresis for 2 weeks but attributes that to not taking her raloxifene hydrochloride (Evista).
Allergies	Sulfa, codeine, phenytoin (Dilantin), and Dilaudid. No food allergies.
Medications	Prednisone, 5 mg QD. Fosinopril sodium (Monopril), 10 mg QD. HCTZ, 25 mg QD. Laxative (Metamucil), BID. Multivitamin (Centrum Silver), 1 QD. Montelukast sodium (Singulair), 100 mg QD. Lansoprazole (Prevacid), 30 mg QD. Zoloft, 50 mg QD. Raloxifene hydrochloride (Evista), 60 mg 1 QD. Albuterol MDI PRN. Salmeterol xinafoate (Serevent) and fluticasone propionate (Flovent) MDIs.
Social	Denies smoking or alcohol. Her husband smoked, so she was exposed to passive smoke, but he passed away in 1996 after a terminal illness. Lives by herself next to her daughter.

(continued)

REQUESTED DATA   DATA ANSWERS

Family history	Husband: died of cancer at age 73. Children: 3 in good health. Parents: not sure what they died of: old age most likely.
Activities	Retired from Ford Motor Company. High school graduate. Likes to take enrichment classes. Enjoys senior outings and bus trips.
Exercise	3 times weekly by walking or stationary bike.
Medical history	HTN; asthma; GERD.
Developmental stage	Erickson ego integrity vs despair: successfully resolving: close to her children, enjoys senior outings, continues to exercise and take care of her health.

Important questions to ask in the ROS are:

SYSTEM   DATA

General	No change in weight. Has had fatigue and night sweats for a couple of months.
ENT	Sore throat, cough, and SOB for 1 month. She relates it to her asthma. Treated with antibiotics.
Respiratory	History of asthma since 1995. She is on multiple medications for her asthma. She states she gets SOB with minimal exertion. She continues to have a productive cough of yellow sputum.
Cardiac	Denies chest pain or palpitations. She has a history of HTN and hypercholesterolemia.
GU	Denies dysuria, frequency, or urgency. She does have stress incontinence. She has gone through menopause.

● PHYSICAL EXAMINATION

What are significant portions of the physical exam that need to be completed for Elizabeth? Identify the rationale for doing each portion of the exam.

SYSTEM	RATIONALE	FINDINGS
Vital signs		T, 97.4 °F; P, 80; BP, 158/72 mm Hg sitting, left arm; Wt, 172 lbs; Ht, 5′6″.
General appearance		Alert and oriented × 3; well groomed; cooperative and communicates easily. She is fidgeting, scratching, and jaundiced in appearance.
Skin		No visible rash; skin dry and jaundiced. No open lesions or deposits.
ENT		Sclera are mildly ecteric. No sinus tenderness; nares erythematous and injected; pharynx injected without exudate. TMs are cloudy with fluid. The left has a lot of scarring, and the right is partially occluded with cerumen. No LA.
Respiratory		CTA; thoracic movement is symmetrical.
Cardiac		RRR. No murmurs or extra heart sounds.
Abdomen		Rounded and soft; nondistended; active bowel sounds; no masses or tenderness upon palpation. Liver WNL; no tenderness.

● DIFFERENTIAL DIAGNOSIS

What are the significant positive and negative data that support or refute your diagnosis?

DIAGNOSIS	POSITIVE DATA	NEGATIVE DATA
1		
2		
3		
4		
5		
6		
7		
8		
9		

● DIAGNOSTIC TESTS

Based on the history and physical assessment, what, if any, diagnostic testing would you do? Identify your rationale for the testing and interpret the results.

TEST	RATIONALE	RESULTS	INTERPRETATION
CBC with differential		WBC, 6,000/mm^3; RBC, 4.39 million/mm^3; HgB 3.3 mg/dL; HCT 38.4%; MCV, 87.6 m^3; MCH, 30.4 pg; MCHC, 39.7 g/dL; platelets 194,000/mm^3.	
Comprehensive metabolic panel		Glucose, 259 mg/dL (random).	
Hepatic function panel		Total bilirubin, 4.5 mg/dL; alkaline phosphatase, 196 U/L; AST, 171 U/L; ALT, 398 U/L.	
Hepatitis screen		Hepatitis A nonreactive. Hepatitis B nonreactive. Hepatitis C nonreactive.	
Abdominal ultrasound		Dilated common bile duct and dilated intrahepatic ducts. Possible common bile duct stone.	
CT of abdomen and pelvis		18–20-mm mass at the head of the pancreas causing biliary and pancreatic duct obstruction	
Endoscopic retrograde cholangiopan-creatography		A biliary stent was placed above the level of the stricture of the distal common bile duct. Brushings of the distal common bile duct were obtained.	

● DIAGNOSIS

What diagnosis do you determine is appropriate for Elizabeth? Identify the supporting data and the pathophysiology of her condition.

● THERAPEUTIC PLAN

1. What are the goals of therapy for Elizabeth?

2. What are the growth and development issues for Elizabeth?

3. What are issues for the patient and her family?

4. What are the family's educational needs?

5. To whom might you refer Elizabeth and her family at this point?

6. What is the role of the NP in this situation?

REFERENCES

Brentnall, T. (2000). Cancer surveillance of patients from familial pancreatic cancer kindreds. *Medical Clinics of North America, 84*(3), 707–718.

Lillimoe, K., Yeo, C., & Cameron, J. (2000). Pancreatic cancer: State-of-the-art care. *CA Cancer Journal for Clinicians, 50*(4), 241–268.

O'Neal, C., & Cleary, J. E. (2000). Pancreatic cancer: A silent killer. *American Journal of Nursing,* (Suppl), 23–26, 52–54.

Sauter, P. K., & Coleman, J. (1999). Pancreatic cancer: A continuum of care. *Seminars in Oncology Nursing, 15*(1), 36–47.

Rosenberg, L. (2000). Pancreatic cancer: A review of emerging therapies. *Drugs, 59*(5), 1071–1089.

Rosewicz, S., & Widenmann, B. (1997). Pancreatic carcinoma. *Lancet, 349*(9050), 485–489.

Ryosch, T., Schusdziarra, V., Born, P., et al. (2000). Modern imaging methods versus clinical assessment in the evaluation of hospital in-patients with suspected pancreatic disease. *American Journal of Gastroenterology, 95,* 2261–2270.

Yeo, C. J. (1998). Pancreatic cancer: 1998 update. *Journal of the American College of Surgeons, 187*(4), 429–442.

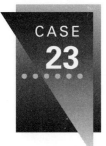

A 36-year-old man with heartburn

SCENARIO

Bill Star is a 36-year-old Caucasian man. He is employed as a stockbroker and works 60–70 hours a week. His job frequently requires that he be out of town on short business trips. Bill presents with a midsternal burning sensation. His discomfort often is worse at night, and he frequently awakens with a bad taste in his mouth. He has experienced no weight loss or change in appetite.

● TENTATIVE DIAGNOSIS

Based on Bill's presentation, what are your differential diagnoses?

● HISTORY

What additional information would you like to obtain from Bill to help with your subjective data collection?

● PHYSICAL ASSESSMENT

Based on the subjective data obtained, what should be included in the objective assessment of Bill and why?

● DIFFERENTIAL DIAGNOSIS

Having collected both subjective and objective data, now link the subjective and objective information to the appropriate differential diagnosis. Identify both positive and negative data that support/refute the diagnosis.

● DIAGNOSTIC TESTS

Are there diagnostic tests that will help to confirm the priority diagnosis or refute the differential diagnosis?

● DIAGNOSIS

Based on the subjective, objective, and diagnostic data you have gathered, what is your diagnosis of Bill? What data support this diagnosis?

● THERAPEUTIC PLAN

1. What lifestyle changes will be important for Bill to adopt?

2. What medications are appropriate for Bill to take?

3. When should Bill return for follow-up?

4. At what point should Bill be referred to a physician or specialist?

5. What resources are available for Bill and the NP?

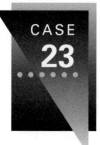

TUTORIAL

A 36-year-old man with heartburn

SCENARIO

Bill Star is a 36-year-old Caucasian male. He is employed as a stockbroker and works 60 to 70 hours a week. His job frequently requires that he be out of town on short business trips. Bill presents with a midsternal burning sensation. His discomfort often is worse at night, and he frequently awakens with a bad taste in his mouth. He has experienced no weight loss or change in appetite.

● TENTATIVE DIAGNOSIS

Based on Bill's presentation, what are your differential diagnoses?

DIAGNOSIS	RATIONALE
Gastric or duodenal ulcer	Bill presents with a midsternal burning sensation, often associated with meals.
GERD	Midsternal burning, associated with meals, waking during the night with a bad taste in his mouth.
Cardiac chest pain	Bill's midsternal pain could contribute to a cardiac etiology.

● HISTORY

What additional information would you like to obtain from Bill to help with your subjective data collection?

REQUESTED DATA   DATA ANSWER

REQUESTED DATA	DATA ANSWER
History of current illness	Midsternal burning has been present for about 4–5 months. It occurs most often after a large meal and often in the middle of the night. There is no radiation of the discomfort, no SOB, no diaphoresis. The discomfort is relieved somewhat by antacids. The discomfort can last for a couple of hours.
Allergies	None.
Medication	ASA as needed. Takes approximately 6/day for H/A. Antacids PRN.
Surgery	Appendectomy, 1974.
Hospitalizations	Appendectomy, 1974. Kidney stones, 1989.
Transfusions	None.
Diet	Regular; no change in appetite; often eats fast food and conducts business over dinner.
24-hour diet recall	B: 3 cups of coffee and danish at 6:30 AM. L: Hamburger, french fries, pop, sometimes a milk shake at 12:00 N. D: Steak, baked potato with butter and sour cream, salad with ranch dressing, coffee at 6–7:00 PM. S: chips, soft drinks, candy bar in the midafternoon.
Sleep	No difficulty sleeping; goes to bed at 11–12:00 P.M. and wakes at 6:00 AM.
Social habits	Smokes 1½ packs of cigarettes QD. ETOH: 3–5 drinks every week. Caffeine: 4–5 cups of coffee and 4–5 caffeinated pops QD. No recreational drugs. No regular exercise.
Social history	Married to wife of 12 years; good relationship; 3 children. Works as a stock broker for 10 years; enjoys his job. Owns his own home. Income: $65,000 a year. Belongs to a country club; plays golf once a week in the summer and fall.
Family history	Father: age 62, living, has HTN. Mother: age 60, living has had breast cancer. Sister: age 33, alive and healthy. Daughter: age 10, alive and healthy. Son: age 8, has epilepsy. Son: age 5, has asthma and allergies.

SYSTEM REVIEWED	DATA ANSWER
General	Current health is good.
Cardiac	Denies chest pain, SOB, orthopnea, history of HTN, edema.
GI	Denies weight gain or loss, vomiting, diarrhea, constipation, blood in stool, change in appetite, history of peptic ulcer disease.
GU	Denies change in pattern of urination, frequency, urgency, burning.
Neurological assessment	C/o tension headaches for past 8 years, mainly during work week. Has associated neck tightness. No N/V, visual problems, or other associated symptoms.
Preventive health	Wears seat belt; has smoke detector in home. No guns in home. Has not had influenza vaccine. Has not had a checkup in past 5 years. Last dental exam 6 months ago. Last vision exam, 10 months ago.

● PHYSICAL ASSESSMENT

Based on the subjective data obtained, what should be included in the objective assessment of Bill and why?

SYSTEM	RATIONALE	FINDINGS
Vital signs	Baseline information	T, 98.4 °F; P, 88; RR, 18; BP, 150/86 mm Hg.
Height/weight	To establish general size and obesity status/weight loss or gain.	Ht, 6′; Wt, 245 lbs.
General appearance	Gives a general overview of Bill's status and urgency of complaint.	Slightly obese; well groomed; in no apparent distress.
HEENT	Not entirely necessary for Bill's problem. Will probably reveal no new information.	PERRLA; EOMI intact; TMs pearly, with + light reflex; nares patent; neck supple; no adenopathy.

(continued)

SYSTEM	RATIONALE	FINDINGS
Cardiac	Prudent for routine exam, and needs to be ruled out as cause of chief complaint.	S1, S2 regular; no murmur; no S4.
Respiratory	Prudent for routine exam.	Respirations even, unlabored. Breath sounds clear throughout.
Abdomen	Allows NP to rule out masses, fluid, ascites, organomegaly, as well as confirm peristalsis with bowel sounds.	Bowel sounds present in four quadrants; abdomen soft, rounded nontender; no HSM; negative CVA tenderness.
Rectal	Prudent to evaluate for GI bleeding.	Prostate unremarkable. Stool hemoccult negative.

● DIFFERENTIAL DIAGNOSIS

Having collected both subjective and objective data, now link the subjective and objective information to the appropriate differential diagnosis. Identify both positive and negative data that support or refute the diagnosis.

DIAGNOSIS	POSITIVE DATA	NEGATIVE DATA
Peptic ulcer disease	Male; often awakened at night with discomfort; smoker; frequent use of ASA.	No family history of PUD; some relief with antacids; no change in weight.
GERD	Heartburn, specifically postprandial. Some relief with use of antacids. Smokes. Large caffeine intake. High-fat diet. Overweight.	Usually does not eat late at night.
Cardiac chest pain	Substernal pain; smokes 1½ packs of cigarettes every day. Blood pressure, 150/86 mm Hg. No knowledge of cholesterol level.	Age, 36 years; nondiabetic; no family history of coronary artery disease; pain is not brought on by exertion; no other associated symptoms.

● DIAGNOSTIC TESTS

Are there diagnostic tests that will help to confirm the priority diagnosis or refute the differential diagnosis?

DIAGNOSTIC TEST	RATIONALE	RESULTS	INTERPRETATION
Barium swallow	The simplest and least expensive test for GERD; 40–60% will have a normal result. It is useful as a screening test; it can identify structural problems of the upper GI tract and aspiration.	Filling of the pharynx and esophagus normal. Esophageal size, contour, and peristaltic motion normal. Mild free reflux present; mucosal irregularities present.	Nondiagnostic test. Suggestive of GERD. Further testing recommended.
Endoscopy	Initially no diagnostic studies are necessary. UGI could help rule out peptic ulcer disease (PUD); however, endoscopy is the preferred test for PUD. The subjective and objective data generally will lead to the diagnosis of GERD. However, physician referral for endoscopy is recommended if any of the following "alarm" symptoms are present: odynophagia, dysphagia, nausea, vomiting, early satiety, weight loss, pulmonary symptoms, blood in stool, or chest pain (Horwitz & Fisher, 1995).	Esophagitis; questionable Barrett's mucosa; biopsies taken. No Barrett's found on biopsy.	GERD.

(continued)

DIAGNOSTIC TEST	RATIONALE	RESULTS	INTERPRETATION
24-hour ambulatory pH monitoring	The diagnosis usually can be made with history and endoscopy; however, if needed, a 24-hour monitoring should be performed. It is helpful in patients with noncardiac chest pain, those with chronic pulmonary or otolaryngologic symptoms suggestive of reflux, or those with typical symptoms when diagnosis is elusive. All patients who are having surgery should have this test done before the procedure. It is extremely reproducible and is the most sensitive and specific diagnostic test for the presence of abnormal acid reflux.	Not done.	Not done.
Electrocardiogram (EKG)	Because the patient is a heavy smoker and is presently hypertensive, an EKG would be an acceptable test to help rule out a cardiac etiology (Uphold & Graham, 1999).	NSR. No indications of ischemia or increased voltage. No acute changes	WNL.
Cholesterol	An increased cholesterol level will help to substantiate a differential diagnosis of a cardiac chest pain. A total cholesterol level check is	Total cholesterol, 158 mg/dL. LDL, 100 mg/dL. HDL, 30 mg/dL.	Low HDL.

(continued)

DIAGNOSTIC TEST	RATIONALE	RESULTS	INTERPRETATION
	recommended every 5 years for persons without symptoms of coronary artery disease (American Academy of Family Physicians, 1992).		
Heliobacter pylori	A test to detect the presence of H. pylori, helpful in the diagnosis of PUD. Biopsy or breath test can be completed in office with appropriate equipment. Usually not a test done for suspected GERD.	Not done.	Not done.

● DIAGNOSIS

Based on the subjective, objective, and diagnostic data you have gathered, what is your diagnosis of Bill? What data support this diagnosis?

GERD

Obesity

Immunization: Needs Tetanus

Rationale: Heartburn and nocturnal reflux of acid are hallmark symptoms of GERD (Horwitz & Fisher, 1995). Alcohol, obesity, smoking, a high-fat diet, and caffeine all lead to decreased lower esophageal sphincter tone and reflux (Hixson, Kelley, Jones, & Tuohy, 1992). Absence of the aforementioned "alarm" symptoms rules out other diagnoses. In addition, Bill's EKG and total cholesterol were within normal limits. This, in addition to the lack of family history of CAD and no associated cardiac symptoms, help to rule out a cardiac etiology.

Pathophysiology

The etiology of GERD is unknown. The most significant defect is an abnormality of the antireflux barrier: the lower esophageal sphincter (LES). There are two major abnormalities associated with the increased frequency of reflux: a low basal LES pressure and a transient LES relaxation unassociated with a swallow. The transient relaxation is the most common cause of an episode of reflux. Obesity contributes to GERD, as do certain foods and lying down after meals.

● THERAPEUTIC PLAN

1. *What lifestyle changes will be important for Bill to adopt?*
   Teaching lifestyle changes will play a large role for the nurse practitioner. Initially, GERD should be addressed nonpharmacologically in the following manner, known as Phase I therapy:

   - Normalize weight.
   - Avoid large meals.
   - Do not eat at least 2 hours before bedtime.
   - Avoid alcohol, tobacco, caffeine, fatty foods, and chocolate.
   - Elevate the head of the bed on blocks.
   - Use antacids as much as seven times a day.
   - Avoid the following medications: theophylline, narcotics, calcium channel blockers, nicotine, anticholinergics, estrogen, B-adrenergic agonists, progesterone, and alpha adrenergic agonists. These medications decrease LES tone and should be avoided when possible (Hixson et al., 1992; Horwitz & Fisher, 1995).

   A 2- to 3-week trial of Phase I therapy is recommended (Horwitz & Fischer, 1995). If no improvement is noted, Phase II therapy should be started.

   Normalizing weight will be helpful for Bill in terms of his cholesterol level. To help with weight control, the NP should discuss with him the need to exercise, which will help with weight loss and increase his HDL level.

   Bill needs a tetanus booster because it has been more than 10 years since he got his last immunization.

2. *What medications are appropriate for Bill to take?*
   Phase II therapy can be initiated after failure of Phase I therapy and is aimed at decreasing gastric acid secretion, augmenting LES pressure, and improving esophageal clearance.

   In Phase II therapy, pharmacologic agents are added to the lifestyle changes. The first drug of choice in Phase II therapy is a histamine 2 (H2) receptor antagonist (Horwitz & Fisher, 1995).

   There are four equally effective H2 antagonists:

   - Cimetidine (Tagamet), 400 mg BID
   - Ranitidine (Zantac) 150 mg BID
   - Famotidine (Pepcid) 20 mg BID
   - Nizatidine (Axid) 150 mg BID (Katz, 1999; Robinson, 1995).

   H2 receptor antagonists should be administered in BID doses, once in the morning and once after dinner. Treatment should be continued for 8 to

12 weeks. The average healing rate with this regimen is approximately 50% (Katz, 1999).

If no improvement is noted with H2 blockers, proton pump inhibitors (PPI) are an option for refractory GERD. Omeprazole (Prilosec), lansoprazole (Prevacid), and rabeprazole sodium (Aciphex) offer significant inhibition of acid secretion on a 24-hour basis. However, these drugs are expensive and once used may prohibit a return to H2 receptor antagonists (Robinson, 1995). Current data suggest this is the most successful treatment of GERD. Healing rates are 80% to 90% at 8 weeks. Using a PPI for initial treatment of GERD has been approved by the FDA, but it is costly (approximately $4–$5 dollars a day).

Antacids are considered second-line treatment for GERD and often are initiated at the same time Phase I therapy is started. They act to neutralize gastric acids and thus increase the pH of refluxed gastric content. However, they offer only temporary symptomatic relief because of their short duration of action (Hixson et al., 1992). If used, dosing is recommended to seven times a day, 1 to 3 hours after meals and at bedtime. Liquid antacids are recommended over chewable ones, and they should not be administered within 2 hours of an H2 receptor antagonist.

Prokinetic drug therapy is another pharmacologic option for patients with GERD. In GERD there are several mechanisms that predispose the patient to excessive esophageal acid exposure. These include: improper tone of the LES, impaired peristaltic contractions, gastric hypersecretion, and impaired gastric emptying, all of which can lead to reflux of stomach content (Hixson et al., 1992; Robinson, 1995). Metoclopramide (Reglan) could be used as a third-line choice for GERD.

Whether H2 receptor antagonists, antacids, or PPI are chosen, if improvement in symptoms is demonstrated, the chosen treatment should be continued for 6 to 8 weeks. The patient will need follow-up after pharmacologic therapy is completed. It needs to be emphasized that the lifestyle changes initiated in Phase I therapy need to become a way of life.

3. *When should Bill return for follow-up?*
Bill should return in 2 weeks to allow for evaluation of his symptoms. If the lifestyle changes have helped with the reduction of symptoms, they should be continued. If there is no improvement in Bill's symptoms, Phase II treatment should be started.

4. *At what point should Bill be referred to a physician or specialist?*
If Bill were to experience any of the mentioned "alarm" symptoms (odynophagia, dysphagia, nausea, vomiting, early satiety, weight loss, pulmonary symptoms, blood in stool, or chest pain), immediate referral is indicated (Horwitz & Fisher, 1995). Referral also is indicated if two different medications have been tried without relief of symptoms. In addition, any patient who does not have a response to therapy with H2 receptor antagonists or PPI should be referred for additional evaluation.

GERD is a chronic disease, and most patients will require long-term therapy. Patients with erosive esophagitis or Barrett's esophagus generally require PPI therapy and regular follow-up endoscopies, whereas those with nonerosive esophagitis can be continue on a regimen of H2 blockers or prokinetic agents.

Surgery is indicated in approximately 5% to 10% of patients with reflux disease. Indications for surgery include strictures unresponsive to medical therapy, hemorrhage secondary to erosive esophagitis, reflux-induced hoarseness, and symptoms refractory to medical management. Barrett's esophagus should be treated aggressively with medical agents before surgery is attempted. A fundoplication around the distal esophagus provides symptomatic improvement in approximately 90% of patients.

5. *What resources are available for Bill and the NP concerning his condition?*

American College of Gastroenterology (ACG)
4900-B South 31st Street
Arlington, VA 22206-1656
703/820-7400
Fax: 703/931-4520
Home page: *http://www.acg.gi.org*

American Gastroenterological Association (AGA) National Office
7910 Woodmont Avenue, 7th Floor
Bethesda, MD 20814
301/654-2055
Fax: 301/654-5920
E-mail: aga001@80l.com
Home page: *http://www.gastro.org*

Digestive Disease National Coalition (DDNC)
507 Capitol Court NE, Suite 200
Washington, DC 20002
202/544-7497
Fax: 202/546-7105

National Digestive Diseases Information Clearinghouse (NDDIC)
Bethesda, MD
301/654-3810
http://www.niddk.nih.gov/health/digest/nddic.htm

National Institute for Diabetes, Digestive and Kidney Disorders (NIDDK)
http://www.niddk.nih.gov/health/digest/digest.htm

Society of Gastroenterology Nurses and Associates, Inc. (SGNA)
401 North Michigan Avenue
Chicago, IL 60611
312/321-5165 or 800/245-SGNA (7462)

Fax: 312/321-5194
E-mail: sgna@sba.com
Home page: *http://www.sgna.org*

REFERENCES

American Academy of Family Physicians, Commission on Public Health and Scientific Affairs, (1992). *Age charts for periodic health exams.* Kansas City, MO: AAFP.

Bailey, M. A., & Katz, P. O. (2000). Gastroesophageal reflux disease in the elderly. *Clinical Geriatrics , 8*(8), 64–72.

Carr, M., Nguyen, A., Nagy, M., Poje, C., Pizzuto, M., & Brodsky, L. (2000). Clinical presentation as a guide to the identification of GERD in children. *International Journal of Pediatric Otorhinolaryngology, 54*(1), 27–32.

Eloubeidi, M., & Provenzale, D. (2000). Health-related quality of life and severity of symptoms in patients with Barrett's esophagus and gastroesophageal reflux disease patients without Barrett's esophagus. *American Journal of Gastroenterology, 95*(8), 1881–1887.

Gordon, D. (2000). New endoscopic strategies offer middle ground for treating GERD. *Gastroenterology, 119,* 611.

Hixson, L. J., Kelley, C. L., Jones, W. N., & Tuohy, C. D. (1992). Current trends in the pharmacotherapy for gastroesophageal reflux disease. *Archives of Internal Medicine, 152,* 717–721.

Horwitz, B. J., & Fisher, R. S. (1995). Intervening in GERD: The phases of management. *Hospital Practice, 15,* 43–52.

Kaplan-Machlis, B., Spiegler, G., Zodet, M., & Revicki, D. (2000). Effectiveness and costs of omeprazole vs ranitidine for treatment of symptomatic gastroesophageal reflux disease in primary care clinics in West Virginia. *Archives of Family Medicine, 9,* 624–630.

Katz, P. (1999). Disorders of the esophagus. In R. Barker, J. Burton, P. Ziever (Eds.), *Principles of ambulatory medicine* (5th ed., pp. 459–470.). Baltimore: Williams & Wilkins.

Middlemiss, C. (1997). Gastroesophageal reflux disease: A common condition in the elderly. *Nurse Practitioner: American Journal of Primary Health Care, 22*(11), 51–52, 55–61.

Nelson, W., Vermeulen, L., Geurkink, E., Ehlert, D., & Reichilderfer, M. (2000). Clinical and humanistic outcomes in patients with gastroesophageal reflux disease converted from omeprazole to lansoprazole. *Archives of Internal Medicine, 160,* 2491–2496.

Richter, J., Peura, D., Benjamin, S., Joelsson, B., & Whipple, J. (2000). Efficacy of omeprazole for the treatment of symptomatic acid reflux disease without esophagitis. *Archives of Internal Medicine, 160,* 1810–1816.

Robinson, M. (1995). Prokinetic therapy for gastroesophageal reflux disease. *American Family Physician, 52,* 957–961.

Uphold, C., & Graham, M. (1999). Clinical guidelines in family practice (2nd ed.). Gainesville, FL: Barmarroe Books.

Wong, R., Hanson, D., Waring, P., & Shaw, G. (2000). ENT manifestations of gastroesophageal reflux. *American Journal of Gastroenterology, 95*(8 Suppl), S15–S22.

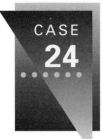

A 31-year-old woman with a fever

SCENARIO

Lee Jenson presents to the health center reporting a fever after undergoing an elective abortion 4 days ago. She works full time in retail and had to miss work today because of her symptoms. She is married and has two children.

● TENTATIVE DIAGNOSES

*What are the potential diagnoses you have identified based on this scenario? What are **red flags** that cannot be missed?*

DIAGNOSIS	RATIONALE
1	
2	
3	
4	
5	
6	
7	

● HISTORY

What are significant questions in the history for Lee? Is all information that is needed requested?

REQUESTED DATA	DATA ANSWER
Temperature	The fever has been constant since last night. The highest temperature has been 100.4° F. Also experiencing chills intermittently.
Has anyone else in your family been sick?	No.
Did you have any problems the first 2 days after the abortion?	No; pregnancy symptoms of tender breasts, nausea, and urinary frequency stopped after the procedure.
Are you experiencing pelvic, lower back, or abdominal discomfort?	Pelvic cramping from the procedure stopped on the second day after abortion. Now complains of a dull ache in lower back and pelvic area. Also has generalized malaise.
What have you done to relieve this discomfort?	Ibuprofen 400 mg orally started this morning has provided minimal relief.
Are you having any vaginal bleeding or discharge?	Vaginal bleeding had decreased to spotting. Now notices a strong foul odor for 1 day.
Are you experiencing any changes in urinary functioning (hematuria, dysuria, oliguria, frequency, etc.)?	Denies any change in urinary functioning.
Length of symptoms	The fever started last night. Also, the onset of lower back and pelvic discomfort was last night.
Medications	Oral contraceptives and ibuprofen.
How has this affected your ADLs?	Did not go to work today because of physical complaints. Her husband took the children to school and will take them to their aunt's home in the evening so she may rest better.
Allergies	NKA.
OB/GYN history	LNMP: 10 weeks ago, normal flow and duration. Elective abortion at 10 weeks estimated gestational age via D&E 4 days ago. Mammogram: none. SBE: regularly for past year. G6P2A4; multiple miscarriages due to early fetal demise.
Medical history and hospitalizations/fractures/ injuries	Chicken pox and measles as child. Left radial fracture from fall as child.
Adult illness	Unremarkable.

(continued)

REQUESTED DATA	DATA ANSWER
Social history	Tobacco: never. Alcohol: 1–2 beers every weekend Caffeine: 2 cups of coffee/1–2 colas/day
Family history	Adopted.
Social organizations	Roman Catholic church; local PTA volunteer.
Relationship with husband	Perceives herself to be in a monogamous relationship. Married 11 years. They have sex about once a week, and both enjoy this. Husband works as construction manager. They both decided they did not have enough money or time to care for another child. In addition, she had many spontaneous miscarriages; she also had DVTs while pregnant so that she had to take heparin while pregnant. This made the quality of life for all family members very poor.
Relationship with children	Values time spent with the children and husband in evenings. Volunteers as a home-room mother at the childrens' school. Helps her elderly parents with their needs.
Income/insurance/home	She and her husband earn middle class wages. Both perceive their jobs to be secure. Health and dental insurance through husband's employer, but they would owe 20% of any health costs incurred. They own their home.

● PHYSICAL ASSESSMENT

What are the significant portions of the physical examination that should be completed for Lee?

SYSTEM	RATIONALE	FINDINGS
Vital signs		BP 108/66 mm Hg right arm; HR, 88 bpm; RR, 20; T, 100.4 °F; Ht, 5′ 3″; Wt, 130 lbs.
General appearance/skin		Generalized discomfort. Skin warm. Color flushed.
HEENT		Normocephalic; no sinus tenderness; TMs gray and WNL. Nose pink and moist with septum. Midline; oral mucosa moist and pink. Uvala midline; no pharyngeal erythema or oral lesions noted.

(continued)

SYSTEM	RATIONALE	FINDINGS
		No LA, supple neck. Thyroid; non-palpable, no masses.
Lungs		CTA.
Heart		S1, S2 WNL; no MRG.
Abdomen		BS +; soft, no splenomegaly. Liver palpable just below right costal margin. Lower abdominal tenderness. No LA. Negative CVAT.
Neurological assessment		Alert and oriented; slow but steady gait. Strength/sensation intact. DTRs 2+.
Pelvic		External: negative. Vagina: bleeding noted. Cervix: bleeding noted as os, . CMT +. Uterus: enlarged, soft with tenderness. Adnexal: slight bilateral tenderness.
Rectal		Normal findings. Small amount brown stool.
Extremities		Pulses 2+. No edema noted.

● DIFFERENTIAL DIAGNOSES

What are the significant positive and negative findings that support or refute your diagnoses for Lee?

DIAGNOSIS	POSITIVE DATA	NEGATIVE DATA
1		
2		
3		
4		
5		
6		

● DIAGNOSTIC TESTS

Based on the history and physical examination, what, if any, diagnostic testing would you obtain? Identify your rationale for the testing and interpret the tests.

DIAGNOSTIC TEST	RATIONALE	RESULTS	INTERPRETATION
Urine HCG		Positive.	
Serum β HCG		Pending.	
Wet prep		Positive for WBC.	
DNA probe for GC and chlamydia		Pending.	
Urinalysis		Negative.	
CBC with differential and ESR		WBC, 13,000. 30.	
Transvaginal ultrasound		Negative for retained products of conception. Positive for inflammation.	

● DIAGNOSES

What diagnosis do you determine as being appropriate after a review of the subjective and objective data?

Data Supporting the Diagnosis

● DISCUSSION OF THE PATHOPHYSIOLOGY OF THE CASE, AND THE ETIOLOGY OF THE PROBLEM

● THERAPEUTIC PLAN

1. What influences must be considered before determining the therapeutic plan?

2. *What will you do to manage Lee's condition?*

3. *Should a physician be consulted for Lee's care?*

4. *What patient education should you discuss with Lee?*

5. *What impact does this event have in terms of Lee's future reproductive health?*

6. *What form should follow-up for Lee take?*

7. *What are community resources that are available for the NP and Lee?*

REFERENCES

Henshaw, S. K. (1999). Unintended pregnancy and abortion: A public health perspective. (p.11–22). In M. Paul, E. S. Lichtenberg, L. Borgatta, & D. A. Grimes, (Eds.), *A clinician's guide to medical and surgical abortion* (pp. 11–22). New York: Churchill Livingston.

Lichtenberg, E. S., Grimes, D. A., & Paul, M. (1999). Abortion complications: Prevention and management. In M. Paul, E. S. Lichtenberg, L. Borgatta, & D. A. Grimes, (Eds.), *A clinician's guide to medical and surgical abortion* (pp. 197–216). New York: Churchill Livingston.

Mattox, J. (1998). Spontaneous abortion and contraception. In J. Mattox (Ed.), *Core textbook of obstetrics and gynecology* (pp. 103–114, 292–296). St. Louis: Mosby.

McConlogue-O'Shaughnessy, L. (2000). Postabortion care. In D. Robinson, P. Kidd, & K. Rogers (Eds.), *Primary care across the lifespan* (pp. 905–907). St. Louis: Mosby.

Robinson, D. L., Dollins, A., & McConlogue-O'Shaughnessy, L. (2000). Care of the woman before and after an elective abortion. *The American Journal for Nurse Practitioners 4*, 17–18, 21–22, 25–26, 29.

Rowland Hogue, C. J., Boardman, L. A., Stotland, N. L., & Peipert, J. F. (1999). Answering questions about long-term outcomes. In M. Paul, E. S. Lichtenberg, L. Borgatta, & D. A. Grimes, (Eds.), *A clinician's guide to medical and surgical abortion* (pp. 217–228). New York: Churchill Livingston.

Sawaya, G. F., Grady, D., Kerlikowske, K., et al. (1996). Antibiotics at the time of induced abortion: The case for universal prohylaxis based on a meta-analysis. *Obstetrics and Gynecology, 87*, 884–890.

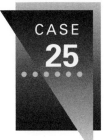

A 70-year-old woman with shortness of breath and cough

SCENARIO

Patricia Anne Bechinski presents to the clinic with a history of a "cold" for more than 2 weeks that has been hanging on. She is now getting short of breath (SOB) and coughing up thick, yellow-green mucus. The SOB increases with exertion and has been worse by nighttime during the last 2 days. Pat has been feeling a little "flushed" for a couple of days. Her chest feels "tight," with chest pain during coughing. "Fits" of coughing have awakened her at night for several nights in a row; now her chest aches all over. She has tried Robitussin cough medicine, but it is not helping, and acetaminophen (Tylenol Extra Strength) twice a day has given her little relief. Pat has really been feeling tired all day for at least the last week, and she has been generally "feeling so lousy" she has lost her appetite. She does not smoke, never did; she gets the flu occasionally.

TENTATIVE DIAGNOSES

*What are the potential diagnoses you have identified based on the scenario presented? Make sure you include any vital **red flag** diagnoses that cannot be missed.*

DIAGNOSIS　　　*RATIONALE*

1

2

3

4

(continued)

DIAGNOSIS	RATIONALE
5	
6	
7	
8	
9	

● HISTORY

What are significant questions in the history for Pat?

REQUESTED DATA	DATA ANSWER
Allergies	NKA to medications or food but has seasonal allergies.
Current medications	Guaifenesin (Robitussin) cough medicine prn. Acetaminophen (Tylenol Extra Strength) twice a day for last 3 days. Only prescription medication is for blood pressure, prescribed 2 years ago: Bisoprolol fumarate 5 mg and HCTZ 6.25 mg (Ziac). Took HCTZ alone for 10 years, but it stopped being effective. Vitamins with extra calcium regularly and calcium carbonate (Tums) for occasional indigestion.
Surgery/transfusions	None.
Immunizations	Flu shot usually yearly but has not had it yet this year. Has never had a pneumonia vaccination.
Medical history and hospitalizations/ fractures/injuries/ accidents	Usual childhood illnesses; no rheumatic fever. Hospitalized only to have her children, vaginal deliveries. No injuries or accidents; states she has led a "charmed" life.
Adult illness	History of HTN diagnosed 12 years ago.
Appetite/weight change	Not really hungry right now, but weight is stable.

(continued)

REQUESTED DATA	DATA ANSWER
Social history	Pat enjoys gardening, reading, attending church socials, and walking. Tobacco: never and never around passive smoke. Alcohol: none. Caffeine: 2–3 cups decaf coffee/day. Illegal drugs: none. Exercise: frequent walks of approximately 1 mile.
Family history	Grandparents history unknown. Mother and father both had HTN, mother died of a stroke at 85 years. Father also had diabetes and bladder cancer and died in his sleep at age 90. Two siblings: one sister, 75 years with diabetes and HTN, had cancer of left breast at age 55 years, which was successfully removed without complication or recurrence; a brother who died young, at age 35 years, from injuries received in an auto accident.
Social organizations	Member of St. Mary's Catholic Church; participates in many church activities; volunteers at the local hospital. Plays cards a few evenings a week with neighborhood friends. Family activities as described below.
Relationship with husband	Widowed, lives in her own home independently.
Relationship with children	Daughter and her husband live in same neighborhood. Patient has two grandchildren who are married and live nearby. Sees her daughter at least three times per week, almost daily since she has been sick. Family comes to visit frequently. Shares evening meals often, exploring new recipes and engaging in healthy conversation while preparing meals and during dinner. Watches rental movies with family at least weekly. Goes shopping with her daughter when she can.
Income/insurance/ home	Financially stable with retirement income, Social Security, and wise investments. Owns home. Medicare Part A and B with supplemental rider for medications.
Length of symptoms	History of a "cold" for more than 2 weeks, now getting SOB and coughing worse by nighttime during the last 2 days. Has been feeling a little "flushed" for a couple of days, and her "fits" of coughing have awakened her at night for several nights in a row.
How has this affected your ADLs?	Fatigue alters energy level—tired all the time now. Has felt so tired that she has been unable to walk outside for about a week now and too tired to exercise inside. Thinks she may have worked too long clearing the garden and raking leaves over 2–3-day period 3 weeks ago. No cooking much. Missed church last week. Too tired to do a good house cleaning—just tidied up a little. Had her daughter get her groceries.

(continued)

REQUESTED DATA	DATA ANSWER
How do you manage stress?	Occasional leisurely walks with daughter, gardening, walking, reading, church, friends, cooking, meditation.
Any evidence of blood loss (hemoptysis stool, urine, etc.)?	No hemoptysis or hematemesis. No changes in stool or urine elimination.
Has anyone else in family been sick?	No family or friends are sick right now.

● PHYSICAL ASSESSMENT

What are the significant portions of the physical examination that should be completed for Pat? Identify the rationale for the portions of the exam you will do.

SYSTEM	RATIONALE	FINDINGS
Vital signs		Temperature, 99.8 °F; P, 102 bpm; RR, 26; BP, 138/82 mm Hg right arm; Ht, 5'6"; Wt, 156 lbs.
General appearance/skin		Alert; NAD; articulate; cooperative; answers questions appropriately; good eye contact. Skin warm and dry; slightly pale; cheeks ruddy; no lesions.
HEENT		Normocephalic; eyes clear without drainage, TMs intact and pearly gray; no bulging; some nasal congestion but nares patent; negative for sinus tenderness; mouth without lesions; mucosa pink; oropharynx slightly reddened; negative LA; negative JVD; negative for carotid bruits; thyroid nonpalpable; trachea midline.
Lungs		Negative chest wall tenderness upon palpation; symmetrical chest expansion; AP and lateral ratio 2:1; no retractions; rate slightly increased but nonlabored; resonance percussed upper airways with dull percussion elicited bilateral bases; bronchovesicular breath sounds heard throughout; diminished sounds bilateral bases, with scattered course inspiratory crackles, positive for egophony with slightly decreased respiratory excursion. Negative for pleural friction rub.

(continued)

SYSTEM	RATIONALE	FINDINGS
Heart		PMI palpated at 5th intercostal space, midclavicular line, heart borders percussed WNL; S1 and S2 strong, without murmurs; negative for S3 or S4 gallop; no extra heart sounds, clicks, or snaps; negative for peripheral edema; all peripheral pulses palpable and strong at 2+/4+.
Abdomen		Rounded without obvious pulsations or masses; bowel sounds present and normoactive times four quadrants times 2 minutes each. Tympany percussed throughout, negative for pain or discomfort upon palpation. Negative for arterial bruits. Negative for LA.
Neurological assessment		Alert and oriented; gait normal. Strength/sensation intact. DTRs 2+/4+. No liver flap.
Extremities		Pulses 2+/4+. No edema noted. See under heart.

● DIAGNOSTIC TESTS

Based on the history and physical examination, what diagnostic testing would you obtain?

Included below are tests that were obtained and some that could/would/should be obtained in some cases, but were not necessary in Pat's case.
What do the test results indicate?
What impact do the labs have on the patient's condition?

DIAGNOSTIC TEST	RATIONALE	RESULTS	INTERPRETATION
CXR, PA and lateral		Mild infiltrates bilateral bases. Negative for masses, cardiomegaly, pleural effusion, or obstruction.	
CBC with differential		Hgb, 12 g/dL; Hct, 40%; WBC, 11.2 × 10³/µL; MCV, 85.3 m³; MCH, 28.3 pg; MCHC, 33.2 g/dL;	

(continued)

DIAGNOSTIC TEST	RATIONALE	RESULTS	INTERPRETATION
		RDW, 14.6; platelets, 385,000/mm^3; neutrophils, 5600 mm^3; lymphocytes, 3800 mm^3; monocytes, 526 mm^3; eosinophils, 310 mm^3; basophils, 43 mm^3.	
Sputum for gram stain		Not done.	
Other microbiologic studies: blood cultures, culture of sputum		Not done.	
Thyroid screen		TSH, 5 μU/mL; T$_4$, 6 U/L.	
Electrolytes, renal panel		Na, 139 mEq/L; K, 4.0 mEq/L; Cl, 101 mEq/L; CO$_2$, 30 mEq/L; BUN, 8 mg/dL; creatinine, 0.7 mg/dL.	
Glucose		Fasting, 107 mg/dL.	
Hepatic enzymes		Alkaline phosphatase 102 U/L; AST, 124 U/L; ALT, 10 U/L.	
PPD		Not done.	

● DIAGNOSIS

What diagnosis(es) do you determine as being appropriate after a review of the subjective and objective data?

● DIFFERENTIAL DIAGNOSES

What are the significant positive and negative findings that support or refute your diagnoses for Patricia?

DIAGNOSIS	POSITIVE DATA	NEGATIVE DATA
1		
2		
3		
4		
5		
6		
7		
8		
9		

Data Supporting the Diagnosis

Brief Discussion of the Pathophysiology and Etiology of Pneumonia

● THERAPEUTIC PLAN

1. How is this diagnosis classified?

   A.

   B.

2. What influences the therapy decisions for treatment of the less serious presentation?

3. What will the management of Pat's diagnosis consist of?

4. Under what circumstances should Pat be admitted to the hospital?

5. When should Pat be referred to a specialist and to whom?

6. What patient education/prevention information should you discuss with Pat?

- Education:

- Prevention:

7. *What impact or potential impact does this illness have in terms of Pat's ADLs?*

8. *What suggestions can you make for Pat for her fatigability?*

9. *What, if any, special considerations must you keep in mind because of Pat's age?*

10. *When should Pat return for follow-up?*

11. *What are community resources that are available for the NP and Pat?*

REFERENCES

Bandyopadhyay, T., Gerardi, D. A., & Metersky, M. L. (2000). A comparison of induced and expectorated sputum for the microbiological diagnosis of community-acquired pneumonia. *Respiration, 67,* 173–176.

Brown, P., & Lerner, S. (1998). Community-acquired pneumonia. *Lancet, 352,* 1295–1302.

Fine, M. J., Auble, T. E., Yealy, D. M., Hanusa, B. H., Weissfeld, L. A., Singer, D. E., Coley, C. M., Marrie, T. J., & Kapoor, W. N. (1997). A prediction rule to identify low risk patients with community-acquired pneumonia. *New England Journal of Medicine, 336,* 243–250.

Irwin, R., & Madison, J. (2000). The diagnosis and treatment of cough. *Journal of the American Medical Association, 343,* 1715–1721.

Kuru, T., & Lynch, J. P. (1999). Nonresolving or slowly resolving pneumonia. *Clinics in Chest Medicine, 20,* 623–651.

Lorente, M., Falguera, M., Nogues, A., Ruiz Gonzalez, A., Merino, M., & Rubio Caballero, M. (2000). Diagnosis of pneumococcal pneumonia by polymerase chain reaction (PCR) in whole blood: A prospective clinical study. *Thorax, 55,* 133–137.

Marrie, T., Lau, C., Wheeler, S., Wong, C., Vandervoot, M., & Feagan, B. (2000). A controlled trial of a critical pathway for treatment of community-acquired pneumonia. *Journal of the American Medical Association, 283,* 749–755.

Meehan, T., Fine, M., Krumholz, H., Scinto, J., Galusha, D., Mockalis, J., Weber, G., Petrillo, M., Houck, P., & Fine, J. (1997). Quality of care, process, and outcomes in elderly patients with pneumonia. *Journal of the American Medical Association, 278,* 2080–2084.

Sopena, N., Sabria-Leal, M., Pedro-Botet, M., Padilla, E., Dominguez, J., Morera, J., & Tudela, P. (1998). Comparative study of the clinical presentation of legionella pneumonia and other community-acquired pneumonias. *Chest, 113,* 1195–1200.

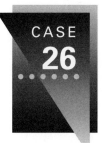

A 49-year-old woman seeking evaluation for possible osteoporosis

SCENARIO

Myoji Otsuka presents asking for an evaluation for possible osteoporosis. She is a full-time homemaker, married, with one child, who became concerned that she has osteoporosis after attending a health fair at which the disorder was discussed.

● TENTATIVE DIAGNOSES

What are the potential diagnoses you have identified on the basis of this scenario? What are red flag diagnoses that you cannot miss?

DIAGNOSIS	RATIONALE
1	
2	
3	

● HISTORY

What subjective data are most significant to elicit in this case? What essential points should be considered in the review of systems?

REQUESTED DATA   DATA ANSWER

Allergies	NKDA.
Medications	OTC for occasional H/A, minor aches/pains; daily multivitamin.
Surgery/transfusion	Emergency abdominal hysterectomy and 2 blood transfusions in 1989 after postpartum hemorrhage.
Medical history/ hospitalizations/ injuries/accidents	Measles, mumps, chicken pox as child. Hospitalized once (for childbirth) in Japan (1978).
History of specific disorders associated with risk for osteoporosis	Denies the following health problems associated with increased risk of osteoporosis: anorexia/bulimia; gastrectomy; intestinal bypass surgery; hyperprolactin levels; diabetes mellitus; thyroid disease; parathyroid disease; liver disease; genetic disorders, metabolic or malabsorption problems; renal failure.
OB/GYN history	G2P1A1(@6 weeks' gestation). Spontaneous vaginal delivery (1978) of female; immediate postpartum hemorrhage related to placenta accreta, necessitating emergency abdominal hysterectomy. LNMP: 1977, prior to pregnancy; menses always irregular. During rigorous ballet training did not menstruate regularly for years. Last Pap: 12 months ago (every 2-year routine). Mammogram: 6 months ago. BSE: routinely.
Family history	Father: deceased, age 40, in MVA. Mother: alive; recovering from fractured hip. Brothers: 3, ages 46, 43, 39, alive and healthy. Spouse: 54, good health; prostate cancer surgery 3 years ago. Child: 22 y/o daughter, good health.
Social history	Tobacco: never. Alcohol: social use, on average 1 drink every 2 weeks. Drugs: never. Social participation: multiple social engagements every week related to husband's executive position: volunteers at local soup kitchen and American Red Cross; active in First Baptist Church. Moved to USA from Tokyo 4 years ago for husband to accept executive position in international company.

(continued)

REQUESTED DATA *DATA ANSWER*

Family relationships	All extended family in Japan. Sees them at least every other year. Frequent communication by telephone.
	Spouse: married 24 years; mutually monogamous relationship with infrequent sex since husband's prostate surgery. Sees him less than in past because of business responsibility.
	Daughter: attends college approximately 1000 miles away. Speaks on phone several times weekly and by email every day; enjoys good relationship and eagerly anticipates college holidays for visits.
Income/insurance/home	Husband earns executive salary in large international corporation; has medical and dental insurance; owns home.
Symptoms	Increasing frequency of backaches and noticeable rounding of shoulders; clothing fits tighter across abdomen, despite no change in weight and "I am hemming clothes which have fit for years. My daughter has started to tease me about shrinking."
Diet	Caffeine: 3 cups brewed coffee daily; 6–8 cups hot tea daily; colas, rare.
	Has lactose intolerance but eats occasional cheese and yogurt. Eats fruits, vegetables, and rice daily, often stir-fry; rarely eats red meat. 24-hour dietary recall indicates < 800 mg calcium.
Exercise	Exercise: swims every other day; walks at least 1 mile daily. Plays tennis occasionally. Rides stationary bike daily. Has always been active; was a ballet dancer throughout school and danced professionally for 2 years.
Evidence of history of medications toxic to bone remodeling	Denies use of following meds known toxic to bone remodeling: glucocorticoids, anticonvulsants, lithium, methotrexate, tetracyclines, thyroid hormone, isoniazid, GnRh agonists, benzodiazepines, anticoagulants.
	Has used these meds known toxic to bone remodeling: occasionally takes aluminum hydroxide (Maalox) for indigestion associated with American cuisine.
Exposure to sunlight	Works in flower garden outside several times each week. Swims outside every other day in summer. Walks outside for 1 mile on sunny days.
History of fractures/ scoliosis	Denies fractures, scoliosis.
Signs/symptoms of menopause	Uncertain; no signs/symptoms. "Having hysterectomy so early has confused that whole picture. My mother went through change about my age now."
Evidence of medical conditions associated with osteoporosis	Denies prolonged immobilization, diabetes, renal failure, liver disease, COPD, rheumatoid arthritis, malabsorption, adrenal disease, thyroid disease, hyperlactenemia, genetic syndromes (Marfan's, osteogenesis imperfecta, Klinefelter's, Turner's, Ehlers-Danlos, homocystinuria).

● PHYSICAL ASSESSMENT

Which portions of the physical examination are essential in Mrs. Otsuka's case to assure a definitive diagnosis?

SYSTEM	RATIONALE	FINDINGS
Vital signs		T, 98.0°F; P, 92; RR, 18; BP, 110/68 mm Hg; Wt, 97 lbs; Ht, 5′4″ (patient gave height as 5′5″).
General appearance/skin		Alert; appears stated age; no acute distress. Skin warm, dry. Color consistent with Asian heritage.
Dentition		WNL; no tooth loss.
Heart		S1, S2; no murmurs.
Thyroid		Nontender without enlargement or nodules.
Lungs		CTA; thoracic excursion WNL; normal position and symmetry of rib cage.
Abdomen		Protruberant; soft; BS+; no organomegaly, tenderness, or ascites.
Back		Both mild cervical lordosis and dorsal kyphosis present. Point tenderness at T 5–6. Normal ROM.
Neurological/ musculoskeletal assessment		Rises easily from chair without using arms to lift off; normal ROM and muscle strength of lower extremities; normal gait; sensation intact; DTRs 2+.

● DIFFERENTIAL DIAGNOSES

What are the significant positive and negative findings that either support or refute your diagnosis for this patient?

DIAGNOSIS	POSITIVE DATA	NEGATIVE DATA
1		
2		
3		

● DIAGNOSTIC TESTS

Based on the subjective and objective data, what diagnostic tests will you order?

DIAGNOSTIC TEST	RATIONALE	RESULTS	INTERPRETATION
CBC		RBC, 4.5 million/ mm³; Hgb, 13.3 g/dL; HCT, 40%; MCV, 88; MCH, 30; MCHC, 34; RDW, 12.5% Bands, 2%; Segs, 66; Eosinophils, 2%; Basophils, 0; Lymphcytes, 22%; Monocytes, 8%.	
ESR		10 mm/hr.	
Serum protein electrophoresis		Not done.	
Serum calcium		8.8 mg/dL.	
Serum phosphorus		3.8 mg/dL.	
Alkaline phosphotase		42 U/L.	
TSH		25 μU/mL.	
Glucose level		106.	
Parathyroid hormone		212 pg/mL.	
Urinary free cortisol		Not ordered.	
25 hydroxy/viatmin D level		Not ordered.	
DXA Dual energy xray absorptionometry		T score, −2.5.	
Dual energy photon absorptionometry (DPA)		Not ordered.	
Single energy photon absorptionometry (SPA)		Not ordered.	
Quantitative computerized tomography (QCT)		Not ordered.	

● DIAGNOSIS

What diagnosis seems most likely for Mrs. Otsuka after a review of both subjective and objective findings?

1.

Data Supporting Diagnosis

● THERAPEUTIC PLAN

1. How is osteoporosis classified? What is the associated pathophysiology for each type, and how does the pathologic cause influence the management?

Osteoporosis

CLASSIFICATIONS OF OSTEOPOROSIS	PATHOPHYSIOLOGIC CAUSE FOR CLASSIFICATION	MANAGEMENT FOR CLASSIFICATION
Primary osteoporosis Type I		
Primary Osteoporosis Type II		
Secondary osteoporosis		

2. How should Mrs. Otsuka's osteoporosis be managed?

*HORMONE REPLACEMENT THERAPY**

DRUG	DOSING IMPLICATIONS FOR NP
1	
2	
3	
4	
5	
6	
7	

*If uterus is present, add progesterone to conjugated estrogens.

Contraindications to hormone replacement therapy

Absolute:

Relative:

Another classification of drugs for osteoporosis is the bisphosphonates. Identify possible medications and dosages for each type.

Bisphosphonates

DRUG	IMPLICATIONS FOR NP
1	
2	
3	

Use of Calcitonin-salmon

Calcitonin-salmon can be used for postmenopausal women who cannot take estrogen. What are the doses and is this patient a candidate?

1

2

3. What patient education should be a part of this patient's plan of care?
Review high calcium foods. Dairy foods provide 300 mg/serving. Explain that food sources are more efficient than supplements. Identify nondairy sources of calcium (see Table 26-9).

Nondairy sources of calcium

FRUITS AND VEGETABLES GROUP   SERVING SIZE   CALCIUM (MG)

Discuss benefits of HRT. Discuss risks and side effects of HRT.

4. *At what point should this woman be referred to a specialist? What kind?*

5. *What impact can this illness have on the quality of Mrs. Otsuka's life?*

6. *What preventive measures can be implemented to prevent fractures?*

7. *When should this patient return for follow-up? What will be done at the follow-up visit?*

8. *What implications, if any, does this disorder have for the Otsuka family?*

9. *What are the community resources available for the NP and for the patient?*

REFERENCES

Alexander, I. M. (1998). Healthy bones: Counseling teens, new mothers, and menopausal patients about osteoporosis risks. *Conversations in Counseling, Winter,* 4–6.

Brager, R. (1997). Alendronate treatment for osteoporosis: Patient education should be part of your treatment plan. *Advance for Nurse Practitioners, 5*(3), 28–34.

Consensus statement on osteoporosis: Prevention, diagnosis, and treatment. *Women's Health in Primary Care, 3*(9), 670–672.

Durst, E. S. (2000). The A, B, Cs of bone building in adolescence. *Journal of the American Academy of Nurse Practitioners, 12*(4), 135–140.

Kessenich, C. R. (2000). Osteoporosis in primary care: The role of biochemical markers and diagnostic imaging. *The American Journal of Nurse Practitioners, 4*(2), 24–29.

Kessenich, C. R. (2000). Risedronate: A new biophosphonate for the treatment of osteoporosis. *The Nurse Practitioner, 25*(3), 106–108.

Kessenich, C. R. (1998). Raloxifene: A new class of anti-estrogens for the prevention of osteoporosis. *The Nurse Practitioner, 23*(9), 91–93.

Kleerekoper, M. (1999). Using bone remodeling markers in osteoporosis treatment. *Patient Care, 33*(4), 121–130.

Licata, A. A. (1999). Update on osteoporosis: Strategies for prevention and treatment. *Women's Health in Primary Care, 2*(3), 229–243.

McClung, B. L. (1999). Using osteoporosis management to reduce fractures in elderly women. *The Nurse Practitioner, 24*(3), 26–47.

McClung, B. L., & Sieber, A. N. (2000). *Nursing practice guide: Clinical management of patients at risk for or diagnosed with osteoporosis.* New York: Medical Information Services, Inc.

Notelovit, M. (1995). Osteoporosis prevention: A lifetime guide. *Women's Health Digest, 1*(1), 34–43.

Osteoporosis. (1999). *Well-Connected.* New York: Nidus Information Services.

Schmidtt, M. (2000). Osteoporosis: Focus on fractures. *Patient Care for the Nurse Practitioner, 3*(2), 61–71.

Siris, E. S., & Schussheim, D. H. (1998). Osteoporosis: Assessing your patient's risks. *Women's Health in Primary Care, 1*(1), 99–106.

Staley, C. A. (2000). Oral biophosphonates: Alendronate and Risedronate. *Women's Health in Primary Care, 3*(9), 662, 669.

Whitmire, S. M. (1998). Rebuilding bone: Renewing lives. *Advance for Nurse Practitioners, 6*(9), 30–35.

Woodhead, G. A., & Moss, M. M. (1998). Osteoporosis: Diagnosis and prevention. *The Nurse Practitioner, 23*(11), 18, 23–24, 26–27.

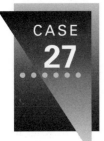

An 8-year-old boy having difficulty in school

SCENARIO

Jared Jones, an 8-year-old white boy was brought by his mother to the well-child clinic for his regular checkup. His mother reports Jared has been in good health since his last checkup. He has always been a picky eater, preferring sweets and snacks to wholesome meals. During the visit, Jared's mother reports that Jared is having a difficult time in school and at home. He has had problems on the playground: he doesn't play games by the rules, often loses interest in games when he has to wait his turn, plays rough, and frequently has accidents. In the classroom he has difficulty following directions and doesn't complete his work. He frequently gets into arguments with and interrupts his teacher and has received two detentions for this behavior this year.

At home Jared refuses to do anything his parents ask. His mother reports that he "just doesn't seem to listen." He bites his nails and is fretful. He blames his 10-year-old brother or 6-year-old sister for everything. Jared always wants to have his way and sulks when he has to compromise. His mother reports his father and she both feel these behaviors have gone on long enough. They have tried to discipline Jared but always wind up feeling ineffective.

● TENTATIVE DIAGNOSES

Based on Jared's presentation, what are your tentative differential diagnoses?

● HISTORY

What additional information should be obtained from Jared and his mother to confirm/rule out the above diagnoses?

● PHYSICAL ASSESSMENT

What components of the physical exam should be done to assist in making the diagnosis?

● DIFFERENTIAL DIAGNOSES

What are the negative/positive data that assist in determining the appropriate diagnoses?

● DIAGNOSTIC TESTS

What diagnostic tests are appropriate to do for Jared to assist in your diagnoses?

● DIAGNOSIS

What is your conclusive diagnosis? What data support this decision?

● THERAPEUTIC PLAN

1. *What are issues to consider in the diagnosis of ADHD?*
2. *What are medications that are considered standard interventions for ADHD?*
3. *What evaluation data would indicate the medications are effective for Jared?*
4. *What counseling should be done for Jared and his family?*
5. *What interventions should be discussed to increase Jared's success at school?*
6. *What is the role of the NP in the care of children with ADHD?*
7. *What are resources that the family can use to adapt to ADHD?*

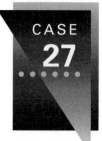

TUTORIAL

An 8-year-old boy having difficulty in school

SCENARIO

Jared Jones, an 8-year-old white boy was brought by his mother to the well-child clinic for his regular checkup. His mother reports Jared has been in good health since his last checkup. He has always been a picky eater, preferring sweets and snacks to wholesome meals. During the visit, Jared's mother reports that Jared is having a difficult time in school and at home. He has had problems on the playground: he doesn't play games by the rules, often loses interest in games when he has to wait his turn, plays rough, and frequently has accidents. In the classroom he has difficulty following directions and doesn't complete his work. He frequently gets into arguments with and interrupts his teacher and has received two detentions for this behavior this year.

At home Jared refuses to do anything his parents ask. His mother reports that he "just doesn't seem to listen." He bites his nails and is fretful. He blames his 10-year-old brother or 6-year-old sister for everything. Jared always wants to have his way and sulks when he has to compromise. His mother reports his father and she both feel these behaviors have gone on long enough. They have tried to discipline Jared but always wind up feeling ineffective.

● TENTATIVE DIAGNOSES

*Based on Jared's presentation, what are your tentative differential diagnoses? What are **red flag** diagnoses that you cannot miss?*

DIAGNOSIS	RATIONALE
Attention deficit hyperactivity disorder (ADHD)	Jared's mother reports problems at school and home: not completing his work, not following directions, not listening, interrupting teacher, not waiting his turn, losing interest in activities, and frequent accidents.

(continued)

DIAGNOSIS	RATIONALE
Learning disability	Jared's mother reports a history of problems in school, especially not completing assignments.
Oppositional defiant disorder (ODD)	Jared's mother gives a history of refusal to do assignments, follow rules, and/or directions, or do anything his parents ask of him. Jared blames his siblings when he gets into trouble at home.
Organic/neurological problems	Jared's mother shares a history of frequent accidents. Frequent accidents may be the cause of or result of a neurological disorder.
Generalized anxiety disorder	Habits such as nail biting and fretfulness could indicate an anxiety disorder.

● HISTORY

What additional information should be obtained from Jared and his mother to confirm/rule out the above diagnoses?

REQUESTED DATA   DATA ANSWER

REQUESTED DATA	DATA ANSWER
Allergies	None.
Medications	None.
Childhood illnesses/diseases	Chickenpox, age 5. Otitis media: several bouts from age 3–5; placement of pneumatic expansion tubes at age 4.
Immunizations	Up to date.
Hospitalizations	None.
Surgeries	Placement of PE tubes, outpatient.
Fractures/injuries/ accidents	Age 2, fell, hitting head on coffee table; mild concussion; no fractures. Age 4, laceration to left temporal area, 5 stitches. Age 6, fell out of a tree, broken clavicle. Mother reports no history of seizures or seizure-like behaviors.
Prenatal history	39-week gestation. Normal vaginal delivery. No complications.
Developmental history	Met developmental milestones within normal range. Described as clumsy and demanding as far back as mother can remember.

(continued)

REQUESTED DATA   DATA ANSWER

REQUESTED DATA	DATA ANSWER
Growth history	Has consistently been at the 25th percentile for height and weight.
Educational history	Attended preschool from age 3 to 5; had difficulty with social skills; not well accepted by peers. Performance in primary grades has been erratic; low achievement scores in 2nd grade reading and language arts. Mother recently met with teacher for midterm report and was encouraged to pursue evaluation of Jared for learning and attention problems. A referral has not been made to the school psychologist.
Has Jared ever been in any type of special educational program, if so, how long?	None.
Have any instructional modifications been made?	None.
Family history	Father: 11th grade education; failed 3rd grade and 6th grade; in good health; changes jobs frequently, short temper. Mother: 12th grade education; currently being treated for depression on fluoxetine (Prozac). FH of substance abuse in PGF and paternal uncle. Brother: age 10, healthy, doing well in school. Sister: age 6, healthy, doing well in school. Mother denies any family stressors at this time.
Marital relationship	Married 12 years. Many arguments about how to discipline the children. Dad loses his temper with Jared and is quick to spank. Mom is not comfortable with this and becomes angry with Dad. She prefers to remove Jared from this situation, but has not found an effective way to do this.
Sibling relationships	Jared is competitive and often frustrated with his brother. He is close to his sister, and they are able to play together with less conflict.
Social history and activities	Jared has one close friend at school. Does not get along with the kids his age in the neighborhood; often comes home crying. He enjoys shooting hoops; does better by himself. Is most content at home playing video games by himself.
Sleeping patterns	Has difficulty settling down and going to sleep. Does sleep through the night once asleep.
Durations of symptoms	Has always had a lot of energy. Slept little as an infant. Active toddler.

(continued)

REQUESTED DATA   DATA ANSWER

Home setting	Jared lives with his biological parents in a three-bedroom home in a working class neighborhood. Jared shares a bedroom with his brother. There is a fenced yard and a basketball hoop in the driveway.
Family financial status	Dad works full time as a carpenter's assistant. Mom works part time at McDonald's while the children are in school. Mom denies financial problems at this time.
Insurance	Father carries health care insurance through his employer. It is a managed care plan that does provide for mental health services requiring precertification and a limited number of visits for outpatient therapy.
How do you feel about yourself?	"I don't have any friends; the kids at school make fun of me; I want to have friends but they don't want to play with me. I never get picked for the team when we play kickball or baseball."
How do you get along with your brother and sister?	"My brother always picks on me and when I get mad he yells for Dad and I get whipped." "My sister lets me do things with her sometimes."
What is school like for you?	"I hate school. It's boring. My teacher never listens to me. I try real hard to do what I am told, but I never seem to remember it all, or do it right." "I never do anything right."
What do you really like about yourself?	"I'm real good at Nintendo."
What do you do that you are proud of?	"I shoot baskets good, but nobody wants to shoot with me; it's no fun to shoot by myself."
What make you happy?	"I love Power Rangers."

● PHYSICAL ASSESSMENT

What components of the physical exam should be done to assist in making the diagnosis?

SYSTEM	RATIONALE	FINDINGS
General appearance	Provides overall view of patient.	Alert, cooperative 8-year-old white boy in NAD. Ht, 28-3/4" (73 cm); Wt, 50 lbs. (23K).

(continued)

SYSTEM	RATIONALE	FINDINGS
Vital signs	Baseline information.	BP 98/64 mm Hg; HR, 88 bpm RR, 20; T, 98.6 °F.
Skin	Well check-up, important to get overall screening exam.	No rash
HEENT	Important to screen for neurological signs that may have an impact on his behavior.	PERRLA; UNL DISC; margin well defined and sharp; TMs thick (old scars) landmarks normal; +mobility. No nodes; neck supple, no masses.
Lungs	Baseline data for well physical.	CTA.
Heart	Baseline data for well physical.	S1, S2 no murmur. Pulses 2+ symmetrical.
Abdomen	Well child exam.	Soft, + BS nontender/nondistended. No masses; no HSM.
GU	Determine sexual growth and development.	Tanner I; circumcision WNL; testes both descended.
Neurological assessment	Emphasis placed here to rule out a neurological/organic cause for behavior.	CN II-XII intact. Toes no clonus; DTR 2+ symmetrical; gait symmetrical; negative Romberg; RAMs normal; equal strength; heel-toe walk; back straight.

● DIFFERENTIAL DIAGNOSES

What are the negative/positive data that assist in determining the appropriate diagnoses?

DIAGNOSIS	POSITIVE DATA	NEGATIVE DATA
ADHD	Has difficulty at home and at school; doesn't play games by the rules; difficulty sustaining interest in games; demonstrates physical clumsiness and frequent accidents;	Does not exhibit the behaviors associated with hyperactive type of ADHD; such as fidgets, often leaves seat in classroom, runs about or climbs excessively in situations in which it is inappropriate, "on the go" or

(continued)

DIAGNOSIS	POSITIVE DATA	NEGATIVE DATA
	difficulty following directions; does not complete his work and doesn't listen; complains of being bored in school. Low self-esteem and poor social skills. School recommending further assessment for attentional difficulties and learning problems. Questionable positive family history.	behaving as if "driven by a motor," and often talks excessively. Jared does not blurt out answers before questions have been completed.
Learning disability	Family history suggestive of learning problems for father, documented problems in school with low achievement scores in reading and language arts, low self-esteem.	Achievement in school to this point has been below expected; however, Jared has low scores on achievement tests but has demonstrated a skill level sufficient to be in his age-appropriate grade.
Oppositional defiant disorder	Argues with adults; actively defies or refuses to comply with adults' requests or rules, and often blames others for his mistakes or misbehavior.	Does not exhibit these behaviors associated with ODD: loses temper, deliberately annoys people, often touchy or easily annoyed by others, often angry and resentful, and often spiteful or vindictive.
Organic/neurological problem	History of repeated minor head traumas. Learning difficulties and behavioral difficulties.	Physical findings show no neurological deficits. No history of seizures.
Generalized anxiety syndrome (GAS)	Difficulty falling asleep and fretfulness and nail biting.	No evidence of excessive anxiety and worry, difficulty controlling worry, restlessness, easily fatigued, irritability, difficulty concentration, and muscle tension.

● DIAGNOSTIC TESTS

What diagnostic tests are appropriate to do for Jared to assist in your diagnoses?

DIAGNOSTIC TEST	RATIONALE	FINDINGS	INTERPRETATION
Clinical interview to assess for DSM-IV-R criteria for ADHD, ODD, GAS, and LD	Good choice. May be completed as part of the interview.	Inattention: careless in work, difficulty in sustaining attention in tasks or play activities, doesn't seem to listen, does not follow through on instruction, fails finish activities, has difficulty organizing tasks and activities. Loses things; easily distracted by stimuli.	Meets DSM IV 9/9 criteria for ADHD, inattention. Was noted to be very distractible during interview. Does not meet DSM IV criteria for ODD, GAS, or LD.
Diagnostic tools: Conners Parent Questionnaire, Conners Teacher Questionnaire, ADHD Rating Scale	Good choices, dependent on length of time you have to spend with the parent and child. These tools could be given to the parent and sent back to you for evaluation. It is helpful to have both parents complete parent questionnaires. Obtain written permission to communicate with the school personnel.	Rated 3 (very much) in the following areas: restless, excitable, fails to finish things he started, fidgeting, inattentive, demands must be met immediately, disturbs other children. In the area of cries, mood changes quickly, and temper outburst, he scored a 2.	Connor score from parents: 28. Normal is < 14 (max, 30). The teacher score was 22. Both scores are indicative of ADHD.
Educational evaluation	Encourage mom to contact school and request that evaluation be carried out there. Have permission in writing for school to send the reports to you.	Reports will be sent to provider.	

(continued)

DIAGNOSTIC TEST	RATIONALE	FINDINGS	INTERPRETATION
MRI or CT scan of the head	Costly and time consuming. No indication that there is a primary organic/ neurological problem. May consider a neurological consult.	Not done at this time.	
Psychiatric evaluation	Good choice. Consultation with child psychiatric clinical nurse specialist to assist in the evaluation of diagnostic information and development of behavior management program. Referral to child psychiatric clinical nurse specialist or child psychiatrist for evaluation of the need for medication. Refer to neuro-psychologist for additional evaluation based on findings reported by the school.	Consultation to assist with holistic treatment plan.	

● DIAGNOSIS

What is your conclusive diagnosis? What data support this decision?

The findings are strongly suggestive of ADHD, inattentive type. Jared meets nine of nine DSM IV criteria for ADHD, inattentive type:

- difficulty sustaining attention in tasks or play activities;
- often does not seem to listen when spoken to directly;
- often does not follow through on instructions and fails to finish schoolwork or chores;
- often avoids, dislikes, or is reluctant to engage in tasks that require sustained mental effort;
- often fails to give close details or makes careless mistakes in school work, work, or other activities;
- often is easily distracted by extraneous stimuli;
- Jared also demonstrates impulsive behaviors:

- difficulty waiting his turn and
- interrupts or intrudes on others.

Has associated features of children with ADHD, including

- family history
- low self-esteem
- poor social skills
- clumsiness
- demanding early temperament
- history of academic difficulty

It would be in the child's best interest to consult with a psychiatric clinical nurse specialist when you receive the screening forms from the school. If the data obtained from the additional sources reinforces the diagnosis of ADHD, the child and family should be referred for appropriate treatment (Barkley, 1990; APA, 1994)

● THERAPEUTIC PLAN

1. What are issues to consider in the diagnosis of ADHD?

- Accuracy of diagnosis. Many children are quickly diagnosed with ADHD and placed on medication without a thorough evaluation. Some changes may be seen in the child's behavior; however, over a long period of time, it will become evident that there are behaviors that are persistent. Many parents and health care providers are quite comfortable with the diagnosis of ADHD and will agree to medication as a quick fix. Many children with a diagnosis of ADHD actually fall within normal limits in terms of their behavior based on their age and developmental level. Parents need education on developmental expectations and parenting skills.
- Coordination of diagnostic data. Look at the data from the various sources, talk with the people who have provided the data, and make sure that all of the data requested have been returned. Begin to build rapport with the school personnel because the care of this child will require participation of individuals from many disciplines.
- A comprehensive multidisciplinary approach will be needed to provide treatment.
- Parental participation will be necessary in various aspects of treatment.
- Clarify what services will be covered by the insurance company before making referrals.
- Be aware of your own limitations in evaluating the diagnostic data.

2. What are medications that are considered standard interventions for ADHD?
The treatment for ADHD is multifaceted. The following treatment options are standard interventions. For additional information, a reliable source is Russell Barkley's *Attention-Deficit Hyperactivity Disorder: A Handbook for Diagnosis and Treatment.*

Stimulants

1. Methylphenidate (Ritalin), a 77% positive response
   Dosage, 5 to 20 mg (0.3 to 0.7 mg/kg)
   BID dose given early morning and mid-day
   TID dose given early morning, mid-day, and after school
   Example, 8 am, 12 noon, and 4 pm
   Maximum dose not to exceed 60 mg daily.
   Ritalin SR one dose/day effect lasts 8 hours. Also, new drug methyl-phenidate (Concerta) once daily.
2. Dextroamphetamine (Dexedrine), a 74% positive response
   Dosage 2.5 to 10 mg BID/TID
   Dosage intervals as for Ritalin
3. Dexedrine Spansules one dose/day
4. Adderall (efficacy unknown)
   Dosage, 5 mg QD/BID

All of the above listed drugs are Schedule II drugs and require a written prescription.

1. Pemoline (Cylert), a 73% positive effect
   Dosage 18.75 mg to start; typical dose 0.5 to 3 mg/kg
   One dose/day

3. *What evaluation data would indicate the medications are effective for Jared?*
   Jared should demonstrate an increase in his attention span and concentration as well as improved peer relations and an increase in compliance if the drug is working for him. Gradually increase the dose weekly until the desired effect is seen. Behavior changes and attentional changes should be noted within the first week of treatment; changes may be more obvious in the school situation. If no improvement is noted after 1 month of treatment, discontinue drug and try another. If no changes are noted even when dose is increased, the child probably does not have ADHD.

4. *What counseling should be done for Jared and his family?*
   Counseling is an integral part of the treatment for ADHD. These children are frustrating to those who interact with them, and the children themselves are frustrated by all of the negatives they receive regarding their behavior. Suggested counseling would include:

   • Parent counseling and education about ADHD
   • Parent training in the area of behavior management
   • Parent counseling and training on environmental modifications or structuring
   • Parent education on medications and the role they play in treatment
   • Individual counseling with the child
   • Family therapy for the whole family
   • Couples/marital therapy for the parents

5. *What interventions should be discussed to increase Jared's success at school?*
   Children with ADHD have difficulty in the area of academic performance and achievement. They demonstrate inattention and impulsive and restless be-

havior in the classroom. They have difficulty staying seated, paying attention, working independently, and following directions and rules. The child with ADHD can be disruptive and interrupt class lessons as well as quiet work periods. Such children also lack organizational skills and have difficulty keeping track of their academic tools (books, pencils, and paper) and assignments.

The initial intervention with the school is to educate the teacher about the disorder. Once the teacher has a working knowledge of the disorder, behavior management programs can be established. The behavior management program at school is an integral part of the overall behavior management program. Weekly or biweekly meetings among the parents, teachers, and therapist are helpful in evaluating and monitoring the behavioral management program.

Needed areas of teacher education:

- Teacher counseling and education about ADHD
- Teacher training in classroom management
- Teacher training in environmental modifications

6. *What is the role of the NP in care of children with ADHD?*
The role of the NP is to coordinate services and implement a comprehensive multidisciplinary treatment program. It is important to collaborate with the school and become knowledgeable of the services that can be provided in the school in the areas of special education, behavior management, and environmental modifications. Nurse practitioners caring for children will be able to provide a higher level of care if there are established relationships with professional peers to enhance the consultation process.

7. *What are resources that the family can use to assist in their adjustment to ADHD?*

Attention Deficit Information Network (AD-IN)
475 Hillside Avenue
Needham, MA 02194
http://www.addinfonetwork.com
Provides up-to-date information on current research and regional meetings. Offers aid in finding solutions to practical problems faced by adults and children with an attention disorder.

ADD Warehouse
300 NW 70th Avenue
Plantation, FL 33317
(800) 233-9273
Distributes books, tapes, and videos on ADHD

National Attention Deficit Disorder Association
1788 Second Street Suite 200
Highland Park, IL 60035
(847) 432-ADDA (2332)
http://www.add.org

Parent Support Associations

Children and Adults with Attention Deficit Disorders (C.H.A.D.D)
8181 Professional Place, Suite 201
Landover, MD 20785
(800) 233-4050, (301) 306-7070
www.chadd.org

ADDA (Attention Deficit Disorder Advocacy Group)
4300 West Park Boulevard
Plano, TX 75093
(303) 690-7548

Attention Deficit Disorder Archive
www.seas.upenn.edu/~mengwong/add

8. *To whom would you refer Jared or consult with to provide him with expert care for his ADHD?*
It is advisable to consult with or refer to a child psychiatric clinical nurse specialist or a child psychiatrist.

REFERENCES

Agerter, D., & Rasmussen, N. (2000). Diagnosing and treating ADHD in children. *Minnesota Medicine, 83*(6), 51–54.

American Academy of Pediatrics. (2000). Clinical practice guideline: Diagnosis and evaluation of the child with attention-deficit/hyperactivity disorder. *Pediatrics, 105*(5), 1158–1170.

American Psychiatric Association. (1994). *Diagnostic and statistical manual of mental disorders* (4th ed.). Washington, DC: American Psychiatric Association.

August, G., & Realmuto, G. (2000). Pharmacotherapy in ADHD. Guidelines for prescribing stimulant medications in young children. *Minnesota Medicine, 83*(6), 45–46.

Baren, M. (1994). Managing ADHD. *Contemporary Pediatrics, 11*(12), 29–30, 33–34, 37–38.

Barkley, R. (1990). *Attention deficit hyperactivity disorder: A handbook for diagnosis and treatment.* New York: Guilford Press.

Barkley, R. A. (1996). Attention deficit hyperactivity disorder. In E. J. Mash, & R. A. Barkley (Eds.), *Child psychopathology* (pp. 63–112). New York: Guilford Press.

Bauchner, H. (2000). ADHD: A new practice guideline from the American Academy of Pediatrics. Attention deficit hyperactive disorder. *Archives of Disturbed Child, 83*(1), 63.

Donovan, D. (2000). An alternative approach to ADHD. *Harvard Mental Health Letter, 16*(11), 5–7.

Evink, B., Crouse, B., & Elliott, B. (2000). Diagnosing childhood attention-deficit/hyperactivity disorder. Do family practitioners and pediatricians make the same call? *Minnesota Medicine, 83*(6), 57–62.

Faraone, S., Biederman, J., Mick, E., Williamson, S., Wilens, T., Spencer, T., Weber, W., Jetton, J., Knaus, I., Pert, J., & Zallen, B. (2000). Family study of girls with attention deficit hyperactivity disorder. *American Journal of Psychiatry, 157,* 1077–1083.

Gephart, H. R. (1999). The ADHD history: 42 questions to ask parents. *Contemporary Pediatrics, 16*(10), 127–128, 130, 133–134.

Gephart, H. R. (1997). A managed care approach to ADHD. *Contemporary Pediatrics, 14*(5), 123–124, 126, 128.

Kwasman, A., Tinsley, B., & Lepper, H. (1995). Pediatricians' knowledge and attitudes concerning diagnosis and treatment of attention deficit and hyperactivity disorders. A national survey approach. *Archives in Pediatric Adolescent Medicine, 149,* 1211–1216.

Murphy, M., & Risser, N. (2000). NP abstracts. Drug trials for ADHD. *Nurse Practitioner: American Journal of Primary Health Care, 25*(5), 102–103.

National Institute of Mental Health. (1994). *Attention deficit hyperactivity disorder: Care and treatment.* Washington, DC: National Institute of Mental Health.

National Institutes of Health. (1998). Diagnosis and treatment of attention deficit hyperactivity disorder (ADHD). *NIH Consensus Statement, 16*(2), 1–37.

Owens, J., Maxim, R., Nobile, C., McGuinn, M., & Msall, M. (2000). Parental and self-report of sleep in children with attention- deficit/hyperactivity disorder. *Archives in Pediatric Adolescent Medicine, 154,* 549–555.

Richters, J. E., Arnold, L. E., Jensen, P. S., Abikoff, H., Conners, C. K., Greenhill, L. L., Hechtman, L., Henshaw, S., Pelham, W., & Swanson, J. (1995). NIMH collaborative multisite multimodal treatment study of children with ADHD: I. Background and rationale. *Journal of the American Academy of Child and Adolescent Psychiatry, 34,* 987–1000.

Seidman, L. J., Biederman, J., Faraone, S. V., Milberger, S., Norman, D., Seiverd, K., Benedict, K., Guite, J., Mick, E., & Kiely, K. (1995). Effects of family history and comorbidity on the neuropsychological performance of children with ADHD: Preliminary findings. *Journal of the American Academy of Child Adolescent Psychiatry, 34,* 1015–1024.

Shrand, J. A., & Jellinek, M. S. (1995). Psychopharmacology in office practice. *Contemporary Pediatrics, 12*(11), 106–110, 112, 114–116.

Smalley, S., McGough, J., Del'Homme, M., New Delman, J., Gordon, E., Kim, T., Liu, A., & McCracken, J. (2000). Familial clustering of symptoms and disruptive behaviors in multiplex families with attention-deficit/hyperactivity disorder. *Journal of the American Academy of Child and Adolescent Psychiatry, 39,* 1135–1143.

Wagner, B. J. (2000). Attention deficit hyperactivity disorder: Current concepts and underlying mechanisms. *Journal of Child and Adolescent Psychiatric Nursing, 13*(3), 113–124.

Young, S. (2000). ADHD children grown up: An empirical review. *Counseling Psychology Quarterly, 13*(2), 191–200.

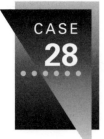

A 28-year-old woman with headache and congestion

SCENARIO

Sophie Hughes is a 28-year-old Caucasian woman complaining of facial pain, fever, headache, congestion, and nasal discharge for 10 days. She states the headache increases in intensity with coughing or bending over.

● TENTATIVE DIAGNOSES

*What are the potential diagnoses you have identified based on the scenario presented? What are **red flag** diagnoses that you cannot miss?*

DIAGNOSIS	RATIONALE
1	
2	
3	
4	
5	
6	

● HISTORY

What are significant questions in the history for Sophie? Is information that is needed not included? Is there information that is not needed for this situation?

REQUESTED DATA	DATA ANSWER
Allergies	NKDA; hay fever in spring and fall.
Current medications	Oral contraceptives; loratadine (Claritin-D) 24 hour 1 po Qd prn.
Surgery/transfusions	Tonsillectomy at age 8; no transfusions.
Medical history/ hospitalizations/ fractures/injuries/ accidents	Healthy except seasonal allergic rhinitis and occasional acute sinusitis.
Adult illness	Acute sinusitis approximately twice yearly.
Social history	Tobacco: 1 pack per day for 10 years. Alcohol: rare. Caffeine: 1 cup coffee in morning. Drugs: none. Exercise: occasional walks of approximately 1 mile.
Family history	Father: age 58, HTN and GERD. Mother: 56, chronic sinusitis. Brother: 30, good health. Sister: 22, depression. No spouse or children.
Income/insurance/home	Employed as a Delta ticket agent. Insurance through Delta. Owns condo.
Stress management	Handles stress well, usually just talks her way through problems

● PHYSICAL ASSESSMENT

What are the significant portions of the physical examination that should be completed for Sophie? Identify what parts of the exam that you would do and why.

SYSTEM	RATIONALE	FINDINGS
Vital signs		BP 120/70 mm Hg, right arm; HR, 72 bpm; RR, 20; T, 100.6°F; Ht, 5'4"; Wt, 116 lbs.

(continued)

SYSTEM	RATIONALE	FINDINGS
General appearance/skin		Appears miserable.
HEENT		Normocephalic, maxillary/frontal sinus tenderness; TMs gray with good light reflex; ery/edema/drainage of bilat nasal turbinates; injection throat, cervical adenopathy.
Lungs		CTA.
Heart		S1, S2 WNL; no MRG.

● DIFFERENTIAL DIAGNOSES

What are the significant positive and negative findings that support or refute your diagnoses for Sophie?

DIAGNOSIS	POSITIVE DATA	NEGATIVE DATA
1		
2		
3		
4		
5		
6		

● DIAGNOSTIC TESTS

Based on the history and physical examination, what, if any, diagnostic testing would you obtain? Interpret the tests that have been done.

DIAGNOSTIC TEST	RATIONALE	RESULTS	INTERPRETATION
Nasal smear for eosinophils		Not done.	

(continued)

DIAGNOSTIC TEST	RATIONALE	RESULTS	INTERPRETATION
Skin testing		Not done.	
Sinus X-rays or CT scan		Not done.	
CBC		WBC, $8.7 \times 10^3/\mu L$; RBC, $4.2 \times 10^6/\mu L$; Hgb, 12.8 g/dL; HCT, 38.2%; MCV, 87.4 m^3; Platelets, 175,000/mm^3.	

● DIAGNOSES

What diagnoses do you determine as being appropriate after a review of the subjective and objective data?

● PATHOPHYSIOLOGY OF THE CASE, AND THE ETIOLOGY OF THE PROBLEM

Describe the pathophysiology and etiology of the problem.

Data Supporting the Diagnosis

Identify the data that support your final diagnosis.

● THERAPEUTIC PLAN

1. *What is the first-line therapy for this condition?*

2. *What are the factors prompting the use of second-line drugs? Identify some of the choices for second-line therapy.*

3. *What are some prevention measures against getting sinusitis?*

4. Does green mucus indicate a bacterial infection?

5. How might Sophie be encouraged to stop smoking? What options are available?

REFERENCES

(2000). Antimicrobial treatment guidelines for acute bacterial rhinosinusitis. *Otolaryngology Head and Neck Surgery, 123*(1 PT 2), Supplement 31–54.

Brook, I. (1998). Microbiology of common infections in the upper respiratory tract. *Primary Care: Clinical Office Practice, 25*, 633–648.

Brook, I., Gooch, W. M., Jenkins, S. G., Sher, L., Pichichero, M., & Yamauchi, T. (2000). Medical management of acute bacterial sinusitis: Recommendations of a clinical advisory committee on pediatric and adult sinusitis. *Annals of Otolaryngology, 109*(5, Suppl 182), 1–20.

Corey, J. P. (1996). Chronic rhinitis: The differential diagnosis. *Hospital Medicine, 32*(3 Suppl), 3–8.

Corey, J., Houser, S., & Ng, B. (2000). Nasal congestion: A review of its etiology, evaluation, and treatment. *Ear Nose Throat Journal, 79*(9), 690–693, 696, 698.

Duchene, T. (2000). Managing sinusitis in children. *The Nurse Practitioner, 25*(9), 42–55.

Engels, E., Terrin, N., Barza, M., & Lau, J. (2000). Meta-analysis of diagnostic tests for acute sinusitis. *Journal of Clinical Epidemiology, 53*, 852–862.

Hamilos, D. (2000). Chronic sinusitis. *Journal of Allergy and Clinical Immunology, 106*(2), 213–227.

Incaudo, G. A., & Wooding, L. G. (1998). Diagnosis and treatment of acute and subacute sinusitis in children and adults. *Clinical Review of Allergy and Immunology, 16*, 157–204.

International Rhinitis Management Working Group. (1994). International consensus report on the diagnosis and management of rhinitis. *Allergy, 49*(19 Suppl), 1–34.

Levinson, S. (2000). Diagnosis and treatment of recurrent sinusitis. *Journal of the American Medical Association, 284*, 1240–1241.

Lieu, J., & Feinstein, J. (2000). Confirmations and surprises in the association of tobacco use with sinusitis. *Archives of Otolaryngology—Head and Neck Surgery, 126*, 940–946.

Montgomery, M. T. (2000). Extraoral facial pain. *Emergency Medicine Clinics of North America, 18*(3), 577–600.

Newton, D. A. (1996). Sinusitis in children and adolescents. *Primary Care: Clinical Office Practice, 23*(4), 701–717.

Nollette, K. A. (2000). Continuing education: Antimicrobial resistance. *Journal of the American Academy of Nurse Practitioners, 12*(7), 286–299.

O'Brien, K. L., Dowell, S. F., Schwartz, B., Marcy, S. M., Phillips, W. R., & Gerber, M. A. (1998). Acute sinusitis: Principles of judicious use of antimicrobial agents. *Pediatrics, 101*(1), 171–174.

Young, S., Dobozin, B., & Miner, M. (1999). *Allergies: The complete guide to diagnosis, treatment, and daily management* (2nd ed.). New York: Plume.

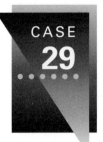

A 43-year-old woman presenting for a wellness exam

SCENARIO

Edna Wilson is a 43-year-old systems analyst with a local telecommunications company. Her employer requires a yearly physical exam. She is married and has two teen-age children.

● TENTATIVE DIAGNOSES

*What are the potential diagnoses you have identified based on this scenario? Make sure you include any vital **red flag** diagnoses that cannot be missed.*

DIAGNOSIS	RATIONALE
1	

● HISTORY

What are significant questions in the history for Edna?

REQUESTED DATA	DATA ANSWER
Allergies	NKA.
Medications	Multivitamin; calcium, 1000 mg; St. John's wort.

(continued)

REQUESTED DATA   *DATA ANSWER*

REQUESTED DATA	DATA ANSWER
Surgery/transfusion	D&C; tubal ligation; no blood transfusions.
Medical history/ Hospitalization/ fractures/injuries/ accidents	Chicken pox as child. Childbirth ×2. Sutures on forehead from sports injury, no sequelae.
Adult illnesses	Mononucleosis, age 22. No sequelae.
OB-GYN history	LNMP: 9 weeks prior, light flow, 3 days duration. Periods are irregular, not unusual to skip 2 or 3 months. Last Pap 18 months previously, normal result. G3P2Ab1 (induced). Mammogram: 0. SBE: occasionally.
Immunization history	No shots since school age.
Appetite/weight change	Appetite same. Weight fluctuates 5–6 lbs between menstrual cycles.
Diet history	Breakfast: coffee, sometimes a bagel or toast. Lunch: sandwich or salad, usually at desk. Dinner: meat, usually chicken or fish, and vegetables. Water and/or wine with dinner. Snacks: salsa and chips, popcorn, rarely sweets.
Social history	Tobacco: never. Alcohol: wine often with evening meal, cocktails at business functions, but never more than 2. Caffeine: 3–4 cups coffee daily. Occasional cola in afternoon. Drugs: marijuana socially until 2 years ago. Exercise: treadmill, 2 miles twice weekly at gym.
Family	Father: deceased at age 66; MI Mother: 68, breast cancer 9 years ago. Brothers: age 45, HTN; age 40, paraplegia, MVA at age 30. Sister: age 46, good health. Spouse: age 45, overweight, hyperlipidemia. Children: son, 17, and daughter, 15, good health.
Sexual history	Monogomous for 18 years; 6–8 partners during high school and college; one elective abortion at age 20. Sexual arousal is delayed, and sexual intercourse is not as pleasurable as it used to be.
Social organizations	Civitan, Pilot clubs; member of Episcopal church; attends at holidays; considers herself a religious person. Sponsor for daughter's cheerleading group.

(continued)

REQUESTED DATA   DATA ANSWER

Relationship with husband	Married 18 years. They have sex about 2 times a week unless work causes one or the other to travel; usually enjoyable, but lately she has been slow to reach arousal. Husband works as a pharmaceutical representative and is occasionally away from home overnight.
Relationship with children	Both she and her husband support their children's sports activities. Yearly family vacations that usually involve a cottage rental at the shore or mountains.
Income/insurance/home	She and her husband make decent wages. Both jobs are in highly competitive companies, but jobs seem secure. Medical and dental insurance through husband's job. They own their home.
Stress management	Works out at the gym twice weekly for 30 minutes.
International travel	Business trip to Mexico 6 months ago.
Birth control	Withdrawal or condoms.
Why taking St. John's wort? How long? Has it helped?	Pressures at work and home made her anger easily or made her dissolve in tears. Began the herb 6 months ago on the recommendation of a friend. Has helped some, but still often teary-eyed for seemingly no reason.
Elimination	BMs every 3–4 days; hard, knotty, and sometimes painful. Voids 4–5 times daily, no discomfort.
Personal safety (abuse, harassment)	No problems with emotional or physical abuse. Incident of sexual harassment at work 2 years ago. Just settled by company committee last month.

● PHYSICAL ASSESSMENT

What are the significant portions of the physical examination that should be completed for Edna?

SYSTEM   RATIONALE   FINDINGS

SYSTEM	RATIONALE	FINDINGS
Vital signs		BP, 138/88 mm Hg right arm; HR, 86 bpm; RR, 20; T, 98.8 °F, Ht, 5'7"; Wt, 155 lbs.
General appearance		Alert, oriented. Skin warm and dry.

(continued)

SYSTEM	RATIONALE	FINDINGS
HEENT		Normocephalic, sinuses nontender. TMs pearly gray; light reflexes sharp in both ears; nasal septum midline; turbinates pink and moist. Uvula midline; no pharyngeal redness.
Lungs		CTA.
Heart		S1, S2 WNL; no heaves or thrills; no murmurs.
Breast		"Grainy" textured breast tissue bilaterally. No masses or nipple discharge.
Abdomen		BS+ all four quadrants; no organomegaly or tenderness to palpation; firm stool palpable in LLQ.
Neurological assessment		Alert and oriented; gait normal. Strength/sensation intact. DTRs 2+.
Extremities		Pulses equal bilaterally, 2+. No peripheral edema.
Pelvic		External: thinning pubic hair. Introitus: pale, dry mucosa. Cervix: pale color, midline, no discharge visible in os. Adnexa: no tenderness. Rectal: hard stool palpable in rectum.
Skin		Deeply pigmented 3 cm placque on left scapula.

● DIFFERENTIAL DIAGNOSES

What are the significant positive and negative findings that support or refute your diagnoses for Edna?

DIAGNOSIS	POSITIVE DATA	NEGATIVE DATA
1		
2		
3		
4		
5		
6		
7		
8		

● DIAGNOSTIC TESTS

Based on the history and physical examination, what, if any, diagnostic testing would you obtain?

DIAGNOSTIC TEST	RATIONALE	RESULTS	INTERPRETATION
Pap smear		Inflammation	
Hgb, lipid panel, basic metabolic panel		Hgb, 11.6 g/dL. Total cholesterol, 230. HDL, 36 mg/dL. LDL, 194 mg/dL. TSH, 8.8 μU/mL. T3, 42 ng/dL. T4, 6 μg/dL. Na, 138 mEq/L. K, 4.0 mEq/L. CL, 101 m Eq/L. CO_2, 30 mEq/L. Glucose, 82 mg/dL. BUN, 8 mg/dL. Creatinine, 0.7 mg/dL.	
PPD		1 cm.	
Urine HCG		Negative.	
Mammogram		No masses identified.	
HIV		Client refused testing.	

● DIAGNOSES

What diagnoses do you determine as being appropriate after a review of the subjective and objective data?

1.

2.

3.

4.

5.

Data Supporting the Diagnosis

● THERAPEUTIC PLAN

1. *What are your immediate therapeutic recommendations?*
2. *What patient education needs to be done based on your discoveries during the history and physical?*
3. *What anticipatory guidance should be given to a person of this age and based on the history?*
4. *What short-term follow-up services need to be provided?*
5. *What long-term follow-up services need to be provided for Edna?*
6. *What are resources for the NP and for Edna?*

REFERENCES

Adkins, S. (1997). Immunizations: Current recommendations. *American Family Physician, 56,* 865–873.

Angard, N., Chez, R. A., & Young, C. (1998). Personal health among midlife women hospital employees. *Journal of Women's Health, 7,* 1289–1293.

(1997). Clinical guidelines: Hepatitis B immunization/prophylaxis. *Nurse Practitioner, 22,* 64–70.

Goroll, A., & Mulley, A. G. (2000). *Primary Care Medicine* (4th ed.). Philadelphia: Lippincott, Williams & Wilkins.

Murray, R. B., & Zetner, J. P. (2001). *Health Promotion Strategies Through the Lifespan* (7th ed.). Upper Saddle River, NJ: Prentice Hall.

Osguthorpe, N. C., & Morgan, E. P. (1995). An immunization update for primary health care providers. *Nurse Practitioner: American Journal of Primary Health Care, 20*(6): 52, 54, 60–65.

Paul, L., & Weinert, C. (1999). Wellness profile in midlife women with a chronic illness. *Public Health Nursing, 16*(5), 341–350.

Poirier, L. (1997). The importance of screening for domestic violence in all women. *Nurse Practitioner, 22,* 105–122.

Robinson, D., Kidd, P., & Rogers, K. M. (2000). *Primary Care Across the Lifespan.* St. Louis: Mosby.

Ruffing-Rahal, M. A., & Wallace, J. (2000). Successful aging in a wellness group for older women. *Health Care for Women International, 21*(4), 267–275.

(1997). Tetanus and diphtheria immunization/prophylaxis in adults and older adults. *Nurse Practitioner, 22,* 116–120.

Treinen, A. (1997). Breast cancer screening: Making sense of controversies. *Nurse Practitioner, 22,* 17–23.

US Preventive Service Task Force. (1996). *Guide to Clinical Preventive Services.* Baltimore: Williams & Wilkins.

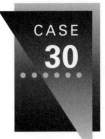

A 55-year-old man with cough, fever, and shortness of breath

SCENARIO

John Kosich is a 55-year-old Russian man who presents with cough, fatigue, fever of 100°F, and increased SOB with activity for 5 days. The cough is productive, with a large amount of thick yellow/green sputum; the cough occurs day and night but is worse at night when supine. The patient needs two pillows to sleep at night. He experiences dyspnea with one flight of steps and intercourse. He has tried OTC cough syrup and Primatene Mist Inhaler with minimal relief.

● TENTATIVE DIAGNOSES

Based on John's presentation, what are your tentative differential diagnoses?

● HISTORY

What questions do you want to ask John to assist you in developing a diagnosis? What are the key points to cover in the review of systems?

● PHYSICAL ASSESSMENT

What are the significant portions of the physical examination that should be completed for John?

● DIFFERENTIAL DIAGNOSES

What are the significant positive and negative data that support or refute your diagnoses for John?

● DIAGNOSTIC TESTS

Based on the history and physical assessment, what, if any, diagnostic testing would you do. Include your rationale for the testing.

● DIAGNOSIS

What diagnoses do you determine as being appropriate for John?

● THERAPEUTIC PLAN

1. *What are the common bacterial etiologies that cause acute exacerbation of bronchitis?*
2. *What are the possible pharmacological treatments for John?*
3. *What are alternative treatments that might be appropriate during the acute exacerbation?*
4. *What long-term treatment might be appropriate for the underlying COPD?*
5. *What are issues of treatment that should be considered for John?*
6. *When should John return for follow-up?*
7. *Based on information given about John, what impact do you think this illness might have on his family?*
8. *What would be appropriate interventions for John's family?*
9. *Where can a nurse practitioner obtain more information concerning bronchitis and COPD?*
10. *What other health care professionals might be involved in a therapeutic plan for John and his family?*
11. *John has improved from the acute exacerbation of bronchitis but continues to smoke 1 pack of cigarettes a day and reports fatigue and dyspnea on exertion. What adjustments would you make in the therapeutic plan based on this information?*

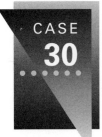

TUTORIAL

A 55-year-old man with cough, fever, and shortness of breath

SCENARIO

John Kosich is a 55-year-old Russian man who presents with cough, fatigue, fever of 100°F, and increased SOB with activity for 5 days. The cough is productive, with a large amount of thick yellow/green sputum; the cough occurs day and night but is worse at night when supine. The patient needs two pillows to sleep at night. He experiences dyspnea when climbing one flight of steps and during intercourse. He has tried OTC cough syrup and Primatene Mist Inhaler with minimal relief. John says he has been smoking a pack of cigarettes a day for 40 years.

● TENTATIVE DIAGNOSES

*Based on John's presentation, what are your tentative differential diagnoses? Identify any **red flags** that you cannot miss.*

DIAGNOSIS	RATIONALE
Pneumonia	John is presenting with productive cough, colored sputum, DOE, SOB, fever, and fatigue. These are all symptoms of pneumonia. Red flag.
Acute bronchitis	John has c/o productive cough, colored sputum, fever, and fatigue.
COPD	John c/o cough, fatigue, and SOB. He has a 40-pack/40 year history of tobacco use.
Asthma	John c/o cough, worse when supine or on exertion. He has a positive tobacco history.
Lung cancer	John c/o cough, SOB, and fatigue. He also has positive smoking history. Red flag.
Tuberculosis (TB)	Complaints of cough, SOB, fatigue, and fever are all symptoms of TB.

(continued)

DIAGNOSIS   *RATIONALE*

Anemia   Fatigue, SOB.

CHF   John's symptoms of SOB, cough, orthopnea, fatigue, DOE, and history of tobacco use could put him at risk for CHF. Red flag.

● HISTORY

What questions do you want to ask John to assist you in developing a diagnosis? What are the key points to cover in the review of systems?

REQUESTED DATA   *DATA ANSWER*

Allergies	No known medical, food, or environmental allergies.
Medications	Lisinopril (Zestril) 10 mg QD; OTC cough syrup; Epinephrine (Primatene Mist) × 5 days.
Surgery	Inguinal hernia repair (1985).
Medical history/ hospitalizations/ fractures/injuries/ accidents	HTN. Tibia/fibula fracture, age 9.
Last complete PE	Not sure when it was.
Immunizations	Has not had any in a long time. He does not think he has ever had the pneumococcal vaccine.
Appetite	Normally good. Has gained pounds in past year, but has not been hungry lately.
24-hour diet recall	B: None. L: Soup/crackers. D: 2 Big Macs, large fries, milkshake.
Sleeping	Difficulty sleeping lately due to SOB/coughing.
Social history	Tobacco: 40 year pack history. Alcohol: Denies.
Family history	Father: died 69; HTN, lung CA, smoker. Mother: living, age 76; CVA, type 2 DM, obese. Daughter: 21 y/o; alive and healthy. Son: 25 y/o, alive and healthy.

(continued)

REQUESTED DATA	*DATA ANSWER*
Relationship with family	Family relationships: married 30 years. Stable relationship with wife. Claims to have a good relationship with daughter who's in college; fair relationship with son, who works at local factory. His mother lives locally. He visits her 2 times a week; considers this a burden on his time.
Income/insurance coverage	Earns $35,000/year as an assembly line worker in a car factory. Has a good insurance coverage through union package.

What are the key points in the review of systems?

SYSTEM REVIEWED	*DATA ANSWER*
HEENT	Unremarkable
Respiratory	C/o a morning cough productive of thick, whitish sputum for 18 months. States he always has a "smoker's" cough in the morning. Also admits to slowly worsening dyspnea and fatigue over the past year. Denies night sweats or hemoptysis. Has 2-pillow orthopnea and PND at night. Admits he has trouble keeping up with peers when walking up stairs or other activities requiring a lot of physical effort.
Cardiac	Unremarkable. Denies any edema.
GI	Denies constipation, diarrhea, or black, tarry or bloody stools.
GU	Denies dysuria, polyuria, retention.
Musculoskeletal	Occasional low-back pain with heavy lifting.
Neurological	Denies syncope or weakness.

● PHYSICAL ASSESSMENT

What are the significant portions of the physical examination that should be completed for John?

SYSTEM	FINDINGS
Vital signs	BP, 138/86 mm Hg; P, 90; RR, 24 shallow; T, 99.8 °F; Ht, 5'10"; Wt, 250 lbs.
General appearance/skin color, character	Skin warm, dry, intact without lesions. Ruddy facial complexion. Early fingernail clubbing.
HEENT	TMs slightly opaque with light reflex and landmarks present. No nasal erythema or exudate; septum midline. Nontender frontal and maxillary sinuses. Pharynx mildly erythematous with no purulent exudate. Negative LA. Neck supple; thyroid symmetrical w/out enlargement; no carotid bruits; no JVD.
Lungs	AP: lateral diameter > 1:2. Moderate use of accessory muscles. Increased intercostal spaces. Bilateral tympany upon percussion; decreased tactile fremitus. Decreased movement of the rib cage with breathing. Diffuse inspiratory coarse crackles and few scattered end expiratory wheezes throughout bilateral lung fields. Diminished breath sounds bilaterally. Negative LA.
Heart	S1, S2 WNL; no MRG.
Abdomen	Abdomen obese; BS +; negative bruits. No tenderness. No HSM or HJR.
Neurological assessment	Alert and oriented.
Extremities	Increased pigmentation bilateral lower extremity with mild varicosities and thickened toenails. PT pulses 1+; DP pulses 2+ bilaterally. No edema. Tobacco stains present on fingers.

● DIFFERENTIAL DIAGNOSES

What are the significant positive and negative findings that support or refute your diagnoses for John?

DIAGNOSIS	POSITIVE DATA	NEGATIVE DATA
Pneumonia	Productive cough for 3 weeks; SOB, fatigue, crackles, wheezes.	No bronchophony, egobronchophony, whispered pectoriloquy, localized adventitious breath sounds, tactile fremitus and percussion symmetrical bilaterally.

(continued)

DIAGNOSIS	POSITIVE DATA	NEGATIVE DATA
Acute bronchitis	Positive tobacco history; increased productive cough; SOB; fever; fatigue; paroxysmal nocturnal dyspnea; 2-pillow orthopnea; use of accessory muscles; diffuse coarse crackles and wheezes in bilateral lung fields.	18 month history of fatigue, dyspnea, and morning cough; increased AP/lateral diameter.
COPD	40-pack year history of tobacco use; morning sputum production; ruddy complexion; clubbing of fingernails; moderate use of accessory muscles; increased AP: lateral diameter; wheezes; coarse crackles.	Acute exacerbation of signs/symptoms; fever.
Asthma	Smoking history, DOE, cough, fatigue; wheezing and use of accessory muscles.	Lack of childhood history, Primatene Mist minimally effective; fever; amount/color of sputum production.
Lung cancer	Family history; tobacco history; 18-month history of fatigue; SOB; cough; diffuse crackles and wheezes	No weight loss or hemoptysis.
Tuberculosis	SOB; cough; fatigue; tobacco history; diffuse crackles and wheezes.	No weight loss, night sweats, or hemoptysis.
Anemia	Fatigue, SOB.	No black or tarry stools; no paresthesia.
CHF	Paroxysmal nocturnal dyspnea.	No JVD; no HJR; no S3; no fine crackles in bases, tan sputum; no peripheral edema.
Immunization deficiency	Has not had immunizations in a while, including pneumococcal.	

● DIAGNOSTIC TESTS

Based on the history and physical examination, what, if any, diagnostic testing would you obtain?

DIAGNOSTIC TEST	RATIONALE	RESULTS	INTERPRETATION
CXR	Good choice. This will help rule out pneumonia, TB, CA, CHF. It's also inexpensive, quick, and noninvasive.	There is flattening of the diaphragms, hypolucency of the lung fields, and increased AP diameter of the chest. No localized pulmonary infiltrates.	COPD
Oxygen saturation	Good choice. Will help identify hypoxemia, and degree of compromise. Quick, inexpensive, and noninvasive.	92%.	WNL.
PPD	Will rule out TB. Inexpensive and quick.	1 cm.	Negative.
Gram's stain	Allows for more accurate treatment as it identifies causative organisms. It often is difficult to obtain adequate specimen and takes several days to get results.	NL flora.	WNL.
Electrocardiogram	Would do if suspicious of cardiac etiology or involvement. Relatively inexpensive; can be done in most offices.	NSR, normal intervals and axis, no acute changes.	WNL.
CBC with differential	Would not do on initial visit as fever is low grade, and patient is not in	Not done at this time.	

(continued)

DIAGNOSTIC TEST	RATIONALE	RESULTS	INTERPRETATION
	marked distress. However, might do on follow-up if John has not improved. Would help differentiate viral from bacterial infection, as well as polycythemia.		
ABGs	Will identify acidosis, chronic CO_2 retention, acid-base imbalance. Provides a more accurate assessment of oxygen level. Invasive, expensive, needs to be done in hospital lab.	Not done this visit.	
Pulmonary function tests	Good choice after acute exarcerbation. Will differentiate restrictive and obstructive disease and identify severity of illness.	FEV_1, 1.5 l. FEV_1/FVC, < 70%.	Diminished FEV_1 indicates COPD. A FEV_1/FVC ratio of < 70% predicts future decline in lung function.
Electrolytes, liver function tests, renal cholesterol	Provides baseline information about current status.	Na, 145 mEq/L. K, 4.0 mEq/L. Cl, 100 mEq/L. CO_2, 30 mEq/L. Alkaline phosphatase, 100 ImU/L. AST, 44 IU/L. ALT, 52 IU/L. BUN, 24 mg/dL. Creatinine, 0.9 mg/dL. Total cholesterol, 210 mg/dL.	S1 elevated AST, ALT, and cholesterol.
Hgb/HCT	Provides information about hemoglobin/hematocrit. Would help rule out anemia	Hgb, 14.3 g/dL.	WNL.

(continued)

DIAGNOSTIC TEST	RATIONALE	RESULTS	INTERPRETATION
Bronchodilator testing	Indicates how the use of a bronchodilator may be helpful in the treatment plan. Even with initial negative results, after a steroid inhaler there may be positive gains in lung function after several weeks.	FEV_1, 1.5 l before bronchodilator. FEV_1 2.0 l after bronchodilator.	Indicates reversible bronchospasm is present and should be treated with bronchodilators or corticosteroid inhalers.

● DIAGNOSES

What diagnoses do you determine as being appropriate after a review of the subjective and objective data?

- COPD with acute exacerbation
- Immunization deficiency

Data Supporting the Diagnosis of COPD With Acute Exacerbation

Forty-year history of tobacco use. Morning sputum production, ruddy complexion, clubbing of fingernails, moderate use of accessory muscles, increased AP (to lateral diameter, and wheezes, and coarse crackles). Spirometry testing and CXR also support the diagnosis of COPD

Pathophysiology: COPD is a disorder characterized by abnormal test results of expiratory flow that do not change markedly over several months. It consists of the following two entities.

1. Emphysema: a pathologic diagnosis based on a permanent abnormal dilation and destruction of the alveolar ducts and air spaces distal to the terminal bronchioles.
2. Chronic bronchitis: a clinical diagnosis based on the presence of a cough and sputum production occurring on most days for at least a 3-month period during 2 consecutive years.

John probably has chronic bronchitis with an acute exacerbation. Very commonly, there are components of both emphysema and chronic bronchitis. In John's case the predominant symptoms seem to be of chronic bronchitis.

Acute exacerbation: increased cough is the hallmark symptom. Client also may report fever, increased sputum production, increased SOB, and fatigue.

The purulent sputum appears to be a reliable sign of acute exacerbations of COPD (Stockley, O'Brien, Pye, & Hill, 2000) as confirmed with cultures and compared with white or clear sputum.

● THERAPEUTIC PLAN

1. *What are the common bacterial etiologies causing an acute exacerbation of bronchitis?*

   Most common etiologies of acute exacerbation of bronchitis:
   - Streptococcus pneumoniae
   - Haemophilus influenza
   - Moraxella catarrhalis
   - Viral

2. *What are the possible pharmacological treatments for John?*

   Acute exacerbation of COPD: inexpensive, broad spectrum drugs are recommended as first line therapy. Cephalosporins, amoxicillin-clavulanic acid, or quinolones should be prescribed if there is evidence of resistant organisms.
   - Antibiotics: Trimethoprim-sulfamethoxazole (Septra DS) 1 BID or doxycycline PO 100 mg BID
   - Erythromycin 500 mg BID
   - Amoxicillin-clavulanic acid (Augmentin) 250 mg PO TID × 10 days
   - Cefixime (Suprax) 400 mg PO QD × 10 days
   - Clarithromycin (Biaxin) 500 mg PO BID × 10 days
   - Azithromycin (Zithromax) 250 mg 2 PO × 1 day, 1 PO × 4 days
   - Ofloxacin (Floxin) 400 mg PO BID
   - Ipratropium bromide (Atrovent) inhaler 2 puffs TID to up to 6 inhalations QID if needed
   - Albuterol sulfate (Proventil) inhaler 2 puffs QID PRN (provides immediate bronchodilation)

3. *What are alternative treatments that might be appropriate during the acute exacerbation?*
   - Subcutaneous epinephrine 0.3 mL PRN
   - Prednisone with tapering dose if marked limitation of air movement; 40 to 80 g daily in divided doses
   - Mucokinetic agent for particularly thick secretions
   - Expectorants
   - Oxygen therapy with oxygen saturation <85% or PaO2 <55

4. *What long-term treatment might be appropriate for the underlying COPD?*
   - Avoidance of irritants (discontinue smoking)
   - Nutrition: maintain adequate intake of calories and protein
   - Pursed lip breathing/consider pulmonary rehabilitation
   - Pneumonia vaccination
   - Develop appropriate exercise program

- Annual influenza vaccination
- Avoidance of respiratory infections
- Possible O_2 at home if O_2 saturation is $< 85\%$

5. *The recommended stepped treatment for COPD is:*
   - Ipratropium bromide (Atrovent)
   - Beta adrenergic agents
   - Theophylline (sustained release product QD or BID) (Its use has diminished recently, but it remains an effective drug as second-line therapy; it is most helpful with nocturnal symptoms.)
   - Inhaled corticosteroids: appear to reduce symptoms, lower health care use, and improve sensitivity of lungs, but do not slow the progression of COPD (National Heart Lung and Blood Institute, press release December 27, 2000; available *www.nhlbi.nih.gov.*

6. *What are issues of treatment that should be considered for John?*
   - Cost of medications: trimethoprim-sulfamethoxazole and doxycycline are the two least expensive antibiotics.
   - Instruction in proper use of inhaler. Patient should perform return demonstration of proper use of inhaler.
   - Adherence: explain to patient that he will notice results from ipratropium inhaler use in 2 to 4 weeks. This treatment modality will help improve and maintain adequate long-term oxygenation levels.

7. *When should John return for follow-up?*
   - Follow up within 24 to 48 hours by phone; follow-up visits weekly until acute exacerbation is stabilized, and then every 3 to 6 months.
   - Give pneumococcal vaccine at next visit and influenza vaccine (depending on time of year).

8. *Based on the information given about John, what impact do you think this illness might have on his family?*
   - Altered roles and responsibilities
   - Financial concerns
   - Emotional issues.

9. *What would be appropriate interventions for John's family?*

   Family counseling regarding the disease process, treatment modalities and lifestyle alterations.

10. *Where can a nurse practitioner obtain more information concerning bronchitis and COPD?*
    - Local smoking cessation classes, community hospital pulmonary rehabilitation
    - American Lung Association: *www.lungusa.org*
    - Heart Lung and Blood Institute: *http://www.nhlbi.nih.gov*
    - American Thoracic Society: *http://www.thoracic.org/*

- Canadian Lung Association: *www.lung.ca*
- American Academy of Allergy, Asthma and Immunology: *http://www.aaaai.org*
- The Asthma and Allergy Network: *http://www.aanma.org*

11. What other health care professionals might be involved in a therapeutic plan for John and his family?

- Pulmonologist/physician for consultation and referral, oxygen supply company for home oxygen if needed.
- Counselor: individual or family as needed

12. John's condition has improved from the acute exacerbation of bronchitis, but he continues to smoke 1 pack of cigarettes a day and reports fatigue and dyspnea on exertion. What adjustments would you make in the therapeutic plan based on this information?

- Obtain ABGs
- Continue to reinforce smoking cessation
- Pulmonary function tests
- Review pursed lip breathing
- Increase ipratropium bromide (Atrovent) to 3 puffs q 4 hours
- May consider steroid inhaler or theophylline oral product

REFERENCES

American Thoracic Society. (1999). Dyspnea mechanisms, assessment, and management: A consensus statement. *American Journal of Respiratory and Critical Care Medicine, 159,* 321–340.

American Thoracic Society. (1995). Standards for the diagnosis and care of patients with chronic obstructive pulmonary disease. *American Journal of Respiratory and Critical Care Medicine, 152*(Suppl), S77–S120.

Fromm, R., & Varon, J. (1994). Acute exacerbations of obstructive lung disease. *Postgraduate Medicine, 95*(8), 101–106.

Gift, A. G., & McCrone, S. H. (1993). Depression in patients with COPD. *Heart Lung, 22,* 289–297.

Hernández, M. T. E., Rubio, T. M., Ruiz, F. O., Riera, H. S., Gil, R. S., & Gómez, J. C. (2000). Results of a home-based training program for patients with COPD. *Chest, 118*(1), 106–114.

Hospers, J., Postma, D., Rijcken, B., Weiss, S., & Schouten, J. (2000). Histamine airway hyper-responsiveness and mortality from chronic obstructive pulmonary disease: A cohort study. *Lancet, 356,* 1313–1317.

Irwin, R., & Madison, J. (2000). The diagnosis and treatment of cough. *New England Journal of Medicine, 343,* 1715–1721.

Jacobs, M. (1994). Maintenance therapy for obstructive lung disease. *Postgraduate Medicine, 95*(8), 87–96.

Johannsen, J. M. (1994). Chronic obstructive lung disease: Current comprehensive care for emphysema and bronchitis. *Nurse Practitioner, 19*(1), 59–67.

Kendrick, K. R., Baxi, S. C., & Smith, R. M. (2000). Usefulness of the modified 0–10

Borg scale in assessing the degree of dyspnea in patients with COPD and asthma. *Journal of Emergency Nursing, 26,* 216–222, 282–288.

Kips, J. (2000). The clinical role of long-acting beta$_2$-agonists in COPD. *Respiratory Medicine, 94*(Suppl E), S1–S5.

Lyotvall, J. (2000). Pharmacology of bronchodilators used in the treatment of COPD. *Respiratory Medicine, 94*(Suppl E), S6–S10.

Manning, H. L., & Schwartzstein, R. M. (1995). Pathophysiology of dyspnea. *The New England Journal of Medicine 333*(23), 1547–1553.

Mapel, D., Hurley, J., Frost, F., Petersen, H., Picchi, M., & Coultas, D. (2000). Health care utilization in chronic obstructive pulmonary disease. A case-control study in a health maintenance organization. *Archives of Internal Medicine, 160*(17), 2653–2658.

Murphy, M., & Risser, N. (2000). NP abstracts. Corticosteroids and COPD. *Nurse Practitioner: American Journal of Primary Health Care, 25*(2), 87–88.

Murphy, T. F., Sethi, S., & Niederman, M. S. (2000). The role of bacteria in exacerbations of COPD: A constructive view. *Chest, 118,* 204–209.

Pauwels, R. A., Lofdahl, C. G., Latinen, L. A., Schouten, J. P., Postma, D. S., Pride, N. B., Ohlsson, S. (1999). Long-term treatment with inhaled budesonide in persons with mild chronic obstructive pulmonary disease who continue smoking. European Respiratory Society Study on Chronic Pulmonary Disease. *New England Journal of Medicine, 340,* 1948–1953.

Stockley, R. A., O'Brien, C., Pye, A., & Hill, S. L. (2000). Relationship of sputum color to nature and outpatient management of acute exacerbations of COPD. *Chest, 117,* 1638–1645.

Vestbo, J., Sorensen, T., Lange, P., Brix, A., Torre, P., & Viskum, K. (1999). Long-term effect of inhaled budesonide in mild and moderate chronic obstructive pulmonary disease: A randomized controlled trial. *Lancet, 353,* 1819–1823.

Weiner, P., Magadle, R., Berar-Yarnay, N., Davidovich, A., & Weiner, M. (2000). The cumulative effect of long-acting bronchodilators, exercise, and inspiratory muscle training on the perception of dyspnea in patients with advanced COPD. *Chest, 118,* 672–678.

Woo, K. (1995). Fatigue in COPD. Nurse Practitioner: American Journal of Primary Health Care, 20(10), 11, 14–15.

A 20-year-old pregnant woman with back pain

SCENARIO

Krista Foster presents to the college health clinic with a history of flank pain for 2 days. She is single and lives with a female roommate in an apartment close to campus. She is a full-time college student, who graduated from high school a year earlier than her peers.

● TENTATIVE DIAGNOSES

Based on the information provided, what are the potential diagnoses?

DIAGNOSIS	RATIONALE
1	
2	
3	
4	
5	

● DIFFERENTIAL DIAGNOSES

What are the significant questions in the history for Krista? Are there any questions that are missing?

REQUESTED DATA   DATA ANSWER

REQUESTED DATA	DATA ANSWER
Allergies	NKA.
Medications	Prenatal vitamins. Tylenol tabs (2) for the back pain. Last dose 1 hour ago.
Surgery/transfusion	Tonsillectomy at age 10, no complications.
Childhood illnesses	Had frequent bladder infections (about 3/year) between the ages of 8 and 13 years.
Have you noticed any changes in or problems with elimination in either stool or urine?	No changes in stool, but urine has strong odor. Has experienced frequency, urgency, nocturia, and suprapubic discomfort with voiding.
Appetite/weight gain	Anorexic yesterday. Nauseated today, no vomiting. Has gained 20 pounds so far during this pregnancy.
Adult illnesses	Frequent URIs since coming to college 8 months ago.
Medical history/ hospitalizations/ fractures/injuries/ accidents	MMR vaccine prior to coming to college, tetanus vaccine 6 months ago, oral polio vaccine as child. Skateboard accident 3 years ago: sutures in right knee and elbow, no complications.
OB/GYN history	LNMP: 30 weeks ago. Regular periods of 5 days' duration with moderate flow, some cramping. Last saw her family provider for a prenatal visit 2 weeks ago in her hometown. Used condoms unsuccessfully for birth control. G1P0A0. Fetus active today with quickening at about 20 weeks' gestation.
Social history	Tobacco: socially, estimates 2 cigarettes per week. Alcohol: none. Caffeine: 2–3 glasses of iced tea/day; 5–6 colas per day. Drugs: denies. Exercise: walks on campus to classes; no other exercise.
Social organizations	First Methodist church at home. Goes home on weekends.
Relationship with family	Strained lately due to unplanned pregnancy and her parents' hope for her education and future. She confides a lot in her brother and her best friend. Plans to move back home when the baby is born and continue school

(continued)

REQUESTED DATA   DATA ANSWER

Relationship with friends	Roomate is somewhat close to her. Boyfriend is not long in the picture (father of the baby). Has few friends on campus due to her young age as a college freshman and being pregnant.
Income/insurance/home	Parents have insurance through her father's job. He is a track coach, and her mother is an executive with a long distance phone company.
Length of symptoms	Back pain for past 2 days. Does not recall any acute infection prior to pain. Anorexic since yesterday. Fatigued. Denies hurting her back with lifting, etc.
How has this affected your ADLs?	Pain interferes with concentration and ability to sit in class. Unable to go to class today due to pain. Roommate has been helpful in bringing her acetaminophen and meals.
How do you manage stress?	Usually talks things out with her brother or best friend. The unplanned pregnancy has been a major stress.
Any evidence of blood loss?	Noticed no blood in stools or urine. No hemoptysis.
Any gush of fluid, a large amount of mucus discharge from vagina, or cramping similar to menstrual cramps in the last few days?	No gush of fluid, although she reports some dribbling of urine 1 week ago. No cramping, but did have some low abdominal pain with urination 1 week ago.
Any history of STDs or vaginitis?	One episode of vaginal itching and thick, white discharge about 6 months ago. Believes it was a yeast infection; treated after vaginal exam.
Family history	Father: age 42, good health. Mother: age 43, HTN. Brother: 20, good health.

● PHYSICAL ASSESSMENT

What are the significant portions of the physical examination that should be completed for Krista? Include your rationale for doing the exam.

SYSTEM   RATIONALE   FINDINGS

SYSTEM	RATIONALE	FINDINGS
General appearance		Alert, face flushed, anxious expression, appears ill, listless. Diaphoretic.

(continued)

SYSTEM	RATIONALE	FINDINGS
Extremities		Pulses 2+. No edema noted in hands. Skin on dorsal surface of hand returns to original position immediately when pinched.
Vital signs		BP, 138/88 mm Hg left arm; HR, 102 bpm; RR, 20; T, 101 °F; Ht, 5′4″; Wt, 165 lbs.
HEENT		Normocephalic; no sinus tenderness; TMs pearly and WNL; nasal mucosa pink and moist with septum midline; oral mucosa moist and pink. Uvula midline. No pharyngeal erythema or oral lesions noted. No obvious facial edema. No LA; supple neck. Thyroid nonpalpable, no masses.
Lungs		CTA.
Heart		S1, S2, WNL; tachycardia. No MRG.
Neurological assessment		Alert and oriented; gait normal. Strength/ sensation intact. DTRs 2+.
Abdomen/Leopold's maneuvers/fetal heart rate, CVAT tenderness		Fetal movement palpated; fetus in cephalic presentation. Fetal heart rate 160 bpm. No suprapubic tenderness. Bladder nonpalpable. No LA. Marked CVAT tenderness on right.

● DIFFERENTIAL DIAGNOSES

What are the significant positive and negative findings that support or refute your diagnoses for Krista?

DIAGNOSIS	POSITIVE DATA	NEGATIVE DATA
1		
2		
3		
4		
5		

● DIAGNOSTIC TESTS

Based on the history and physical, what, if any, diagnostic testing would you do? What is your rationale for doing the testing, and what is your interpretation of the results?

DIAGNOSTIC TEST	RATIONALE	RESULTS	INTERPRETATION
Urine microscopic examination		RBCs and WBCs are present. See Figure 31-1.	

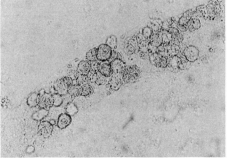

Figure 31–1. (500x).

DIAGNOSTIC TEST	RATIONALE	RESULTS	INTERPRETATION
Dipstick urine sample		Nitrites, 2+; leukocytes, 3+; moderate blood.	
Urine specimen for culture and sensitivity		E. coli, 10^5.	
CBC		WBC, 18,00/μL. RBC, 4.27/μL. Hgb, 12.1 g/dL. HCT, 36.5%. MCV, 85.3 m^3. Platelets, 385/μL.	
Electronic uterine contraction and FHR monitoring		Mild uterine contractions.	
BUN, creatinine, creatinine clearance		BUN, 9 mg/dL. Creatinine, 0.7 mg/dL. Creatinine clearance, 84 mL/min.	

● DIAGNOSIS

What diagnoses do you determine as being appropriate after a review of the subjective and objective data? Discuss the pathophysiology of the condition. How does pregnancy affect the pathophysiology?

Data Supporting the Diagnosis?

1. *How are urinary tract infections classified?*

Classification of UTIs

	SYMPTOMATIC CYSTITIS	ASYMPTOMATIC BACTERIURIA	PYELONEPHRITIS
Symptoms			
Management			
Chronic state			

2. *How serious are UTIs during pregnancy?*
3. *What influence does the pregnancy have on the therapeutic treatment plan?*
4. *How will the management of Krista's problem be handled?*
5. *When should Krista be referred, and to whom?*
6. *What patient education should you discuss with Krista?*
7. *What impact does this illness have on the fetus?*
8. *What information can you offer Krista if she asks you what caused the problem?*
9. *When should Krista return for follow-up?*
10. *What are resources that are available for the NP and Krista?*

REFERENCES

Connolly, A., & Thorp, J. (1999). Urinary tract infections in pregnancy. *Urologic Clinics of North America, 26*(4), 779–787.

Garite, T., & Walker, C. (1997). Outpatient management of pyelonephritis: A reasonable option during pregnancy? *Contemporary OB/GYN, 5,* 57–69.

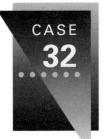

A 48-year-old woman with muscle pain

SCENARIO

Regina Lynn presents to the medical office with a 3-month history of generalized muscle pain that has interfered with sleep. She is married and works part time as a cook and housekeeper.

● TENTATIVE DIAGNOSES

*What are the potential diagnoses you have identified based on the scenario presented? Make sure you include any vital **red flag** diagnoses that cannot be missed.*

DIAGNOSIS   *RATIONALE*

1

2

3

4

5

6

7

8

● HISTORY

What are the significant questions to the history of Regina?

REQUESTED DATA	DATA ANSWER
Allergies	Sulfa drugs, cause a rash. NSAIDs, cause hand and pedal edema.
Current medications	Chlordiazepoxide and clidinium (Librax), for IBS. Omeprazole (Prilosec), for GERD. Calcium polycarbophil (FiberCon), for diverticulosis and IBS. Lo Ovral, for ovarian cyst reduction. Loratadine (Claritin), for allergic rhinitis.
Surgeries	BTL (1976).
Transfusions	No transfusions.
Past Medical History & Hospitalizations/Major injuries	Usual childhood illnesses. Chickenpox and measles as a child. No major hospitalizations or injuries.
Adult illnesses	HEENT: Allergic rhinitis. GI: GERD, IBS, diverticulosis. Repro: ovarian cyst.
Ob/Gyn history	LNMP: 1 week ago; normal flow and duration. Last pelvic exam: 3 weeks ago. Mammogram: 2 months ago. BSE: performs monthly on a regular basis. G3P3A0.
Appetite/weight change	Denies changes in appetite. Denies recent changes in weight, with the exception of small fluctuations (<3%) on a quarterly basis.
Social history	Tobacco: never. Alcohol: never. Caffeine: uses decaffeinated tea and coffee; caffeine-free soft drinks. Drugs: never. Exercise: sporadically walks.
Family history	Father: age 72, DM Type II, CAD, CVA, thyroid mass (benign), sleep apnea, depression. Mother: age 69, hypothyroidism, OA, depression. 3 Brothers: ages 37, 40, and 45, good health. Sister: 52, DM Type II, CAD, angioplasty, depression.
Social organizations	Turner Ridge Baptist Church; Kincaid Lake State Park Association member.

(continued)

REQUESTED DATA   DATA ANSWER

Relationship with husband	Both are monogamous. Married 30 years. They have sex about 1–2 times a week and both enjoy the act. Husband is in management at a job near home on first shift.
Relationship with children	This couple has three adult male children, 2 are married and living on their own, and 1 remains at home. Both value making family-oriented plans with their sons, daughters-in-law, and 1 grandchild.
Income/insurance/home	She and her husband make above-average wages. Both jobs are secure. Both carry their own medical, vision, and dental insurance. They own their home.
Length of symptoms	Widespread muscle pain and sleep disturbances (she primarily is able to nap for only short intervals) for 3 months. Myalgias are fairly constant but worse in the morning and at the latter part of a workday. Denies recent known injuries.
How has this affected your ADLs?	Continues to be able to do her work; however, the quantity of her work is decreased. Also, work around the home has diminished. Poor nocturnal sleeping has led to daytime napping. This has resulted in a lesser degree of daily social activities. Also, inadequate sleep has led to lower energy levels.
How do you manage stress?	Enjoys activities with one of her daughters-in-law (e.g., shopping, board games, television). She feels she also is able to communicate well with her spouse. Church also is a method of relieving stress.
Any weakness or fatigue?	Denies weakness or significant fatigue. She has a c/o diminished energy levels, but denies actual fatigue that prevents carrying out ADLs.
Any associated symptoms?	Regina states that she at times feels as though the joints in her hands are swollen and tight. Tends to be worse in the morning. Denies H/A and feelings of depression. Denies infectious symptoms (e.g., fever).

● PHYSICAL ASSESSMENT

What are the significant portions of the physical examination that should be completed for Regina?

SYSTEM	RATIONALE	FINDINGS
Vital signs		BP, 118/78 mm Hg right arm; HR, 76 bpm; RR, 20; T, 97.8°F; Ht, 5'7"; Wt, 192 lbs.
General appearance		Alert; NAD. Well-groomed. Pleasant and smiling.
HEENT		EOMs intact; no nystagmus. Thyroid nonpalpable. No LA.
Hair, skin, nails		Hair clean, slightly thinning. Skin clean w/some dryness and slight flaking noted. Nails clean and non brittle. No rashes. No ecchymosis.
Lungs		CTA.
Heart		S1, S2 w/o murmurs, rubs, clicks, heaves, or thrills.
Musculoskeletal		No muscular atrophy. Tone WNL, bands nonpalpable, nontaut. Negative twitch response. Bilateral equal strength. FROM. No weakness noted. + Tender points (16/18, occiput, low cervical, trapezius, 2nd rib, supraspinatus, lateral epicondyle, gluteal, knee.) No trigger points.
Neurological assessment		Alert and oriented X3. Gait normal. Strength/sensation intact. DTRs 2+.
Extremities		Pulses X4 are 2+, bilaterally equal. No edema noted.

● DIFFERENTIAL DIAGNOSES

What are the significant positive and negative findings that support or refute your diagnoses for Regina?

DIAGNOSIS	POSITIVE DATA	NEGATIVE DATA
1		
2		
3		
4		
5		
6		
7		

● DIAGNOSTIC TESTS

Based on the history and physical examination, what, if any, diagnostic testing would you obtain? Are all of these tests appropriate to do at this time?

DIAGNOSTIC TEST	RATIONALE	RESULTS	INTERPRETATION
CBC		Hgb, 14.2 g/dL; HCT, 42.4%;	
Metabolic panel/ Electrolytes		WBC, 7.2 × 10³/μL; glucose, 81 mg/dL; BUN, 8 mg/dL; creatinine, 0.8 mg/dL; Na, 139 mEq/L; K, 4.3 mEq/L; Cl, 98 mEq/L; CO_2, 32 mEq/L; calcium, 9.5 mg/dL; protein (total), 6.7 g/dL; albumin, 4.0 g/dL; globulin, 2.7 g/dL; bilirubin (total), 0.3 mg/dL; alkaline phosphatase, 102 U/L; AST, 14 U/L; ALT, 10 U/L;	
TSH		TSH, 3.1 μU/mL.	
RF (Rheumatoid factor)		Negative.	
Antinuclear antibody		Negative.	
Creatinine phosphokinase		35 U/L.	
ESR		12 mm/hour	
EMG		Not done.	
Muscle biopsy		Not done.	

● DIAGNOSIS

What diagnosis do you determine as being appropriate after a review of the subjective and objective data?

Data Supporting the Diagnosis

● PATHOPHYSIOLOGY OF DIAGNOSIS

● THERAPEUTIC PLAN

1. What will the management of Regina's problem consist of?

2. When should Regina be referred to a specialist and to whom?

3. What patient education should be discussed with Regina?

4. What suggestions can you make for Regina for her myalgias?

5. When should Regina return for follow-up?

6. What community resources are available for the NP and Regina?

REFERENCES

Bernard, A. L., Prenie, A., & Edsall, P. (2000). Identification of the health educator's role in the management of fibromyalgia syndrome through an examination of patients' needs. *International Electronic Journal of Health, 3,* 19–27.

Bernard, A. L., Prenie, A., & Edsall, P. (2000). Quality of life issues for fibromyalgia patients. *Arthritis Care and Research, 13,* 42–50.

Creamer, P. (1999). Effective management of fibromyalgia: Exercise, drugs, and cognitive behavior therapy are all helpful. *Journal of Musculoskeletal Medicine, 11,* 622–624, 634–637.

Gowans, S. E., deHueck, A., Voss, S., & Richardson, M. (1999). A randomized, controlled trial of exercise and education for individuals with fibromyalgia. *Arthritis Care and Research, 12,* 120–128.

Kaplan, R. M., Schmidt, S. M., & Cronan, T. A. (2000). Quality of well-being in patients with fibromyalgia. *Journal of Rheumatology, 27,* 785–789.

Leslie, M. (1999). Fibromyalgia syndrome: A comprehensive approach to identification and management. *Clinical Excellence for Nurse Practitioners, 3,* 165–171.

Millea, P. J., & Holloway, R. L. (2000). Treating fibromyalgia. *American Family Physician, 62,* 1575–1582.

Mosely, B. (2000). Fibromyalgia. In D. Robinson, P. Kidd, & K. Rogers (Eds.), *Primary care across the lifespan* (pp. 453–458). St. Louis: Mosby.

Nicassio, P. M., Weisman, M. H., Schieman, C., & Young, C. W. (2000). The role of generalized pain and pain behavior in tender point scores of fibromyalgia. *Journal of Rheumatology, 27,* 1056–1062.

Okifuji, A., Turk, D. C., & Sherman, J. J. (2000). Evaluation of the relationship between depression and fibromyalgia syndrome: Why aren't all patients depressed? *Journal of Rheumatology, 27,* 212–219.

Rogers, J. L., & Maurizio, S. J. (2000). A needs assessment as a basis for health promotion for individuals with fibromyalgia. *Family and Community Health, 22,* 66–77.

Yunus, M. (1996a). Fibromyalgia syndrome: Blueprint for a reliable diagnosis. *Consultant, 36*(6), 1260–1274.

Yunus, M. (1996b). Fibromyalgia syndrome: Is there any effective therapy? *Consultant, 36*(6), 1279–1285.

Yunus, M. B., Inanici, F., Alday, T. C., & Mangold, R. F. (2000). Fibromyalgia in men: Comparison of clinical features with women. *Journal of Rheumatology, 27,* 485–490.

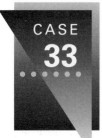

A 9-year-old girl with red, scaling, annular lesions on arm, neck, and chest, and a recent history of inattention at school.

SCENARIO

Cindy Gregg presents to the health center with a history of itching lesions for 2 weeks and an inability to concentrate at school. She lives with her mother and maternal grandmother. She has no siblings. She is in the third grade and has always been an average to above average student.

● TENTATIVE DIAGNOSES

*What are the potential diagnoses you have identified based on this scenario? Make sure you include any vital **red flag** diagnoses that cannot be missed.*

DIAGNOSIS	RATIONALE
1	
2	
3	
4	
5	
6	
7	
8	
9	

● HISTORY

What are significant questions in the history for Cindy and her mother? Are there any questions that are missing that are needed to help with the diagnosis of this case?

REQUESTED DATA	DATA ANSWER
Allergies	NKA.
Medications	Diphenhydramine (Benadryl) 25 mg orally every 6 h PRN for itching. Has been taking it regularly the past couple of weeks, before school, upon returning home in the afternoon, and at bedtime. OTC hydrocortisone cream on lesions BID or TID. Daily multivitamin.
Medical history	PE tubes and adenoidectomy, age 3, for recurrent acute otitis media. Immunizations current and up to date, including Hib, varicella and Hep B. No recent fevers. No recent illness. No recent insect bites or stings. Passed recent vision and hearing screenings at school. No history of rash.
Appetite/sleep	No changes in appetite No changes in sleep pattern; 8–9 hours of sleep per night.
Family history	Mother in good health; grandmother HTN, CAD, "bad nerves," and is on disability due to a back injury 10 years ago. Neither has any rashes, acute illness, or lesions. No siblings. Father lives in another state, does not have contact with Cindy.
Social history	Mother works 2nd shift. Grandmother watches Cindy after school, in the evenings, and on weekends. Neither reports behavior changes at home. Plays outdoors in yard and on sidewalk with 2 neighborhood children on nice days. No wooded areas nearby. No known rashes, lesions on playmates. No changes in soaps or detergents. No new clothing, jewelry, toys, or pets. Regular 3rd grade class. Good grades until 2 weeks ago. Failed 2 spelling tests. Gets along with teacher, family, and peers. Likes school. Sometimes feels sleepy at school lately.

(continued)

REQUESTED DATA   DATA ANSWER

	Teacher reports inattention in class, has fallen asleep twice in past few days. School nurse has requested evaluation of lesions before returning to school.
History of lesions	2 weeks ago, small dime size lesion developed on left antecubital space. Oval with red border. Itchy. Has increased to quarter size, skin in center is scaly. 1 week ago, grandmother noticed lesion on left side of neck, smaller than dime size and also multiple lesions on chest. Treating with topical hydrocortisone cream and liquid diphenhydramine when c/o itching. Itching does not increase at night.

● PHYSICAL ASSESSMENT

What are the significant portions of the physical examination that should be completed for Cindy? What is your rationale for doing the parts of the exam that you do?

SYSTEM   RATIONALE   FINDINGS

SYSTEM	RATIONALE	FINDINGS
Vital signs		BP, 110/60 mm Hg right arm; HR, 88 bpm; RR, 20; T, 98.4 °F; Ht, 54″; Wt, 60 lbs.
General appearance		Alert, NAD, calm, cooperative demeanor during examination. Skin warm and dry, color natural.
HEENT		Normocephalic; TMs gray and WNL; no lymphadenopathy; uvula midline; no pharyngeal erythema or oral lesions; neck supple; no bruits.
Lungs		CTA.
Heart		Regular rate and rhythm. No murmurs.
Neurological assessment		CN 2–12 intact.
Skin		Multiple lesions found. 2½–3 cm left antecubital space and 1-½ cm on left cheek and numerous lesions on chest. Annular, with red, raised border and central clearing. No pustules or vesicles.

(continued)

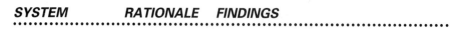

SYSTEM *RATIONALE* *FINDINGS*

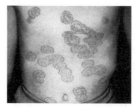

Extremities   No LA; all pulses palpable. Reflexes intact.

● DIFFERENTIAL DIAGNOSES

What are the significant positive and negative findings that support or refute your diagnoses for Cindy?

DIAGNOSIS	POSITIVE DATA	NEGATIVE DATA
1		
2		
3		
4		
5		
6		
7		
8		
9		

● DIAGNOSTIC TESTS

The following tests were done. What do the test results indicate? What impact do the lab results have on Cindy's treatment plan?

DIAGNOSTIC TEST	RATIONALE	RESULTS	INTERPRETATION
Woods lamp		A yellowish fluorescence was seen.	
Potassium hydroxide preparation (KOH prep)		Hyphae appeared as long, translucent, branching filaments of uniform width.	
Fungal culture		Not done.	
ELISA and Western blot		Not done.	
Microscopic exam of skin scraping		Not done.	
DSM IV criteria		Cindy did not meet the APA's DSM IV criteria for ADHD.	
CT scan		Not done.	

● THERAPEUTIC PLAN

1. How is this skin lesion classified?

2. What will the management of Cindy's lesion consist of? How will her school problems be addressed?

3. When should Cindy be referred to a specialist and to whom?

4. What patient education should you discuss with Cindy and her mother?

5. What impact does this illness have in terms of being contagious to Cindy's family, friends, and schoolmates?

6. *What suggestions can you make for Cindy's problems at school?*

7. *When should Cindy return for follow-up?*

8. *What community resources are available for the nurse practitioner, Cindy, and her mother?*

REFERENCES

(2000). Photoclinic: Foresee your next patient. Two feet-one hand syndrome. *Consultant, 40,* 1377.

American Academy of Pediatrics. (2000). *2000 Red book: Report on infectious diseases* (24th ed.). Elk Grove Village, IL: American Academy of Pediatrics.

American Psychiatric Association. (1994). *Diagnostic and statistical manual of mental disorders* (4th ed.). Washington, DC: American Psychiatric Association.

Chin, J. (2000). *Control of communicable diseases manual* (17th ed.). Washington, DC: The American Public Health Association.

Drake, L. A., Dinehart, S. M., Farmer, E. R., et al. (1996). Guidelines of care for superficial mycotic infections of the skin: Tinea corporis, tinea cruris, tinea faciei, tinea manuum, and tinea pedis. Guidelines/Outcomes Committee. American Academy of Dermatology. *Journal of American Academy of Dermatology, 34,* 282–286.

Fitzpatrick, T., Johnson, R., & Wolff, K. (1996). *Color atlas and synopsis of clinical dermatology: Common and serious diseases* (3rd ed.). New York: McGraw-Hill Inc.

Goldstein, A., Smith, K., Ives, T., & Goldstein, B. (2000). Mycotic infections. Effective management of conditions involving the skin, hair, and nails. *Geriatrics, 55*(5), 40–42, 45–47, 51–52.

Kaplan, D. L. (2000). Dermclinic: Cutaneous conundrums, dermatologic disguises. *Consultant, 40,* 989–993, 996–998, 1000.

Monroe, J. R. (1999). Dermatology digest. This child has ringworm—or does he? *JAAPA/Journal of the American Academy of Physician Assistants, 12*(4), 48, 50, 52.

Noble, S. L., Forbes, R. C., & Stature, P. L. (1998). *American Family Physician, 58*(1), 163–174.

Nopper, A., Markus, R., & Esterly, N. (1998). When it's not ringworm: Annular lesions of childhood. *Pediatric Annals, 27*(3), 136–148.

Robinson, D., Kidd, P., & Rogers, K. M. (2000). *Primary care across the lifespan.* St. Louis: Mosby.

Rupke, S. J. (2000). Fungal skin disorders. *Primary Care: Clinics in Office Practice, 27* (2), 407–421.

Steele, R. W. (1997). Sizing up the risks of pet-transmitted diseases. *Contemporary Pediatrics, 14*(9), 43–44, 49, 54.

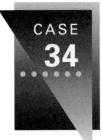

A 55-year-old man with LUQ abdominal pain, nausea, and vomiting

SCENARIO

Ralph Turner is a 55-year-old Indian man who presents with c/o severe sharp LUQ abdominal pain associated with nausea and vomiting. He states the pain started approximately 2 days ago after he ate chili. The pain seems to come on as a spasm/cramping that is quite sharp, then either goes away or turns into a burning sensation that goes to the chest. He states that during the past 7 years he has taken Mylanta for indigestion, and it tends to offer some relief, but it is not helping now.

● TENTATIVE DIAGNOSES

Based on the information provided, what are potential differential diagnoses?

● HISTORY

What are significant questions in the history for Ralph? What are the key points to cover on the review of systems?

● PHYSICAL ASSESSMENT

What are the significant portions of the physical examination that should be completed for Ralph?

● DIFFERENTIAL DIAGNOSES

What are the significant positive and negative data that support or refute your diagnoses for Ralph?

● DIAGNOSTIC TESTS

Based on the history and physical assessment, what, if any, diagnostic testing would you do? Include your rationale for the testing.

● DIAGNOSIS

What diagnoses do you determine as being appropriate for Ralph?

● THERAPEUTIC PLAN

1. *What are lifestyle changes that are recommended for this illness?*
2. *What are the pharmacological treatments for this condition?*
3. *What side effects of the regimen would you warn Ralph about?*
4. *What suggestions would you make for Ralph and his family in terms of family stresses?*
5. *When should Ralph return for follow-up?*
6. *What are resources for the NP and Ralph related to his condition?*

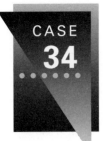

TUTORIAL

A 55-year-old man with LUQ abdominal pain, nausea, and vomiting

SCENARIO

Ralph Turner is a 55-year-old Indian man who presents with c/o severe sharp LUQ abdominal pain associated with nausea and vomiting. He states the pain started approximately 2 days ago after he ate chili. The pain seems to come on as a spasm/cramping that is quite sharp, then either goes away or turns into a burning sensation that goes to the chest. He states that during the past 7 years he has taken Mylanta for indigestion, and it tends to offer some relief, but it is not helping now.

● TENTATIVE DIAGNOSES

What are the potential diagnoses you have identified based on the scenario presented?

DIAGNOSIS	RATIONALE
Gastric cancer	Ralph presents with abdominal pain, nausea, and vomiting. These may be presenting signs of gastric cancer.
PUD	Ralph describes abdominal pain that comes and goes, with a burning sensation in his chest. An antacid offers some relief. These are characteristic symptoms of PUD
Angina	Angina can present as indigestion and burning in the chest.
Cholecystitis	Ralph presents with nausea, vomiting, and chest discomfort after eating spicy foods. These symptoms could be caused by cholecystitis.
Pancreatitis	Nausea and vomiting along with abdominal pain are symptoms of possible pancreatitis.
GERD	Indigestion and burning in the chest are common symptoms seen with GERD.

(continued)

DIAGNOSIS   RATIONALE
••

Gastritis	Gastritis is nonspecific diagnosis that refers to inflammation of the mucosa. It can occur after taking NSAIDs or after heavy alcohol ingestion.

● HISTORY

What are significant questions in the history for Ralph? Is there any information that is missing from this history?

REQUESTED DATA   DATA ANSWER
••

REQUESTED DATA	DATA ANSWER
Allergies	None known.
Current medications	Ibuprofen (Advil)/acetaminophen (Tylenol) prn. Antacid (Mylanta) 1–2 tablespoons every 3–4 hours. Fluoxetine (Prozac), 20 mg QD Laxative as needed.
Surgery/transfusions	Appendectomy at age 15.
Medical history/ hospitalizations/ fractures/injuries/ accidents	+ depression, controlling anger. Gastritis. Measles. Chickenpox.
Immunizations	TB last year negative. Tetanus, 6 years ago.
Appetite/wt loss/gain	Spontaneous wt loss of 10 lbs in last 3 weeks.
24-hour diet recall	B: cold cereal or coffee. L: sandwich, usually tuna, bologna, or peanut butter. Beer or glass of soda. D: Chili, cole slaw, soda or beer.
Relationship of indigestion/abdominal pain to eating	Usually symptoms start 2–3 hours after eating. "If I rest after eating the symptoms do not seem as bad."
Sleeping	No problems falling asleep. Sleeps 6 hours at night. Sometimes has indigestion at night, too. Antacid helps.
Social history	Tobacco: 1½ packs per day. Alcohol: ~ a 12-pack of beer/day shared with friends. Caffeine: 7–8 cups coffee or soda/day. Drugs: none. Exercise: rarely.

(continued)

REQUESTED DATA   DATA ANSWER

Family history	Father: alive, unsure of health, history of alcohol abuse. Mother: 59, deceased stroke. Siblings: 2 sisters, 1 good health, 1 with psychiatric problems; 1 brother, healthy.
Relationship with family	Has girlfriend. She recently had a baby. He finds this very stressful because he is unemployed and has no income, except for working on cars in the neighborhood. Lost his job about 3 months ago. Feels like all he and his girlfriend do now is shout at each other.
Home	Lives in one-bedroom apartment.
Last complete PE	2 years ago when he started a new job.
Income/insurance	Makes about $1,200/month. Health insurance and unemployment will end in 3 months.
Depression history: How do you usually handle stress?	Strike out at those around me.
Have you ever thought of harming yourself?	No.
Describe how you feel now	I feel sad, down in the dumps, and I want to get a job. In 3 months I won't be able to support myself.
CAGE questionnaire	States he sometimes feels guilty about how much beer he drinks, especially when he yells at his girlfriend. He gets angry when she suggests he should not drink as much now since he is a father. Usually does not drink in the morning. After a bad hangover he sometimes feels he should not drink since he feels so bad, but never seems to follow through.

What are the key points on the review of systems?

SYSTEM REVIEWED DATA ANSWER

General	Overall right now feels stressed and not healthy.
GI	Denies black, tarry, or bloody stools or emesis. Sometimes he has constipation.
GU	Denies problems urinating, burning or frequency. No problem with emptying bladder.

(continued)

SYSTEM REVIEWED DATA ANSWER

Lungs   Denies SOB, except when going up lots of steps or carrying the
                     baby. Has a "typical" morning smoker's cough.

Cardiac   Denies sweating, radiation of pain into arm or neck. No SOB or
                     palpitations.

● PHYSICAL ASSESSMENT

What are the significant portions of the physical examination that should be completed for Ralph?

SYSTEM	RATIONALE	FINDINGS
Vital signs	Provides baseline data.	BP, 110/70 mm Hg; HR, 96 bpm; RR, 28; T, 97.8°F; Ht, 5'10"; Wt, 175 lbs.
General appearance/skin	Provides overall indication of status.	Neatly dressed, well developed, anxious. Hair thinning, dull, pale in color. Turgor fair, no jaundice.
Mouth	Gives indication of hydration status.	Lips dry, cracked, oral mucosa pale pink. Tongue dry and tender to touch.
Lungs	Baseline data, checking for fluid or COPD, asthma signs.	CTA.
Heart	Need to evaluate because symptoms are similar to angina. Provides baseline data.	S1, S2 WNL. No MRG.
Abdomen	Area where pain is occurring. Important to conduct complete, thorough exam of abdomen, checking for pain, masses, organomegaly, and peritoneal symptoms.	5-cm well-healed scar RLQ. No venous distention or striae. Symmetrical without obvious bulging. No visible peristalic waves. High pitched, hyperactive BS, no bruits or venous hums. Liver percussed ~ 13 cm in MCL. C/o tenderness in epigastric area. Negative Murphy's sign, psoas and rebound.
Rectal	Evaluate for hemorrhoids, get stool specimen to check for blood.	Small noninflamed external hemorrhoids. No rashes or irritation. No tenderness on palpation. Normal sphincter function. Prostate smooth. No masses. Hard brown stool.

● DIFFERENTIAL DIAGNOSES

What are the significant positive and negative findings that support or refute your diagnoses for Ralph?

DIAGNOSIS	POSITIVE DATA	NEGATIVE DATA
Gastric cancer	History of gastritis; male; age; diet; epigastric discomfort; vomiting.	No family history of cancer; no anorexia, abdominal mass, or ascites.
PUD	Age; male; gnawing, burning pain in epigastric area after meals. Heartburn; diet high in irritating foods; history of NSAID use; food helps relieve pain; smoker.	No tarry, blac or bloody stools; not awakened by pain at night
Angina	Chest discomfort, increased stress, age, male, smokes.	Pain not relieved by rest; no FH; no radiation; diaphoresis.
Cholecystitis	Age; low-fiber, high-fat diet; indigestion; nausea.	No peritonitis; no obesity; gender; no RUQ pain or shoulder pain; negative Murphy's sign.
Pancreatitis	Alcohol consumption; diet; nausea and vomiting, abdominal pain.	Severe abdominal pain that bores through to back, not accentuated by coughing or deep breathing; afebrile.
GERD	Indigestion relieved by antacids; alcohol intake; high-fat intake.	No increase in indigestion with lying down after meals.
Gastritis	High-alcohol intake; burning pain in abdomen.	None, nonspecific diagnosis.

● DIAGNOSTIC TESTS

Based on the history and physical examination, what, if any, diagnostic testing would you obtain?

DIAGNOSTIC TEST	RATIONALE	RESULTS	INTERPRETATION
Hgb/HCT	Able to see decrease in H/H with bleeding with hypochromic, microcytic anemia.	Hgb, 13.8 g/dL; HCT, 41%.	Low normal.

(continued)

DIAGNOSTIC TEST	RATIONALE	RESULTS	INTERPRETATION
Albumin	Helpful to determine nutritional status.	3.3 g/dL.	Low normal.
Electrolytes, liver function/ renal tests	Baseline information of renal and liver functioning, especially important with alcohol intake.	Na, 138 mEq/L; K, 4.3 mEq/L; Cl, 100 mEq/L; CO_2, 30 mEq/L; alkaline phosphatase, 123 U/L; AST, 49 U/L; ALT, 50 U/L; GGT, 45 U; BUN, 23 mg/dL; Creatinine, 0.9 mg/dL.	All WNL, except GGT, which is high, confirming high alcohol intake described in history.
Stool hemoccult	Test for occult blood.	Positive.	Some blood loss in stool.
H. pylori	Confirming presence of H. pylori is important because elimination of the bacteria is likely to cure PUD. Blood, breath, and stomach tissue tests may be performed to detect its presence. Tests highly accurate in detecting the bacteria. In this case the test was done via rapid urease test, along with the endoscopy.	Positive.	Confirms H. pylori as probable cause of PUD.
Abdominal x-ray	Noninvasive study that provides considerable information about the GI system. Helps rule out perforation. Not usually done now because of accuracy of endoscopy.	Not done.	

(continued)

DIAGNOSTIC TEST	RATIONALE	RESULTS	INTERPRETATION
Upper GI series	Used to diagnose esophageal lesions, gastric ulcers, and tumors, small bowel obstruction, and small bowel lesions. Detects 90% of peptic ulcers. Used less frequently because endoscopy allows for biopsy of the mucosa.	Not done.	
Endoscopy	Good choice if barium studies are negative. More expensive but more sensitive and specific than barium. Becoming test of choice in many settings. Can diagnose up to 95% of ulcers.	1.5-cm ulcer located in duodenal bulb.	Duodenal ulcer.
Gastric analysis	Not very helpful in clinical usefulness. Many patients may have normal acid secretion and production. Main indication for gastric analysis is if Zollinger-Ellison syndrome.	Not done.	
Serum gastrin	Useful to screen for Zollinger-Ellison syndrome.	145 pg/mL.	WNL.

● DIAGNOSES

What diagnoses do you determine as being appropriate after a review of the subjective and objective data?

- Peptic ulcer disease (PUD), duodenal
- Alcohol abuse

- Tobacco abuse
- Depression/anxiety by history

● DATA SUPPORTING THE DIAGNOSIS

Abdominal pain with indigestion, age, male, alcohol intake, increased stress, and history of NSAID use. The National Digestive Disease group recognized three major causes of PUD:

- Infection with *Helicobacter pylori*
- Use of NSAIDs
- Pathologic hypersecretory states, such as Zollinger-Ellison syndrome

● PATHOPHYSIOLOGY

Duodenal ulcers occur as a result of imbalance between the normal duodenal protective mechanisms and the amount of acid delivered to the duodenum from the stomach. The imbalances are likely caused by hypersecretory states, ingestions of NSAIDs, and most importantly H. pylori *infection. Risk factors for PUD are male gender (men are more prone to PUD development), stress, and cigarette smoking.*

● THERAPEUTIC PLAN

1. *What are factors that contribute to gastric acidity?*
   - Psychogenic factors
   - Drug therapy
   - Trauma
   - Exposure to irritants
   - Genetic factors
   - Normal aging
   - Certain illnesses (pancreatitis, hepatic disease, Crohn's disease, etc.)
   - Blood type (gastric, type A; duodenal, type O)

2. *What are issues to consider when deciding on treatment for PUD?*
   - Patient ability to afford medication
   - Education of patient and significant other
   - Visits frequently enough to monitor compliance of regimen
   - Careful assessment of outcome radiology/endoscopy results

3. *What are lifestyle changes that are recommended for PUD?*
   In the past, doctors advised people with ulcers to avoid spicy, fatty, or acidic foods. However, a bland diet is now known to be ineffective for treating or avoiding ulcers. No particular diet is helpful for most patients with ulcer. People who find certain foods irritating should avoid those foods.

Smoking has been shown to delay ulcer healing and has been linked to ulcer recurrence; thus, persons with ulcers should not smoke.

4. What are the pharmacological treatments for PUD?
The most effective therapy, according to the NIH panel, is a 2-week, triple therapy. This regimen eradicates the bacteria and reduces the risk of ulcer recurrence in 90% of people with duodenal ulcers. People with stomach ulcers that are not associated with NSAIDs also benefit from bacteria eradication.

Initial treatment for 2 weeks with:

- Tetracycline 500 mg TID
- Bismuth subsalicylate 30 mL QID
- Metronidazole 250 TID/QID
- Amoxicillin 250 to 500 mg TID/QID may be tried as an alternative treatment instead of tetracycline.

Alternative to triple therapy:

- Amoxicillin 250 to 500 mg 2 to 4 times a day or clarithromycin 500 mg TID
- Omeprazole BID for 4 weeks

A treatment (proton pump inhibitor triple therapy) that appears to have become favored, especially by gastroenterologists is:

- Omeprazole 20 mg BID for 14 days
- Metronidazole 500 mg BID for 14 days
- Clarithromycin 500 mg BID for 14 days

If this therapy is used, no treatment beyond 14 days is needed. If *H. pylori* is successfully eradicated, maintenance therapy will not be needed. If Ralph has symptoms that recur, he should be tested again for *H. pylori*. If positive, it probably is incomplete treatment, and another course of treatment should be prescribed.

Compliance is an issue because more than 60% of the doses must be completed to eradicate the organism.

5. What side effects of the regimen would you warn Ralph about?
Inform the patient of the potential side effects of the regimen (superinfection, diarrhea, constipation).

6. What suggestions would you make for Ralph and his family in terms of dealing with the family stresses?
Appropriate interventions for Ralph's' family would be:

- Education about PUD and the therapeutic management.
- Family counseling to learn ways to reduce stress and defuse potentially abusive situations.
- Have emergency telephone numbers close by, including the number for NP/MD as crisis hotlines.
- Nutritional counseling for dietary/financial concerns.

7. Where can an NP obtain more information concerning PUD?
Local library should have a lot of information concerning gastrointestinal diseases.

National Digestive Diseases Information Clearinghouse (NDDIC)
Bethesda, MD
(301) 654-3810
http://www.niddk.nih.gov/health/digest/nddic.htm

National Institute for Diabetes, Digestive and Kidney Disorders
(NIDDK)
http://www.niddk.nih.gov/health/digest/digest.htm

American College of Gastroenterology (ACG)
4900-B South 31st Street
Arlington, VA 22206-1656
Tel: (703) 820-7400
Fax: (703) 931-4520
Home page: *http://www.acg.gi.org*

American Gastroenterological Association (AGA)
National Office
7910 Woodmont Avenue, 7th Floor
Bethesda, MD 20814
Tel: (301) 654-2055
Fax: (301) 654-5920
E-mail: aga001@80l.com
Home page: http://www.gastro.org

Digestive Disease National Coalition (DDNC)
507 Capitol Court NE, Suite 200
Washington, DC 20002
Tel: (202) 544-7497
Fax: (202) 546-7105

Society of Gastroenterology Nurses and Associates, Inc. (SGNA)
401 North Michigan Avenue
Chicago, IL 60611
Tel: (312) 321-5165 or (800) 245-SGNA (7462)
Fax: (312) 321-5194
E-mail: sgna@sba.com
Home page: *http://www.sgna.org*

8. When should Ralph return for follow-up?
Management is essentially symptomatic, emphasizing drug therapy, physical rest, dietary changes, and stress reduction. The goal is to reduce gastric secretions, protect the mucosa from additional damage, and relieve pain. Providing emotional support and offering reassurance will optimize adherence to the treatment regimen. A small precentage of patients with duodenal ulcers require surgical intervention because of hemorrhage, obstruction, perforation, or intractability.

Follow up in 2 to 4 weeks to check on symptoms (response to medications, GI bleeding, adverse reaction to medications). For those with gastric ulcers, document healing with UGI barium radiograph or endoscopy: in 6 weeks for small ulcers; 12 weeks for large. This is imperative in gastric ulcers; unnecessary in uncomplicated duodenal ulcers.

REFERENCES

Childs, S., Roberts, A., Meineche-Schmidt, V., de Wit, N., & Rubin, G. (2000). The management of *Helicobacter pylori* infection in primary care: A systematic review of the literature. *Family Practice, 17*(Suppl 2), S6–S11.

Cutler, A. F., Prasad, V. M., & Santogade, P. (1998). Four-year trends in *Helicobacter pylori* IgG serology following successful eradication. *American Journal of Medicine, 105*(1), 18–20.

Ganga-Zandzou, P. S., Michaud, L., Vincent, P., Husson, M., Wizla-Deram Bure, N., Delassale, E., Turck, D., & Gottrand, F. (1999). Natural outcome of *Helicobacter pylori* infection in asymptomatic children: A two-year follow-up study. *Pediatrics 104*(2, part 1), 216–221.

Howden, C. W., & Hunt, R. H. (1998). Guidelines for the management of *Helicobacter pylori* infection. *American Journal of Gastroenterology, 93*(12), 2330–2338.

Laine, L., Knigge, K., Faigel, D., Margaret, N., Marquis, S., Vartan, F., & Fennerty, M. (1999). Fingerstick *Helicobacter pylori* antibody test: Better than laboratory serological testing? *American Journal of Gastroenterology, 94*, 3464–3467.

McManus, T. J. (2000). *Helicobacter pylori:* An emerging infectious disease. *Nurse Practitioner: American Journal of Primary Health Care, 25*(8, part 1), 40, 43–44, 47–48.

Misra, S. P., Misra, V., Dwivedi, M., Suph, P., Bhargava, V., & Jaisural, P. (1999). Evaluation of the one-minute ultra-rapid urease test for diagnosing *Helicobacter pylori. Journal of Postgraduate Medicine, 75*(881), 154–156.

National Institutes of Health. (1995). *Stomach and duodenal ulcers* (NIH publication No. 95-38). Bethesda, MD: National Digestive Diseases Information Clearinghouse.

National Institutes of Health Conference. (1994). *Helicobacter pylori* in peptic ulcer disease. *Journal of the American Medical Association, 272*, 65–69.

Navuluri, R., & Yue, S. (1999). Understanding peptic ulcer disease pharmacotherapeutics. *Nurse Practitioner, 24*(3), 128–132.

Ofman, J. J., Etchason, J., Fullerton, S., Kahn, K., & Soll, A. (1997). Management strategies for *Helicobacter pylori* seropositive patients with dyspepsia: Clinical and economic consequences. *Annals in Internal Medicine, 126*, 280–291.

Walsh, J. H., & Peterson, W. L. (1995). The treatment of *Helicobacter pylori* infection in the management of peptic ulcer disease. *New England Journal of Medicine, 333*, 984–991.

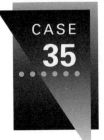

A 7-year-old boy with cough with exercise

SCENARIO

Brennen is a 7-year-old African-American boy accompanied by his mother. He presents with complaints of a nighttime cough and wheezing after playing outside. The cough and wheezing occur 2 to 3 times per week and have persisted for the past couple of weeks. Brennen's mother says the coughing generally occurs in the early morning hours.

● TENTATIVE DIAGNOSES

*What are the potential diagnoses you have identified based on this scenario? Indicate which of the following diagnoses are appropriate for Brennen. List the rationale for each possible diagnosis. What are the **red flag** diagnoses that you cannot miss?*

DIAGNOSIS	RATIONALE
1	
2	
3	
4	
5	
6	

What questions are pertinent in this case for Brennen? Select the items that you would choose to ask about Brennen? Are there any areas that are missing that would contribute important information to the case?

REQUESTED DATA   DATA ANSWER

REQUESTED DATA	DATA ANSWER
Identifying data	Date of birth: 03-03-93. Place of birth: University of Kentucky Medical Center. Parent's names and occupations: Jack, medical technologist; Cindy, registered nurse.
Chief complaint	Increase in coughing at night. In the past couple of weeks, Brennen becomes SOB and wheezy after playing outside. Mother denies chest discomfort, fever, or cold symptoms.
Current illness	Mother states the symptoms of SOB and wheezing begin right after physical activity (if the SOB and wheezing begin during activity, mother is not aware). The symptoms occur about 2–3 times per week. After resolution of symptoms, Brennen is able to play and function without difficulty. The coughing seems to occur at night when he has had difficulties that day. Mother denies chest tightness, fever, cold symptoms (runny nose or sore throat), nausea, or diarrhea. She also states no one else in the home or at school is sick at this time. His appetite and fluid intake are adequate. He denies any problems with bladder or bowels. No one in the household smokes cigarettes.
Parent's perceptions	Mother is very concerned that Brennen's cough is becoming worse. Mother also states that his father feels the same way. The cough interrupts his sleeping habits, which makes him very hard to wake up for school the next morning.
Birth history	Brennen was delivered vaginally at 34 weeks gestation. His birth weight was 5 pounds 2 ounces. He was able to go home with mother at the time of discharge. He experienced no birth trauma and had no medical problems after delivery. Mother experienced no complications during pregnancy. Mother did not smoke, drink alcohol, or take any type of medication throughout the pregnancy except prenatal vitamins. Mother experienced a long and difficult delivery.
Childhood illness	None except for strep throat 2 months ago.
Operations/ hospitalizations	At 8 months of age, Brennen was hospitalized for pneumonia and reactive airway disease. At 9 months, he was placed in the hospital with reactive airway disease. A sweat chloride test was performed, and the result was negative, ruling out cystic fibrosis.

(continued)

REQUESTED DATA   DATA ANSWER

Allergies/medications	Brennen has no allergies to medication or food. He is allergic to mold and pollen, which was confirmed by allergy testing at age 3. Brennen has periods of eczema, which seem to be the worst in early spring and early fall. Mother states the eczema appears to be getting better the older he becomes. Mother states he occasionally takes acetaminophen for fever or HA.
Nutrition	Brennen eats 3 meals a day plus an after-school snack. Mother states Brennen is not a picky eater and will eat whatever is placed in front of him. Drinks juice and milk with the occasional soft drink. Snacks are low-fat and nutritious.
Growth and development	Mother states she is unable to give exact dates for developmental milestones. Mother states that Brennen has gained weight and increased in height. Mother feels Brennen is growing and developing "like a typical 7 year old should."
Social	Development: Brennen sleeps on average 9–10 hours a night. However, lately his sleep habits have been interrupted due to his coughing. Brennen is able to communicate without difficulty. Brennen is a pleasant, well-liked first grader, who likes to attend school and has many friends. Mother states Brennen gets along with others. Relationships with parents and sister are good. Brennen is disciplined by making him sit in his room and the taking away of toys. Brennen is doing fine in school and is left-handed.
Immunizations	Brennen's immunizations are up to date and current until June 2008. He completed his DTaP, OPV, MMR, Hib, Hep B, and varicella series. His last PPD was in April 1997 and negative.
Screening	Brennen's last set of screening procedures (urine, CBC, vision, and hearing) was performed during his first grade physical. No abnormalities were noted.
Safety/injury prevention	Mother states Brennen wears his seat belt and wears a bike helmet when riding his bicycle. Brennen is currently taking swimming lessons.
Family history	Brennen lives with both parents and one sister. No health problems noted within family. Maternal and paternal grandparents are still alive and appear to be in good health.
Review of systems	General: mother believes that overall Brennen is in good health. No recent history of weight loss, weakness, or fever. Skin: no c/o redness, dryness, or sores. Nails are cut short and well trimmed. Head: no complaints of headache or dizziness. EENT: Does not wear glasses. Last eye exam (August 1999); results normal. Denies redness, itching, or watery eyes. Results of last hearing exam in June 1999 were normal. Denies

(continued)

REQUESTED DATA   *DATA ANSWER*

pain or problems with hearing. Mother states that during early spring, Brennen experiences a runny nose with clear drainage. States it is self-limiting in nature. Currently, denies runny nose, nasal congestion, or stuffiness. Denies complaint of a sore throat or hoarseness. Denies difficulty in swallowing or speaking. Last dental exam October 1999. Denies pain or stiffness in neck.

Respiratory: complaints of coughing (dry hacky) at night for past several weeks. Shortness of breath and wheezing is noted after playing outside. Mother states this starts approximate 20 minutes after playing and resolves after a dose of albuterol. Denies chest tightness. Last chest x-ray at 30 months of age. Has never had a pulmonary function test.

Cardiac: mother states no history of heart murmur.

Gastrointestinal: good appetite. Denies upset stomach after eating and late at night. No complaints of indigestion, nausea, or vomiting. Bowel habits are normal. Denies abdominal pain.

Urinary: States bladder habits normal.

Given Brennen's history, what are elements in his exam that are important for you to include with this chief complaint. Remember he is an established patient in your practice.

● PHYSICAL EXAMINATION

SYSTEM   *RATIONALE*   *FINDINGS*

System	Rationale	Findings
Vital signs		T, 98.1 °F (oral); HR, 90 bpm; RR, 20; Pulse ox., 98% on room air; Wt, 44 lbs.
General survey		Brennen is a well-groomed, healthy looking 7-year-old boy. Brennen was sitting in a chair reading a book.
Skin		Without signs of redness or excessive drying. Skin pink and moist with capillary refill < 3 seconds. No edema noted.
EENT		Bilateral TMs pearly with landmarks present. Conjunctiva pink without signs of infection or tearing. Nares pink without signs of congestion. Throat without erythema or cobblestoning. Neck supple without palpable nodes.

(continued)

SYSTEM	RATIONALE	FINDINGS
Lungs		Clear bilaterally. No evidence of wheezes, rhonchi, or rales noted. Respiratory effort easy and regular.
Heart		S1, S2 noted. Regular rate and rhythm. No murmur noted.
Abdomen		Bowel sound ×4. Soft and nontender to palpation. No masses, CVAT, or HSM.

● DIFFERENTIAL DIAGNOSES

Which of the following diagnoses make sense given the history and physical exam that you have completed?

DIAGNOSIS	POSITIVE DATA	NEGATIVE DATA
1		
2		
3		
4		
5		
6		

DIAGNOSTIC TESTS

Which of the following lab tests would you order based on Brennen's history and physical exam data? Interpret the lab results given and identify your rationale for doing each test.

DIAGNOSTIC TEST	RATIONALE	RESULTS	INTERPRETATION
O$_2$ saturation		98%	
PFT or PEFR		150, 240 after bronchodilation	

(continued)

DIAGNOSTIC TEST	RATIONALE	RESULTS	INTERPRETATION
CXR		Not done.	
Exercise challenge testing		Not done.	
CBC		Not done.	
Tissue x-ray of neck		Not done.	

DIAGNOSIS

What diagnoses do you determine as being appropriate after a review of the subjective and objective data?

Pathophysiology of diagnoses?

● THERAPEUTIC PLAN

1. *What are the key issues related to treatment for Brennen based on the identified diagnosis?*
2. *What are the goals of therapy for Brennen?*
3. *Are there any national guidelines or recommendations that pertain to Brennen?*
4. *What medications are available for treatment, and how do they work?*
5. *What is the role of exercise in the treatment for Brennen?*
6. *What education is necessary for Brennen and his mother?*
7. *When should Brennen return for follow-up?*
8. *What community resources are available for Brennen and his family?*

REFERENCES

Amirav, I., & Newhouse, M T. (1997). Metered-dose inhaler accessory devices in acute asthma: Efficacy in comparison with nebulizers: A literature review. *Archives in Pediatric Adolescent Medicine, 151,* 876–882.

Asch-Goodkin, J. (2000). Caring for diverse populations. Eliminating disparities in asthma management. *Patient Care Nurse Practitioner, 3*(5), 68–70, 72, 74.

Autio, L., & Rosenow, D. (1999). Effectively managing asthma in young and middle adulthood. *Nurse Practitioner: American Journal of Primary Health Care, 24*(1), 100–103, 105–106, 108–113.

Bisgaard, H. (2000). Role of leukotrienes in asthma pathophysiology. *Pediatric Pulmonology, 30*(2), 166–176.

Cabana, M., Ebel, B., Cooper-Patrick, L, Powe, N., Rubin, H., & Rand, C. (2000). Barriers pediatricians face when using asthma practice guidelines. *Archives in Pediatric Adolescent Medicine, 154,* 685–693.

Cohen, H. A., Neuman, I., & Nahum, H. (1997). Blocking effect of vitamin C in exercise-induced asthma. *Archives in Pediatric Adolescent Medicine, 151,* 367–370.

Feinstein, R. A., LaRussa, J., Wang-Dohlman, A., & Bartolucci, A. (1996). Screening adolescent athletes for exercise-induced asthma. *Clinical Journal of Sports Medicine, 6*(2), 119–123.

Hansen-Flaschen, J., & Schotland, H. (1998). New treatments for exercise-induced asthma, editorial. *New England Journal of Medicine, 339,* 192–193.

Hunter, J. (2000). Nurse practitioner intervention to improve the use of metered-dose inhalers by children with asthma. *Nurse Practitioner Forum, 11*(1), 32–37

Jones, J. S., Holstege, C. P., Riekse, R., White, L., & Bergquist, T. (1995). Metered-dose inhalers: Do emergency health care providers know what to teach? *Annals in Emergency Medicine. 26,* 308–311.

Kaplan, T. A. (1995). Exercise challenge for exercise-induced bronchospasm. *Physicians in Sportsmedicine, 23*(8), 47–57.

Kosseim, L. M., & Neuman, W. R (2000). Exercise-induced asthma. *Patient Care, 34*(13), 55–57, 61.

Leff, J. A., Busse, W. W., Pearlman, D., et al. (1998). Montelukast, a leukotriene-receptor antagonist, for the treatment of mild asthma and exercise-induced bronchoconstriction. *New England Journal of Medicine, 339,* 147–152.

Milgrom, H., & Taussig, L. (1999). Keeping children with exercise-induced asthma active. *Pediatrics, 104*(3), 38.

Nastasi, K. J., Heinly, T. L., & Blaiss, M. S. (1995). Exercise-induced asthma and the athlete. *Journal of Asthma, 32*(4), 249–257.

National Asthma Education and Prevention Program. (1997). *Expert Panel Report 2: Guidelines for the diagnosis and management of asthma* (NIH Publication No. 97-4051). Bethesda, MD: National Institutes of Health.

Nelson, J. A., Strauss, L., Skowronski, M., Ciuto, R., Novak, R. & McFadden. (1998). Effect of long-term salmeterol treatment on exercise-induced asthma. *New England Journal of Medicine, 339,* 141–146.

Nicol, N. H. (2000). Managing atopic dermatitis in children and adults. *Nurse Practitioner: American Journal of Primary Health Care, 25*(4), 58–59, 63–64, 69–70.

Rosenstreich, D. L., Eggleston, P., Kattan, M., et al. for the National Cooperative Inner-City Asthma Study. (1997). The role of cockroach allergy and exposure to cockroach allergen in causing morbidity among inner-city children with asthma. *New England Journal of Medicine, 336,* 1356–1363.

Rupp, N. (1996). Diagnosis and management of exercise induced asthma. *Physician and Sports Medicine, 24*(1), 77–86.

Schoene, R. B., Giboney, K., Schimmel, C., Hagen, J., Robinson, J., Sato, W., Sullivan, K. (1997). Spirometry and airway activity in track and field athletes. *Clinical Journal of Sports Medicine, 7,* 257–261.

Smith, B. W., & LaBotz, M. (1998). Pharmacologic treatment of exercise-induced asthma. *Clinical Sports Medicine, 17*(2), 343–363.

Storms, W., & Joyner, D. (1997). Update on exercise-induced asthma: A report of the Olympic Exercise Asthma Summit Conference. *Physician and Sports Medicine, 25*(3), 45–55.

Tan, R. A., & Spector, S. L. (1998). Exercise-induced asthma. *Sports Medicine, 25,* 1–6.

Umeki, S. (1994). Allergic cycle: Relationships between asthma, allergic rhinitis, and atopic dermatitis. *Journal of Asthma, 31,* 19–26.

Volcheck, G. (2000). In-office diagnosis of exercise-induced asthma. *Postgraduate Medicine, 107*(2), 48.

Weiler, J. (1996). Exercise-induced asthma: A practical guide to definitions, diagnosis, prevalence, and treatment. *Allergy and Asthma Proceedings, 17,* 315–323.

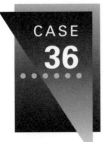

A 65-year-old woman with difficulty sleeping, shortness of breath, and palpitations

SCENARIO

Linda Dryer presents to the clinic complaining of difficulty sleeping during the past month and palpitations. She also has noted an increase in fatigue and an increase in SOB.

● TENTATIVE DIAGNOSIS

*What are the tentative diagnoses that you would identify for Linda? What are the **red flag** diagnoses that you cannot miss?*

DIAGNOSIS	RATIONALE
1	
2	
3	
4	
5	
6	

● HISTORY

What are significant questions in the history for Linda? What are the key points to cover in the review of systems?

REQUESTED DATA	DATA ANSWER
Allergies	PCN.
Medications	Digoxin, 0.125 mg QD; lisinopril, 40 mg QD., furosemide (Lasix), 40 mg BID; potassium chloride, 20 mEq QD; carvedilol (Coreg), 12.5 mg BID; amiodarone, 200 mg QD.
Surgery/transfusion	Automatic internal defibrillator placed 1 year ago
Medical history/ hospitalizations	Normal childhood illnesses; no trauma. Idiopathic cardiomyopathy diagnosed 18 months ago; sustained ventricular arrhythmia 1 year ago.
OB/GYN history	LNMP: menopausal. Last pelvic exam 11 months ago. No mammograms. SBE: approximately every other month. G3P2A1.
Social history	Tobacco: 1 pack per day for 10 years. Stopped 5 years ago. Alcohol: occasional use until 3 years ago. Caffeine: none. Drugs: none. Exercise: no regular exercise.
Family history	Father: died at 56, HTN. Mother: 94, "thyroid trouble." Brothers (2): age 58, HTN, Type 2 DM; age 55, healthy. Sister: none. Spouse: none. Children: 2 sons: age 38, good health; age 34, good health.
Social organizations	None
Marital status	Not married. Not in contact with children's father. No relationships at present.
Relationship with children	38-year-old son lives out on own, comes by often to help. 34-year-old son lives overseas.
Hobbies	Working puzzles, reading, and watching TV. Remains interested in these.
Insurance/income/home	Medicare, disabled, rents apartment.
Length of symptoms	SOB first began 2 years ago. Was doing fine until approximately 1 month ago. More SOB in past month. Difficulty sleeping

(continued)

REQUESTED DATA *DATA ANSWER*

	began approximately 2 months ago but noticeably worse past few weeks. Palpitations began approximately 1 month ago and are becoming more frequent with longer durations. No discharges from her defibrillator. No syncopal episodes or dizziness.
Diet	2-g sodium diet. Avoids caffeine. No alcohol. Appetite good; no early satiety.
Elimination	No urinary problems; frequent bowel movements 4–5/day; no diarrhea.
Sleep	Goes to bed at 10 p.m. but often unable to get to sleep for an hour or more. Awakens often during night. Sleeps on 2 pillows and has for past 2 years. No PND or cough.
Weight	Weighs self each morning, and weight has been stable past few months.
Activity	No regular exercise. Increased activity intolerance. SOB of breath with ADLs.
How has this affected daily life	Fatigued in morning and all day. Tries to nap during day but cannot. Can do only minimum of household chores, then has to stop to catch breath. Older son does most of grocery shopping now.
How do you manage stress	Worries a lot more now. Cries often. More irritable lately. Watches TV for distraction.
Any evidence of blood loss	No hemoptysis or hematemesis.
Any changes in skin	Some darkening noted. Dryer lately.

● PHYSICAL ASSESSMENT

What are the significant portions of the physical exam that should be completed for Linda?

SYSTEM *RATIONALE* *FINDINGS*

Vital signs	BP, 134/56 mm Hg; T, 98.6 °F, HR, 112 bpm; RR, 22; Ht, 5′4″; Wt, 128 lbs (stable)
General	Alert and oriented ×3; nervous; African-American female. Skin warm/very dry, color good. Extensor surface knees and elbows darker pigmentation.

(continued)

SYSTEM	RATIONALE	FINDINGS
HEENT		Normocephalic; eyes clear; sclera white; lid lag noted; PERRLA. Nasal mucosa pink, moist; no discharge, no sinus tenderness. TM gray and WNL. Oral mucosa WNL; no erythema noted in oropharnyx. Hair fine and thin. Palpable goiter. Positive bruit. JVD 10 cm. HJR noted; no LA.
Chest		Lungs, CTA = bilateral. Heart tones, S1, S2, S3; + SEM. IV/VI left sternal border radiating to axilla. RRR.
Abdomen		BS +; no masses. Liver 2 cm below costal margin with slight tenderness. Spleen nonpalpable.
Neuro		Tremor noted in hands.
Rectal		Normal. Brown stool.
Extremities		Nail ridges noted. No edema.

● DIFFERENTIAL DIAGNOSIS

What are the significant positive and negative data that support or refute your diagnosis for Linda?

DIAGNOSIS	POSITIVE DATA	NEGATIVE DATA
1		
2		
3		
4		
5		
6		
7		

● DIAGNOSTIC TESTS

Based on the history and physical assessment, what, if any, diagnostic testing would you do. Include your rationale for the tests, and interpret the results identified.

TEST	RATIONALE	RESULTS	INTERPRETATION
H/A		Hgb, 14.1 g/dL. HCt, 42%.	
Renal panel		Na, 136 mEq/L. K, 4.2 mEq/L. Cl, 102 mEq/L. CO_2, 26 mEq/L. BUN, 26 mg/dL. Creatinine, 0.9 mg/dL. Mg, 1.8 mEq/L.	
Electrocardiogram		Sinus tachycardia with rate of 120; normal intervals and axis; no acute changes; LVH.	
TSH		0.2 μU/mL.	
Free T4		27 μg/dL.	
Hemoccult		Negative	
CXR		Slightly rotated film with good penetration; soft tissue and bone unremarkable; lung fields clear, without evidence of acute infiltrate; heart size enlarged, consistent with cardiomyopathy.	

● DIAGNOSIS

What diagnosis do you determine as being appropriate for Linda?

1.

2.

Data Supporting the Diagnosis

Pathophysiology

Briefly describe the pathophysiology behind Linda's condition and symptoms.

● THERAPEUTIC PLAN

1. What treatment should be used for Linda?

2. How does this new condition affect Linda's previous cardiac problems?

3. What patient education is important for Linda?

4. When should Linda return for follow-up?

5. What resources are available for Linda?

REFERENCES

American Association of Clinical Endocrinologists (AACE). (1996). *AACE practice guidelines for evaluation and treatment of hyperthyroidism and hypothyroidism.* http://www.aace.com/clinguideindex.html.

American College of Physicians (ACP). (1998). Screening for thyroid disease: Clinical guideline, part 1. *Annals of Internal Medicine, 129,* 141–143.

Barker, R. L., Burton, J. R., & Zieve, R. D. (1999). *Principles of ambulatory medicine* (5th ed.). Baltimore: Williams & Wilkins.

Behnia, M., & Gharib, H. (1996). Primary care diagnosis of thyroid disease. *Hospital Practice, 31*(6), 121–124.

Bhattacharyya, S., & Bhattacharyya, A. (2000). Hyperthyroidism in an elderly patient [letter]. *Postgraduate Medicine Journal, 76,* 597–598.

Braverman, L. E., & Dworkin, H. J. (1997). Thyroid disease: When to screen, when to treat. *Patient Care, 31*(6), 18–20, 29–34.

Brody, M. B., & Reichard, R. A. (1995). Thyroid screening: How to interpret and apply the results. *Postgraduate Medicine, 98*(2), 54–66.

Daniels, G. H. (1995). Thyroid function tests: The pivotal role of sensitive TSH measurements. *Consultant, 35*(2), 209–213.

Dong, B. J., Houck, W. W., Gambertollio, J. G., Gee, L., White, J. R., Bubp, J. L., Greenspan, F. (1995). Bioequivalence of generic and brand name levothyroxine products in the treatment of hypothyroidism. *Journal of the American Medical Association, 277,* 1205–1213.

Gittoes, N. J., & Franklyn, J. A. (1998). Hyperthyroidism: Current treatment guidelines. *Drugs, 55,* 543–553.

Haddad, G. (1998). Is it hyperthyroidism? *Postgraduate Medicine, 104*(1), 42–59.

Heitman, B., & Irizarry, A. (1995). Hypothyroidism: Common complaints, perplexing diagnosis. *The Nurse Practitioner, 20,* 54–60.

Helfand, M., & Redfern, C. C. (1998). Screening for thyroid disease: Clinical guideline, part 2. *Annals of Internal Medicine, 129,* 144–158.

Kaiser, F. E. (1995). Thyroid function tests. *Clinics in Geriatric Medicine, 11*(2), 171–178.

Klee, G. G., & Hay, I. D. (1997). Biochemical testing of thyroid function. *Endocrinology and Metabolism Clinics of North America, 26,* 763–774.

Larson, J., Anderson, E. H., & Koslawy, M. (2000). Thyroid disease: A review for primary care. *Journal of the American Academy of Nurse Practitioners, 12*(6), 226–232.

Lazarus, J. H. (1996). Antithyroid drug treatment. *Clinical Endocrinology, 45,* 517–518.

Okamoto, T., Iihara, M., & Obara, T. (2000). Management of hyperthyroidism due to Graves' and nodular diseases. *World Journal of Surgery, 24,* 957–961.

Scripture, D. L. (1998). Case report: hyperthyroidism: an unusual case presentation. *The Nurse Practitioner, 23*(2), 50–55.

Singer, P. A., Cooper, D. S., (1995). Treatment guidelines for patients with hyperthyroidism and hypothyroidism. *Journal of the American Medical Association, 273,* 808–817.

Toft, A., & Boone, N. (2000). Thyroid disease and the heart. *Heart, 84,* 455–460.

Waldstein, S. S. (1998). Replacement and suppressive treatment with thyroid hormone. In Falk SA (Ed.), Thyroid disease endocrinology, surgery, nuclear medicine, and radiotherapy (2nd ed., pp. 475–494). New York: Lippincott-Raven.

Wallace, K., & Hofmann, M. T. (1998). Thyroid dysfunction: How to manage overt and subclinical disease in older patients. *Geriatrics, 53*(4), 32–34, 36–38, 41.

Woeber, K. (2000). Update on the management of hyperthyroidism and hypothyroidism. *Archives in Family Medicine, 9,* 743–747.

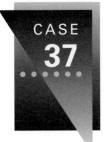

A 65-year-old man with nocturia

SCENARIO

Blake Thomas is a 65-year-old African-American man who has noticed increased nocturnal urination for approximately 4 months. He had expressed concern to his wife, who insisted he should see his health care provider.

● TENTATIVE DIAGNOSIS

*Based on the information provided so far, what are the potential differential diagnoses? What are the **red flags** you cannot miss?*

DIAGNOSIS   ***RATIONALE***

1

2

3

4

5

● HISTORY

What are the significant questions in Mr. Thomas' history? Are there any data missing that are important to his case?

REQUESTED DATA	DATA ANSWER
Allergies	None but intolerance to mycins; they cause GI upset.
Medications	None.
Surgery/transfusion/ hospitalizations/ accidents	Vasectomy 20 years ago.
Medical History	Treated for hypertension 12 years ago with a diuretic for 4 years. Lost 30 pounds, with return to normal blood pressure. No known problem since that time.
Adult illnesses	Asthma since the age of 20. Flares rarely.
Family history	Father: died at age 42, MVA. Mother: died at age 75, CVA. Sister: age 48; alive and healthy. Sister: age 51; HTN. Brother: age 59; HTN and history of prostate cancer treated with seed implants. Daughter: age 28; alive and healthy. Daughter: age 33; obese.
Appetite	Lactose intolerance. Good appetite, with weight steady last 8 years.
24-hour diet history	B: 2 cups coffee, toast w/jelly, 1 egg. L: tuna sandwich, chips, diet cola. D: steak, baked potato, salad, bread. S: popcorn.
Sleeping pattern	Sleeps well for 7 hours. Nocturia 2–3 times a night for 4 months.
Personal/social history	Works assembly line at local auto plant. Wife works as LPN (PT) in local hospital. Live in 3-bedroom house that will be paid off in 2 years. Youngest daughter is in law school, and they help with tuition.
Alcohol	Approximately 2–3 beers/weekend.
Tobacco	Smoked < 1 pack per day × 10 years; quit 20 years ago.
Caffeine	2 cups coffee/day, approximately 3 colas/week. Minimal chocolate intake.
Drugs	None.
Exercise	Walks dog approximately 0.5 miles/day.
Relationship with spouse	Married for 37 years. Loving relationship; sexual activity mutually satisfying.

(continued)

REQUESTED DATA   DATA ANSWER

REQUESTED DATA	DATA ANSWER
Community activities	Attends Methodist church weekly and involved in Sunday school. No time for other social organizations.
Income	Both Mr. and Mrs. Thomas are working with income adequate to meet their needs and financial obligations. Both have life insurance through their work for $5,000. In addition, Mrs. Thomas has a $25,000 life insurance policy, and Mr. Thomas has a life insurance policy for $50,000. Both policies' premiums have been paid.
Home	Three-bedroom home of 1700 sq. ft. to be paid off in 2 years.
Safety measures	Smoke detectors (4) in home. No CO detectors; a rifle locked in gun cabinet and shells locked in closet. Hot water heater at 135 °F.
Coping measures	Family, friends, strong faith, and prayer.
Have you ever had urgency, hematuria, urinary retention, incontinence, hesitancy, decreased caliber of urinary stream, dysuria, discharge, retention?	Occasional back pain related to job; occasional urgency; no incontinence; some hesitancy; decreased caliber of stream. No dysuria, hematuria, urgency, or discharge.
Last dental exam?	Approximately 8 months ago.
Last eye exam?	Wears bifocals and last exam < 1 year ago.

● PHYSICAL ASSESSMENT

What are the significant portions of the physical examination that should be performed? What is the rationale for doing the parts of the exam identified?

SYSTEM   RATIONALE   FINDINGS

SYSTEM	RATIONALE	FINDINGS
Vital signs		BP, 138/88 mm Hg; RR, 18; HR, 90; Ht, 68"; Wt, 168 lbs.
General appearance		Alert, NAD. Skin warm and dry.
HEENT		Normocephalic. Cerumen in left ear. TMs clear. Weber and Rinne WNL. Fundi benign.

(continued)

SYSTEM	RATIONALE	FINDINGS
Lymphatics		No cervical or inguinal LA.
Lungs		CTA.
Heart		RRR at 84; S1, S2 WNL; no MRG.
Abdomen		Soft; flat; no HSM; no tenderness. BS active all 4 quadrants; no aortic, renal, or iliac bruits.
GU		Uncircumcised male; no signs of infection noted. No lesions or masses.
Rectal		Prostate smooth, asymmetric, no nodules, induration. Slightly enlarged.
Neurological assessment		Alert and oriented × 3; appropriate speech and dress. Gait intact. CN II–XII intact. DTRs 2+. Strength and sensation intact.
Musculoskeletal		No joint deformities. Full ROM all joints.
Extremities		No lesions, edema. Peripheral pulses equal bilaterally.

● DIFFERENTIAL DIAGNOSES

What are the significant positive and negative data that support or refute your diagnoses for Mr. Thomas?

DIAGNOSIS	POSITIVE DATA	NEGATIVE DATA
1		
2		
3		
4		
5		

● DIAGNOSTIC TESTS

Based on the history and physical examination, what, if any, diagnostic tests would you order? Include your rationale and interpretation.

DIAGNOSTIC TEST	RATIONALE	RESULTS	INTERPRETATION
Fasting blood sugar		92 mg/dL.	
Complete metabolic panel		Glucose, 92 mg/dL. BUN, 21 mg/dL. Creatinine, 1.0 mg/dL. BUN/creatinine ratio: 11. Na, 143 mEq/L. K, 4.4 mEq/L. Cl, 101 mEq/L. CO_2, 25 mEq/L. Calcium, 10.1 mg/dL. Protein, total 8.3 g/dL. Albumin, 4.7 g/dL. Globulin, 3.9 g/dL. Bilirubin total, 1.3 mg/dL. Alkaline phosphatase, 89. AST, 40 U/L. ALT, 42 U/L.	
Lipids		Triglycerides, 245 mg/dL. Cholesterol (total), 204 mg/dL. HDL, 47 mg/dL. LDL, 128 mg/dL. Chol/HDLC ratio, 4.77.	
CBC		WBC, 5.9 1000/mm³ RBC, 5.06 million/mm³. Hgb, 15/8 g/dL. Hct, 46.3%. MCV, 92.1 μm³. MCH, 31.5. MCHC, 34.2%. RDW, 11.8. Platelets, 236 μL.	
Fecal occult blood testing		Negative.	
Urinalysis		Appearance, clear. Bilirubin, negative. Glucose, negative. Ketones, negative. Nitrite, negative. Blood, negative.	

(continued)

DIAGNOSTIC TEST	RATIONALE	RESULTS	INTERPRETATION
		pH 5.2. Protein, negative. SG, 1.018. Urobilinogen, negative.	
Electrocardiogram		NSR at rate of 92; normal intervals and axis; no acute changes.	
PSA		6.8 μg/L	
AUA-SI (American Urological Association Symptom Index)		5.	

● DIAGNOSES

What diagnoses do you determine are appropriate for Mr. Thomas?

Data Supporting the Diagnoses

● THERAPEUTIC PLAN

1. *What is the plan that you will develop for Mr. Thomas related to discussing the results of his physical examination?*

2. *What is the plan that you will develop for Mr. Thomas related to his diagnostic tests?*

3. *What is the plan that you will develop for Mr. Thomas related to the concern about ruling out prostate cancer?*

4. *What health promotion measures would you suggest to Mr. Thomas?*

5. *How do you think the potential diagnosis of prostate cancer might affect Mr. Thomas and his family?*

6. *What community resources might be of assistance to Mr. Thomas and his family?*

American Prostate Society
7188 Ridge Road
Hanover, MD 21076
(410) 859-3735
www.ameripros.org
American Cancer Society (local): *www.acs.org*
American Cancer Society (National): 800-ICS-2345
For general medical/health information on the Internet:
www.webmd.com
www.oncolink.upenn.edu

REFERENCES

Bates, B. (1999). *Bates' guide to physical examination and history taking* (pp. 722–728). Philadelphia: Lippincott Williams & Wilkins.

Catalona, W. J., Oesterling, J. E., & Resnick, M. I. (1998). Current recommendations on PSA testing. *Patient Care, 32*(9), 59–83.

Catalona, W. J., Resnick, M. I., & Williams, R. D. (1999). Treating early prostate cancer: Difficult decisions abound. *Patient Care, 33* 82–105.

Cookson, M. S., & Smith, J. A. (2000). PSA testing: Update on diagnostic tools. *Consultant, 40*(4), 670–676.

Heil, B. J. (1999). Treatment of benign prostatic hyperplasia. *Journal of the American Academy of Nurse Practitioners, 11,* 303–310.

Morton, R. A., & Witte, M. N. (1998). Prostate cancer: Who's at risk? *Patient Care, 32*(10). 150–158.

Potter, S. R., & Partin, A. W. (2000). What you can learn from percent free PSA testing. *Patient Care, 34*(3). 94–108.

Professional guide to signs & symptoms. (1996). (2nd ed.). Springhouse, PA: Springhouse Publishers, 98, 739, 741, 745, 747.

Stutzman, R. E. (1999). Bladder outlet obstruction. In L. R. Barker, J. R. Burton, & P. D. Zieve (Eds.), *Principles of ambulatory medicine* (pp. 605–607). Baltimore: Williams & Wilkins.

U.S. Preventive Services Task Force. (1996). *Guide to clinical preventive services* (2nd ed., p. 95). Alexandria, VA: Williams & Wilkins.

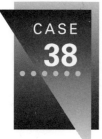

CASE
38

A 62-year-old woman with a facial rash and a red eye

SCENARIO

Saundra Wright is a 62-year-old Caucasian woman who complains of a painful red eye. She first noticed the red eye on Sunday, with a few red bumps on her face 1 or 2 days later. Since then the rash has spread to the tip of her nose. Several of the spots under her eye look like blisters and are crusting over. Her eye continues to hurt, and she complains of blurry vision.

● TENTATIVE DIAGNOSIS

Based on the information provided so far, what are the potential differential diagnoses?

● HISTORY

What are significant questions in the history for Saundra? What are the key points to cover in the review of systems?

● PHYSICAL ASSESSMENT

What are the significant portions of the physical examination that should be completed for Saundra?

● DIFFERENTIAL DIAGNOSES

What are the significant positive and negative data that support or refute your diagnoses for Saundra?

● DIAGNOSTIC TESTS

Based on the history and physical assessment, what, if any, diagnostic testing would you do? Include your rationale for the testing.

● DIAGNOSIS

What diagnoses do you determine as being appropriate for Saundra?

● THERAPEUTIC PLAN

1. *What are the goals of management for this condition?*
2. *What treatment would you begin immediately for Saundra?*
3. *What referral should be made immediately for Saundra?*
4. *What self-care measures can you recommend for Saundra?*
5. *Saundra complains of severe pain in her eye and face. What explanation would you give her regarding the pain, and what treatment would you recommend?*
6. *Saundra's husband has heard this rash is contagious. What explanation and teaching would you give him concerning this rash?*
7. *Are there any sequelae that may occur as a result of this rash?*
8. *What resources are available for the NP and Saundra?*

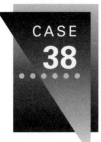

CASE
38

TUTORIAL

A 62-year-old-woman with a facial rash and a red eye

SCENARIO

Saundra Wright is a 62-year-old Caucasian woman who complains of a painful red eye. She first noticed the red eye on Sunday, with a few red bumps on her face 1 or 2 days later. Since then the rash has spread to the tip of her nose. Several of the spots under her eye look like blisters and are crusting over. Her eye continues to hurt, and she complains of blurry vision.

● TENTATIVE DIAGNOSES

What are the potential diagnoses you have identified based on the above scenario?

DIAGNOSIS	RATIONALE
Contact dermatitis	Saundra could have been exposed to a substance, and having a subsequent dermatologic reaction to it.
Herpes simplex	Herpes simplex presents with vesicles, and can occur on the face.
Herpes zoster	Herpes zoster presents with painful vesicles.
Impetigo	A bacterial infection which can affect the face.
Conjunctivitis, uveitis	Saundra's red eye could be caused by a viral or bacterial infection, based on his complaints of a painful, red eye.
FB of the eye	Saundra's complaint of a painful, red eye could be caused by a FB in the eye.

● HISTORY

1. What are significant questions in the history for Saundra?

REQUESTED DATA   *DATA ANSWER*

REQUESTED DATA	DATA ANSWER
Allergies	NKDA
Current medications	Indapamide (Lozol) 2.3 mg day for HTN Many types of vitamins Albuterol (Proventil) MDI 2 puffs QID as needed Beclomethasone (Beclovent) 2 puffs BID
Surgery	Thoracotomy 8 years ago for lung cancer Numerous bronchoscopies for radiation/evaluation of lung cancer
Past medical history and hospitalizations/ fractures/injuries/ accidents	Childhood: chicken pox, mumps, measles HTN for 15 years, treated with diuretics, well controlled Diagnosed with large cell lung cancer in 1995.
Appetite	Good. Lost approximately 25 lbs. after initial treatment of lung cancer, then started eating again—wanted to make sure he was not emaciated. Gained back about 40 lbs.
24 hour diet history	B: eggs, bacon, toast L: sandwich, with coffee or soda D: meat, vegetable, bread, dessert S: popcorn, desserts
Social history	Tobacco: smoked 2½ ppd for 40 years Alcohol: drinks approx 2–4 beers/day (12 oz) Drugs: denies Caffeine: drinks 3–6 cups of coffee, rarely soda Exercise: no regular
Family history	Father: died at 48, DM Mother: died 76, obesity, heart problems Siblings: sister, died at 58, has been in poor health for a long time Children: 6 children, 3 girls—all smoke, 3 boys—2 smoke. All healthy except 1 boy with alcohol abuse, and vocal cord nodules. Spouse: 1st husband deceased of lung cancer, 2nd HTN, otherwise healthy.
Income/insurance/home	Works full time at Ford assembly plant, 6 days/week. Insurance carried through employer. Owns home.
Present illness: has he put anything on rash, what makes it better or worse, exposure to any chemical or irritant	Eye redness began on Sunday (now Wed). Then rash began 1–2 days later. Tried hydrocortisone, with little effect. No itching. Rash becoming more painful and irritating as the days go on. No previous rash like this in past. No exposure to chemicals or change in routine or medicines. Wife does not have a rash. Denies any problems with eyes before rash began.

2. What are the key points on the review of systems?

SYSTEM REVIEWED	DATA ANSWER
General	Feels fatigued much of the time. Usually takes a nap after work.
Skin	Pale skin. No other lesions anywhere else, just on face.
HEENT	Has noticed blurry vision since rash. Has reading glasses for near vision.
Lungs	Coughs frequently. Takes antibiotics frequently for infection. Some SOB with activity.
Cardiac	Unremarkable, denies chest pain or discomfort.
GI/GU	Unremarkable.

● PHYSICAL EXAMINATION

What are the significant portions of the physical examination that should be completed for Saundra?

SYSTEM	RATIONALE	FINDINGS
Vital signs	Provides baseline	BP, 138/84; HR 96; RR 20; T 99.2 Ht., 5'4"; Wt., 185 lbs.
General appearance/ skin	Provides overall description of patient	Pale, obese female sitting on exam table with red rash visible on tip of nose and below eye Rt. Papular/vesicular rash, erythematous bases with pustules and crusts of 1 or 2 lesions. No honey colored discharge. No involvement of left eye or side of face. Rash in somewhat linear pattern around Right side of face into hair line

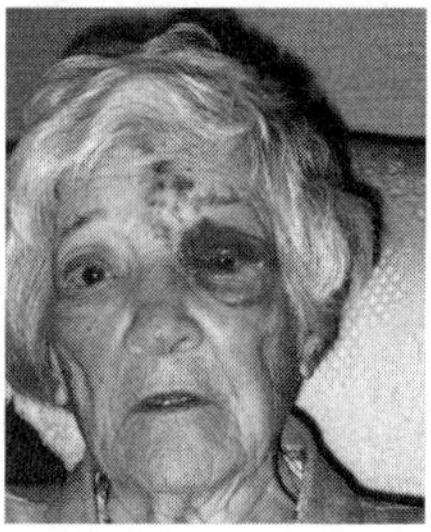

FIGURE 38–1. Herpes zoster (shingles).

(continued)

SYSTEM	RATIONALE	FINDINGS
HEENT	Need to evaluated eye, lymph nodes	VA: 20/60 OD, 20/30 OS Rt. Eye with injected conjuctiva, tearing. Rt. Upper eyelid edematous. Photophobia. No FB visible with lid eversion. Fluorescein revealed no corneal abrasions. Unable to complete fundus exam due to light sensitivity.
Lungs	Given PMH of lung cancer, need to obtain check pulmonary status	Clear, with occasional expiratory wheezes in posterior chest
Heart	Baseline data	RRR, no MRG

● DIFFERENTIAL DIAGNOSES

What are the significant positive and negative findings that support or refute your diagnoses for Saundra?

DIAGNOSIS	POSITIVE DATA	NEGATIVE DATA
Contact dermatitis	Papular/vesicular erythematous rash on face.	No history of contact with chemical irritants, or change in medication/exposure.
Herpes simplex	Papular/vesicular erythematous rash on face.	No previous history of herpes simplex, no contact with anyone who had herpes simplex, no disseminated pattern of distribution.
Herpes zoster		No prodromal symptoms.
Impetigo	Papular/vesicular erythematous rash on face, involving one side of face only/dermatome–opthalmic branch of the trigeminal nerve, painful rash, involvement of eye: conjunctivitis, photophobia, over 50 years of age, history of chicken pox, depressed immunity secondary to lung cancer.	No honey colored discharge, not a child, no crowded living condition, poor hygiene.

(continued)

DIAGNOSIS	POSITIVE DATA	NEGATIVE DATA
Conjunctivitis, uveitis	Red, injected painful conjunctiva with photosensitivity.	Red eye was prodrome for rash, no exposure to viral or bacterial conjunctivitis.
FB of eye	Red, injected painful conjunctiva with photosensitivity.	No recollection of FB going into eye. No FB visible.

● DIAGNOSTIC TESTS

Based on the history and physical examination, what, if any, diagnostic testing would you obtain?

DIAGNOSTIC TEST	RATIONALE	RESULTS	
Tzanck smear	Smear that confirms presence of herpes zoster.	Smear shows giant and or multinucleated epidermal cells.	Herpes zoster
Varicella zoster virus (VZV) antigen detection	Direct fluorescent antibody (DFA) detects VZV antigen in smear of vesicle base or fluid. Specific and very sensitive.	Not done.	
Viral culture	Isolation of VZV.	Not done.	
Dermatopathology	Lesional skin biopsy which shows vesicle formation and giant or multinucleated keratinocytes.	Not done.	

● DIAGNOSES

What diagnoses do you determine as being appropriate after a review of the subjective and objective data?

Herpes Zoster (Shingles) of the ophthalmic branch of the trigeminal nerve

Large cell cancer of the lung

Obesity
Alcohol dependence

Data Support

Progression of rash from papules/vesicles initially changing to crusts/pustules. Dermatome involvement of right side of face including eye, tip of nose, cheek and into hairline (ophthalmic branch of trigeminal nerve), decreased immunity due to lung cancer, age > 50, painful rash, eye symptoms

● PATHOPHYSIOLOGY

Reactivation of the varicella-zoster virus that has been dormant in a dorsal root gan-glion. At any point there after latent virus can be reactivated and produce the char-acteristic rash. Over 66% of patients with herpes zoster are over 50 years of age.

● THERAPEUTIC PLAN

1. *What are the goals of management for HZ?*
   • The goals of management include
     ○ minimize pain
     ○ reduce viral shedding
     ○ speed crusting of lesions and healing
     ○ ease physical, psychological and emotional discomfort
     ○ prevent viral dissemination or other complications
     ○ prevent or minimize postherpetic neuralgia (PHN)

2. *What treatment would you start Saundra on immediately?*
   Use of antiviral agents within 72 hours helps decrease the duration of the acute pain, accelerates the healing of the lesions, and may decrease the in-cidence of PHN. Choices of antiviral agents include:

   • Acyclovir (Zovirax) 800mg 5× day for 7 to 10 days
   • Valacylovir (Valtrex) 1000 mg TID for 7 days
   • Famciclovir (Famvir) 500mg TID × 7 days

   The use of cortisone is controversial. It is felt by some that use of Pred-nisone early in the course of HZ may reduce the likelihood of PHN, how-ever, this has not been shown in controlled studies (Fitzpatrick, 1997). Saundra was started on Famiclovir (Famvir)

3. *What referral should be made for Saundra immediately?*
   Since Saundra has eye involvement, referral to an ophthalmologist is im-perative. It is also a good idea to refer Saundra back to his oncologist, since he can be considered immunosuppressed and may need IV acyclovir and recombinant interferon to prevent dissemination of the herpes zoster.

4. *What self-care measures can you recommend for Saundra?*

Application of moist dressings (water, saline, Burow's solution) may be soothing and alleviate pain. Topical antibacterial ointment promotes healing and prevents secondary bacterial infection as the lesions begin to crust (Barker, 1995).

5. *Saundra complains of severe pain in her eye and face. What explanation would you give her regarding the pain, and what treatment would you recommend?*
The HZ virus gains access to the body during an episode of chicken pox. The HZ virus remains dormant in the sensory ganglia, until a person's immunity decreases. The virus then replicates, and travels down the sensory nerve causing pain in the location of the nerve, and then the painful skin lesions follow. Pain is caused by nerve inflammation, nerve infection during the acute reactivation, and then nerve inflammation and scarring with post-herpetic neuralgia (PHN) (Fitzpatrick, 1997).

Early control of pain is indicated with narcotic analgesics. Failure to manage pain can result in failure to sleep, fatigue and depression.

6. *Saundra's husband has heard that this rash is contagious. What explanation and teaching would you give him concerning this rash?*
Herpes zoster itself does not cause HZ or shingles in exposed individuals. However, since HZ is caused by the varicella virus, people who have not had chicken pox are susceptible to transmission of the virus via the airborne route. Steve should avoid being around people who are immunosuppressed, such as those on chemotherapy or persons with +HIV status.

7. *Are there any sequalae that may occur as a result of this rash?*
HZ can cause chronic problems. This is also classified as PHN, characterized by burning, ice-burning, shooting or lacinating pain which can last weeks, months and years after the skin involvement has resolved. Antidepressants may be helpful for chronic pain of HZ. Capsaicin cream also may be helpful. Topical analgesics as well as nerve blocks may assist in the reduction of pain.

If the eye is involved, as in Saundra's case, there may be a permanent loss of vision depending on the extent of the lesions. Ramsay Hunt syndrome is HZ affecting the facial and auditory nerves so that facial palsy occurs, usually within 2 weeks of the initial outbreak. Tinnitus, vertigo or deafness may result (Barker, 1999).

REFERENCES

Alper, B., & Lewis, P. (2000). Does treatment of acute herpes zoster prevent or shorten postherpetic neuralgia? *Journal of Family Practice, 49* (3), 255–264.

Barker, R., Burton, J., & Zieve, P. (1999). *Principles of ambulatory medicine*, (5th ed.). Baltimore, MD: Williams & Wilkins.

Brunton, S. (1995). Herpes Zoster: A management update. *Family Practice Recertification, 17*(9), 14–25.

Colin, J., Presant, O., Cochener, B., Lescale, O., Rolland, B., & Hoang-Xuan, T. (2000). Comparison of the efficacy and safety of valaciclovir and acyclovir for the treatment of herpes zoster ophthalmicus. *Ophthalmology, 107* (8), 1507–1511.

Fitzpatrick, T., Johnson, R., Wolff, K., Polano, M., & Suurmond, D. (1997). *Color Atlas and Synopsis of Clinical Dermatology,* (3rd ed.). New York: McGraw Hill.

Landow, K. (2000). Acute and chronic herpes zoster: an ancient scourge yields to timely therapy. Symposium: Fourth of four articles on troublesome skin problems. *Postgraduate Medicine, 107*(7), 107– 108, 113–114, 117–118.

Lee, V. K., Simpkins, L. (2000). Herpes zoster and postherpetic neuralgia in the elderly. *Geriatric Nursing: American Journal of Care for the Aging, 21*(3): 132–137.

Newman, K., & Herman, L. (2000). Dermatology digest. Tingling rash in an older man . . . herpes zoster ophthalmicus. *Journal of the American Academy of Physician Assistants, 13*(8): 21–22, 75–76.

Reifsnider, E. (1997). Common adult infectious skin conditions. *Nurse Practitioner: American Journal of Primary Health Care, 22*(11), 17–18, 20, 23–24.

Saunders, C. S. (1999). Case & comment. Neck pain and arm weakness in an older woman. *Patient Care Nurse Practitioner, 2*(9): 54–55.

Shiuey, Y., Ambah, B., & Adamis, A. (2000). A randomized, double-masked trial of topical ketorolac versus artificial tears for treatment of viral conjunctivitis. *Ophthalmology, 107* (8), 1512–1517.

Stankus, S., Dlugopolski, M., & Packer, D. (2000). Management of herpes zoster (shingles) and postherpetic neuralgia. *American Family Physician, 61*(8), 2437–2444, 2447–2448.

Wu, C., Marsh, A., & Dworkin, R. (2000). The role of sympathetic nerve blocks in herpes zoster and postherpetic neuralgia. *Pain, 87*(2), 121–129.

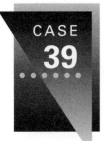

A 65-year-old man with elevated blood pressure

SCENARIO

Denzel Armstrong is an obese 65-year-old African-American man who is new to the clinic. His previous physician retired 1 year ago, and Mr. Armstrong is now seeking care for his hypertension. He complains of getting up frequently at night to urinate lately. His only medical problem is high blood pressure, for which he takes hydrochlorothiazide 25 mg/day.

● TENTATIVE DIAGNOSES

Based on Mr. Armstrong's presentation, what are your tentative differential diagnoses? What are red flags that you cannot miss?

DIAGNOSIS	RATIONALE
1	
2	
3	
4	
5	

● HISTORY

What questions do you want to ask Mr. Armstrong to assist you in developing a diagnosis?

REQUESTED DATA   DATA ANSWER

REQUESTED DATA	DATA ANSWER
Allergies	None.
Medications	HCTZ, 25 mg QD; albuterol MDI, 2 puffs QID PRN; denies OTC medications.
Childhood diseases	Measles; chicken pox.
Immunizations	Yearly influenza vaccine. Can not remember last tetanus shot. Had negative TB test at age 20 (military). No pneumonia vaccination.
Surgery	None.
Transfusions/ Hospitalizations	None.
Fractures/injuries	None.
Adult illness	Bronchitis every winter.
Last physical exam	One year ago with retired MD. BP was okay using medicine. No rectal exam.
Dental exam	2 years ago.
Vision exam	2 years ago. Denies blurring, wears reading glasses.
Weight	Denies change in weight.
Appetite	Hungry all the time; has a sweet tooth.
Thirst	C/o of dry mouth, drinks pop, lemonade, and sweetened ice tea all day long (10–15 glasses).
Urination	C/o increased urination and having to urinate several times at night. Denies dysuria, hematuria, foul odor, or cloudy urine. States this has occurred over the past year and worsened in the past 2 weeks. Denies prior UTI or STD; no history of prostate exam or problems. Worried that he has "sugar" diabetes because of all the urination.
Past history of HTN	Diagnosed with HTN 12 years ago, on HCTZ for past 4 years. Has BP checked at senior center 2–3 times each year, and it has been good. One BP was 160/96.

(continued)

REQUESTED DATA   DATA ANSWER

REQUESTED DATA	DATA ANSWER
24-Hour diet recall	B: 2 eggs, bacon, 3 pieces of toast with jelly, oatmeal with sugar, juice. L: cheese sandwich, cookies, grapes, juice, lemonade. S: Chocolate candies (whole bag), chips, pop (4–6), sweetened ice tea (3–4). D: Pork chops (3), rice, gravy, corn, bread, ice tea, banana. S: cake and ice cream before bed. Eats what he wants; no diet followed.
Describe breathing problems you have had	SOB increases with exertion; able to walk 4–5 blocks before SOB. No paroxysmal nocturnal dyspnea. Morning cough with production 4–5× per year when sick; no hospitalization; no children with asthma. Denies occupational exposure to asbestos, chemicals, dust, or second hand smoke. Smoked 1 pack/day for 25 years; quit smoking 20 years ago.
Family history	Father: died 59 of heart problems. Mother: died age 68 of stroke and "sugar." Never took insulin. Brother: age 57 with HTN. Sister: age 59 with "sugar" and breast cancer. Sister: age 63 living and healthy. Cousin with type 1 diabetes. Children: 4, all living and healthy.
Social history	Married 43 years. Wife does all cooking and shopping. Wife is good, supportive, and monogamous. She is in good health. Retired chemist. 4 children; 10 grandchildren. Close family with grandchildren visiting frequently. Has lots of candy around for the children. Social activity is full with family. Feels his life is happy.
Lifestyle	No exercise: walks dog once a day. No alcohol except special occasions. Smoked 25 years; quit 20 years ago.
Sleep	Sleeps about 6 hours/night; interrupted only to urinate. Occasional naps in front of TV.
Religion/spirituality	"Church-going" Christian.
Income/insurance	Retired on fixed income < $45,000; owns home. Medicare A and B.
Preventive measures	Wears seat belt; smoke detector in home and changes battery each Christmas. No guns in house; railings on steps; no scatter rugs. House in good repair.
Review of systems	Denies numbness/tingling/swelling in hands/feet. Denies chest pain

● PHYSICAL ASSESSMENT

Based upon the subjective data you have obtained, what parts of the physical exam should be performed and why?

SYSTEM	RATIONALE	FINDINGS
Vital signs		BP, 160/100 mm Hg right arm sitting and standing, large cuff and 164/92 mm Hg left arm sitting; P, 72; RR, 18; Height, 5'10"; Wt, 221 lbs; T, 97.8 °F.
Skin		Warm, dry, without lesions, scars.
HEENT		Normocephalic, PERRLA, EMOI intact. Fundoscopic: red reflex present, no nicking or hemorrhage. TM intact bilaterally. Pharynx: swallows without difficulty; no erythema. Neck: thyroid nonpalpable; no carotid bruits.
Lungs		AP/lateral diameter WNL; slight wheeze on forced expiration; CTA; no prolonged expiration; resonance to percussion.
Cardiovascular		Regular rate and rhythm; no murmurs or gallops; peripheral pulses 2+; no peripheral edema.
Abdomen		BS present; obese; no organomegaly or masses. No abdominal bruits.
Rectal		Prostate firm, without nodule; no masses.
Neurological assessment		Alert and oriented; gait coordinated; perceives light touch and pain in extremities bilaterally; vibratory sense intact; no apparent neurological deficits. Brachial and patellar DTRs 2+.
Feet		No open areas, no excessive callus formation. Nails in good repair.

● DIFFERENTIAL DIAGNOSES

Examine all the data available to this point. Link the subjective and objective data to the appropriate differential diagnosis. Identify both positive and negative data that support or refute the diagnoses.

DIAGNOSIS	POSITIVE DATA	NEGATIVE DATA
1		
2		
3		
4		
5		
6		

● DIAGNOSTIC TESTS

What diagnostic tests need to be performed to confirm the diagnosis so plan of care can be developed? What is your interpretation of the results? (These tests were all done fasting.)

DIAGNOSTIC TEST	RATIONALE	RESULTS	INTERPRETATION
CBC		Hgb, 14 g/dL. HCT: 45%. WBC, 6,200/mm^3. RBC, 4.5 million/mm^3. Platelets, 323,000.	
Glycosylated hemoglobin		HgbA1C, 9.8%.	
Renal panel, including FBS, BUN, creatinine		Glucose, 175 mg/dL. Na, 143 mEq/L. K, 3.8 mEq/L. Cl, 101 mEq/L. CO_2, 23 mEq/L. BUN, 11 mg/dL. Creatinine, 0.8 mg/dL.	
Calcium/ Magnesium		Calcium, 9.0 mg/dL. Magnesium, 2.1 mEq/L.	
Uric acid		Uric acid, 5.3 mg/dL.	

(continued)

DIAGNOSTIC TEST	RATIONALE	RESULTS	INTERPRETATION
Thyroid function (T_4 and TSH)		T_4, 10 μg/dL. TSH, 3μU/mL.	
Lipids		Cholesterol, 250 mg/dL. Triglycerides, 244. HDL, 36 mg/dL. LDL, 166 mg/dL.	
Prostate specific antigen (PSA)		PSA, 2.0 ng/mL.	
Urinalysis		Hazy appearance; pH 5.5; protein negative; glucose, 500 mg/dL; ketone, negative; bilirubin, negative; blood, negative; no leukocytes, no nitrites; urobilinogen 0.2 mg/dL, specific gravity: 1.010.	
Liver function tests		Alkaline phosphatase, 124 ImU/mL. AST, 40 U/mL. ALT, 41 U/mL.	
Electrocardiogram		NSR; minimal voltage criteria for LVH.	
CXR		No evidence of cardiomegaly; early changes associated with COPD.	

● DIAGNOSIS

What is your conclusive diagnosis? What was your rationale to support the diagnoses?

DIAGNOSIS	SUPPORTING DATA
1	
2	
3	
4	
5	

● THERAPEUTIC PLAN

1. What are issues that need to be considered when deciding on treatment?

2. What BP is optimum?

3. What choices are available relative to pharmacologic therapy? What is the rationale behind choosing the antihypertensive agent?

4. What counseling should be done relative to dietary changes that need to be made?

5. What recommendations would you give before Mr. Armstrong begins an exercise regimen?

6. What other preventive medications would you prescribe for Mr. Armstrong?

7. What is the influence of his other diagnoses relative to his HTN? Discuss each diagnosis and indicate your plan of care for each.

8. What alternative treatments might be appropriate to assist Mr. Armstrong in the overall treatment plan?

9. When should Mr. Armstrong be seen for follow-up?

10. On a return visit 1 week later, Mr. Armstrong's BP is 146/90 mm Hg sitting and standing. His fasting blood glucose is 142 mg/dL. What changes would you make to the plan of care based on this information?

11. What would a long-term therapeutic plan look like for Mr. Armstrong?

12. What impact might the diagnoses of HTN and type 2 DM have for Mr. Armstrong's family?

13. What resources are available for Mr. Armstrong related to his HTN and DM?

14. What other health care professionals might be consulted to develop a holistic treatment plan for Mr. Armstrong?

REFERENCES

Ammon, P. K. (1999). Individualizing the approach to treating obesity. *Nurse Practitioner: American Journal of Primary Health Care, 24*(2), 27–28, 31, 36–38.

Appel, L., Moore, T., Obarzanek, E., Vollmer, W., Svetkey, L., Sacks, F., Bray, G., Vogt, T., Cutler, J., Windhauser, M., Lin, P., & Karania, N. (1997). A clinical trial of the effects of dietary patterns on blood pressure. *New England Journal of Medicine, 336,* 1117.

Berlowitz, D. R., Ash, A. S., Hickey, E. C., Friedman, R., Glickman, M., Kaden, B., & Moskowitz, M. (1998). Inadequate management of blood pressure in a hypertensive population. *New England Journal of Medicine, 339,* 1957–1963.

Buppert, C. (2000). Measuring outcomes in primary care practice. *Nurse Practitioner: American Journal of Primary Health Care, 25*(1), 88–92, 95–98.

Bushnell, K. L., & Smith, L. A. (1998). Hypertension clinical outcomes in a nurse practitioner managed care setting. *Seminars for Nurse Managers, 6*(3), 155–160.

Hansson, L., Aznchetti, A., & Carruthers, S. (1998). Effects of intensive blood pressure lowering and low dose aspirin in patients with hypertension: Principal results of the Hypertension Optimal Treatment (HOT) randomized trial. *Lancet, 351,* 1755–1762.

Hines, S. E. (2000). Caring for diverse populations. Intelligent prescribing in diverse populations. *Patient Care Nurse Practitioner, 3*(5), 47–48, 51–52, 55–56.

Jamerson, K., & DeQuattro, V. (1996). The impact of ethnicity on response to antihypertensive therapy. *American Journal of Medicine, 101*(Suppl 3A), 22S–32S.

Johnson, M. J., Williams, M., & Marshall, E. S. (1999). Adherent and nonadherent medication-taking in elderly hypertensive patients. *Clinical Nursing Research, 8*(4), 318–335.

Joint National Committee. (1997). *The sixth report of the Joint National Committee on Detection, Evaluation, and Treatment of High Blood Pressure.* Bethesda, MD: National Institutes of Health.

Joint National Committee on Prevention, Detection, Evaluation, and Treatment of High Blood Pressure. (1997). The sixth report of the Joint National Committee on Prevention, Detection, Evaluation, and Treatment of High Blood Pressure (JNC VI). *Archives of Internal Medicine, 157,* 2413–2446.

Kaplan, N. M. (1998). *Clinical hypertension* (7th ed.). Baltimore: Williams & Wilkins.

Kaplan, N. M., & Gifford, R. W. (1996). Choice of initial therapy for hypertension. *Journal of the American Medical Association, 275,* 1577–1580.

LoBuono, C. (2000). Clinical clips. Are newer antihypertensive therapies necessarily better? *Lancet,* 1999;354:1751–1756. *Patient Care Nurse Practitioner, 3*(3), 99.

Mundinger, M., Kane, R., Lenz, E., Totten, A., Tsai, W., Cleary, P., Friedwald, W. (2000). Primary care outcomes in patients treated by nurse practitioners or physicians: A randomized trial. *Journal of the American Medical Association, 283,* 59–68.

National High Blood Pressure Education Program Working Group. (1994). National High Blood Pressure Education Program Working Group Report on hypertension in diabetes. *Hypertension, 23,* 145–150.

Noel, H., Saunder, E., & Smolensky, M. (2000). Hypertension, chronotherapy, and patient management. *Nurse Practitioner, 25*(3Suppl), 2–10; quiz 10-SP10-1.

Sadowski, A., & Redeker, N. (1996). The hypertensive elder: A review for the primary care provider. *Nurse Practitioner, 21,* 99.

Saunders, C. S. (2000). Aiming for lower than 140/90 mm Hg. *Patient Care Nurse Practitioner, 34,* 60–62, 65–66, 69–70.

Saunders, C. S., & Pennachio, D. L. (2000). Medicine in the news. An update to JNC VI . . . Joint National Committee on Prevention, Detection, Evaluation, and Treatment of High Blood Pressure. *Patient Care Nurse Practitioner, 3*(7), 7–8.

SHEP Cooperative Research Group. (1998). Influence of long-term, low-dose, diuretic-based, antihypertensive therapy on glucose, lipid, uric acid, and potassium levels in older men and women with isolated systolic hypertension: The Systolic Hypertension in the Elderly Program. *Archives of Internal Medicine, 158,* 741–751.

Staessen, J. A., Thijs, L., Fagard, R., O'Brien, E., Clement, D., deLeeuw, P., Mancia, G., Nacher, C., Palatini, P., Parati, G., Toumilehto, J., & Webster, J. (1998). Predicting cardiovascular risk using conventional vs ambulatory blood pressure in older patients with systolic hypertension. Systolic Hypertension in Europe Trial Investigators. *Journal of the American Medical Association, 282,* 539–546.

Summary of the 2nd Report of the National Cholesterol Education Program (NCEP) Expert Panel on Detection, Evaluation, and Treatment of high blood cholesterol in adults. (1993). *Journal of the American Medical Association, 269,* 3009–3014.

Tobin, L. J. (1999). Evaluating mild to moderate hypertension. *Nurse Practitioner: American Journal of Primary Health Care, 24*(5), 22, 25–26, 29–230.

Vanchieri, C. (1998). Hypertension guidelines promote aggressive therapy. *Annals of Internal Medicine, 128,* 162–164.

Wood, M. H. (1996). Current considerations in patients with coexistent diabetes and hypertension. *Nurse Practitioner: American Journal of Primary Health Care, 21*(4), 19–20, 27–28, 30–31.

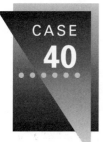

An 18-month-old boy presents for a well-child exam

SCENARIO

Austin is an 18-month-old boy here for a well-child exam. His birth date is 12/30/98. His last visit to see you was 8/13/99.

● TENTATIVE DIAGNOSES

*Based on the information provided, what are potential differential diagnoses? What are **red flag** diagnoses that you cannot miss?*

DIAGNOSES	RATIONALE
Well child exam	No complaints of acute illness.

● HISTORY

What are significant questions in the history for Austin?

REQUESTED DATA	INFORMATION
Health, concerns	Mom states he has had a little cold, but he is doing well
Medical history	He has been healthy. No hospitalizations or surgeries.
Immunizations	2 DtaP, 2 Hib, 2 IPV, 3 Hep B.
Allergies	Denies food, drug, or environmental allergies.

(continued)

REQUESTED DATA   INFORMATION

Medications	Gives one dropper full of acetaminophen (Tylenol) for comfort and fever when needed.
Prenatal history	Mom had four prenatal visits. Mom had gestational diabetes, and the umbilical cord was wrapped around his neck when he was born. Wt at birth: 8 lbs 3 oz. Mom denies smoking, drugs, or drinking alcohol during pregnancy. Bottle fed. Mom does not know APGAR scores. Born 1 week before term.
Developmental information	Does OK. At 4 months, did not support weight on forearms when prone and was behind in most developmental expectations prior to 1 year. He currently can walk, run, uses sipper cup, points to some body parts, can follow one-step command, climbs on chairs, and throws a ball. He can not identify animals, except a dog, rarely uses a spoon, and rips pages out of books. He has not used blocks, and they do not give him anything to write with since he scribbled on the wall.
Habits	Pacifier much of waking time, especially if tired/irritable. If pacifier is not available, does not use thumb.
Family history	Mother: 21; obesity. Father: 24, healthy, smoker. Two brothers: one is 6, has another father, healthy; one is 4, healthy.
Diet	Eats a variety of foods: fruits, vegetables, meat. Drinks milk. Has bottle at bedtime. Drinks lots of fruit juice.
24-hour recall	B: ½ cup cereal, ½ cup milk, ½ cup orange juice. S: ½ cup punch. L: ½ hot dog, ½ banana, 1 cup Juicy Juice. S: 2 peanut butter cookies. D: ¼ bologna sandwich, ½ cup applesauce, ½ cup milk. S: ½ cup milk, ½ cup Juicy Juice.
Sleep	Goes to bed between 9 and 10 pm. Gets up at 8:30 am. Takes one nap during the day.
Day care/baby-sitter	Grandmother watches him.
Dental care/bottle to bed	Yes, has given him a bottle to go to bed. He has a fit unless he gets the bottle when he goes to bed.
Safety concerns	Car seat most of the time. Hot water heater, unable to control. Electrical outlets, some are covered. Walker, no. Gates at stairways, yes. Guns in home, no. Choking hazards, tries to, but the older kids have lots of things on the floor.

(continued)

REQUESTED DATA   INFORMATION

	Water safety, no access to pool.
	Poison control, has number.
	Bike helmet, no bike.
	Can child call 911, not applicable.
	Stranger safety and pedestrian safety, not applicable.
Relationship with parents/siblings	The kids are so close in age that they fight a lot. The oldest boy goes to kindergarten. Mom has to watch the other boys with Austin. She is afraid they will hurt him. Grandmother lives in an apartment in the same complex. Grandfather's whereabouts are unknown.
Temperament of child	Cranky and irritable when he does not get his own way but generally happy.
Discipline	Mom tries to do time out and distract him but often is not successful.
Environment	Lives in subsidized housing, so all apartments have number next to phone; rough neighborhood. Known for its crime and drugs.

What are the key points to cover in the review of systems?

SYSTEM   INFORMATION

System	Information
General	Denies any physical concerns at this time.
HEENT	Pulls at ears sometimes; runny nose frequently. Denies problems with clumsiness or falling or visual problems. Seems to hear OK. Otitis media $\times$ 3 over past year.
Chest	Mom notices him wheezing at times when he coughs or has a cold. No SOB.
Heart	No problems.
GI	No problems. Has BM every day.
GU	No problems; circumcised.
Neurological assessment	No problems with gait, balance, coordination, or weakness.
Skin/endocrine	Denies unusual skin discoloration or pigmentation. Denies itching, dry, or scaling skin.

● PHYSICAL ASSESSMENT

What are areas of the physical examination that should be included? What is your rationale for including this portion of the exam?

SYSTEM	RATIONALE	FINDINGS
General		Wt, 22-¾ lbs; Ht, 28½ inches; head circumference, 18 ½ in; T, 98°F; HR, 128 bpm; skin is warm and dry. Behavior and appearance consistent with age. Mildly wary of examiner.
HEENT		Normocephalic, hair light brown, evenly distributed. Anterior fontanel closed, trachea midline, shoddy tonsilar nodes. Full ROM of neck. Peripheral eye structures unremarkable. Red reflex present. Small ears, normal alignment. TMs intact, pearly gray, 16 deciduous teeth.
Lungs		CTA; breathing easy and regular.
Cardiac		Sinus tachycardia; no murmurs.
Abdomen		Protuberant, umbilicus midline, no herniation. No vascular patterns noted. Active bowel sounds. No masses or HSM.
Genitalia		Unremarkable male anatomy. Circumcised; testicles descended bilaterally; moderate scrotal rugae.
Neurological assessment		Displays characteristic behaviors for age. DTR 2+. Babinski negative.
Extremities		Gross AROM is symmetrical and without obvious weakness or discomfort. Slightly wide based gait with medial weight bearing and mild pronation. No visible or palpable joint swelling. Pulses 2+.

● DIFFERENTIAL DIAGNOSIS

What are the significant positive and negative data that support or refute your diagnoses for Austin?

DIAGNOSIS	POSITIVE DATA	NEGATIVE DATA
1		
2		
3		
4		

● DIAGNOSTIC TESTS

Based on the history and physical examination, what, if any, diagnostic tests will you do? Include your rationale for the testing and interpret the tests done.

TEST	RATIONALE	RESULTS	INTERPRETATION
Lead Level		3 μ/dL.	
Hgb, HCT		12 g/dL; 38%.	

● DIAGNOSIS

What is the final diagnosis you identify for Austin? What are the supporting data for this diagnosis?

● THERAPEUTIC PLAN

1. *What will you include in your treatment plan for Austin?*
2. *What anticipatory guidance will you include for Austin and his mother?*
3. *When should Austin return for follow-up?*
4. *What are resources for the NP and parents related to well care and immunizations?*

REFERENCES

Adkins, S. (1997). Immunizations: Current recommendations. *American Family Physician, 56,* 865–873.

American Academy of Pediatrics, Committee of Infectious Diseases. (2000). *2000 Red book: Report of the Committee on Infectious Diseases* (23rd ed., pp. 224). Elk Grove Village, IL: Author.

Holt, E., Guyer, B., Hughart, N., Keane, V., Vivier, P., Ross, A., Strobimo, D. (1996). The contribution of missed opportunities to childhood under immunization in Baltimore. *Pediatrics 97,* 474–480.

Houseman, C., Butterfoss, F. D., Morrow, A. L., & Rosenthal, J. (1997). Focus groups among public, military, and private sector mothers: Insights to improve the immunization process. *Public Health Nursing, 14*(4), 235–243.

Kuensting, L. L., & Albers, A. (2000). Second opinion. Should childhood immunizations be given when children have a pediatric visit to the emergency department? . . . Writing for the pro position . . . Writing for the con position. *American Journal of Maternal/Child Nursing, 25*(3), 118–119.

McGrath, N. E., & Mink, C. (2000). Pediatric update. Pediatric immunizations: Are you up-to-date? *Journal of Emergency Nursing, 26*(3), 264–267, 282–288.

Simpson, D. M., Suarez, L., & Smith, D. R. (1997). Immunization rates among young children in the public and private health care sectors. *American Journal of Preventive Medicine, 13*(2), 84–88.

Society of Pediatric Nurses. (1998). *Position statement on immunizations.* Denver, CO: Author.

Suarez, L., Simpson, D. M., & Smith, D. R. (1997). Errors and correlates in parental recall of childhood immunizations. *Pediatrics, 99*(5), 3.

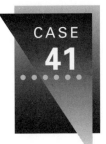

A 44-year-old man with chronic low back pain

SCENARIO

Bill is a 44-year-old Asian man who comes to your office asking for a re-fill of Tylenol with codeine for back pain. His severe pain began 8 months ago. The initial back injury was caused by a MVA 3 years ago. He reports obtaining his last two refills from different emergency departments. Since Bill has separated from his family, he is staying in a friend's apartment. He says he is having trouble keeping his job and paying his bills. He has not seen his wife and three children for several months.

● TENTATIVE DIAGNOSES

Based on the information provided so far, what are the potential differential diagnoses?

● HISTORY

What are significant questions in the history for a man reporting chronic back pain? What additional information do you need in terms of pain assessment?

● PHYSICAL ASSESSMENT

What are the significant portions of the physical examination that should be completed for Bill?

● DIFFERENTIAL DIAGNOSES

What are the significant positive and negative data that support or refute your diagnoses for Bill?

● DIAGNOSTIC TESTS

Based on the history and physical assessment, what, if any, diagnostic testing would you do? Include your rationale for the testing.

● DIAGNOSIS

What diagnoses do you determine as being appropriate for Bill?

● THERAPEUTIC PLAN

1. *What are the issues to consider for Bill when deciding on treatment?*
2. *List short-term and long-term goals appropriate to include in a health care contract with Bill.*
3. *What is the necessary first step in treatment for Bill?*
4. *What other health care providers should be included on the interdisciplinary team to assess Bill and help manage the therapeutic plan?*
5. *If Bill did not have a substance dependence problem, how might the management of his pain differ?*
6. *Based on the information given so far about Bill, what impact do you think this situation has had on his family?*
7. *Bill returns in 6 weeks with reports of successful withdrawal from opiates and participation in a recovery program. Bill says he is feeling better in general, but he still needs help with pain relief. Lab work reveals no anemia and normal liver and renal function. What adjustments could you make to the therapeutic plan?*
8. *What are the principles of pain management?*
9. *Where can a nurse practitioner obtain more information concerning substance abuse and pain management and/or additional resources for assisting affected clients?*

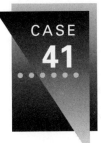

TUTORIAL

A 44-year-old man with chronic low back pain

SCENARIO

Bill is a 44-year-old Asian man who comes to your office asking for a refill of Tylenol with codeine for back pain. His severe pain began 8 months ago. The initial back injury was caused by a MVA 3 years ago. He reports obtaining his last two refills from different emergency departments. Since Bill has separated from his family he is staying in a friend's apartment. He says he is having trouble keeping his job and paying his bills. He has not seen his wife and three children for several months.

● TENTATIVE DIAGNOSIS

*What are the potential diagnoses you have identified based on the above scenario? What are the **red flags** that you can not miss?*

DIAGNOSIS	RATIONALE
Chronic pain disorder	Bill complains of chronic back pain.
Opiate withdrawal	Bill has sought refills on pain medicine from the ED instead of a primary provider.
Opiate abuse	Bill has sought refills on pain medicine from the ED instead of a primary provider.
Opiate dependence	Bill has sought refills on pain medicine from the ED instead of a primary provider.
Malingering	Always a concern when a patient seeks pain medicine from EDs for a problem such as back pain, especially when the accident occurred 3 years ago.
Back pain	C/o of back pain from MVA 3 years ago, but pain increased in last 8 months.

● HISTORY

What are significant questions in the history for a man complaining of chronic back pain from a MVA? Are there any questions that are missing that you need to know?

REQUESTED DATA   DATA ANSWER

Allergies	None.
Medications	Tylenol with codeine 2 tabs orally PRN for pain (admits to self-medication of 4–10 tabs/day); laxative every week; methocarbamol (Robaxin) 750 mg as needed for muscle spasm.
Immunizations	Tetanus-diphtheria toxoid 1994 (sutures left arm from MVA). No Hep B or pneumococcal vaccines.
Surgery/transfusion	Septoplasty, 1991 status post nasal fracture. Concussion, 1994 after MVA. Alcohol treatment program, 1994 after DUI arrest.

Medical history/
  hospitalizations/
  fractures/injuries/
  accidents
	Chicken pox as child.
	Left shoulder dislocation, 1982.
	Right ankle sprain × 2, 1985, 1989.
	Rib fracture from MVA, 1994.

Adult illness	Chronic bronchitis for 5 years. PUD, asymptomatic. No history of GI bleed.
Last complete physical exam	1994, during alcohol treatment.
Appetite	Decreased for 3 months. Intermittent nausea, no vomiting. Lost 15 lbs. in past 3 months after separating from wife.
24-hour diet recall	B: 2 slices bacon, 1 fried egg, 1 piece toast, 3 cups coffee. L: None. D: Fried hamburger, french fries, 16-oz cola.
Sleeping	Back pain awakens him 2–3 times a night. Increased difficulty when runs out of medicine. Feels tired in morning. Muscle aches in back and legs all day.
Social history	Tobacco: Smokes 1 pack per day for 25 years. Alcohol: history of problem drinking. Received treatment in 1994; no drinking for 1 year. Now drinks when pain medication is unavailable. Caffeinated beverages: 4 cups coffee, 2 colas/day.

(continued)

REQUESTED DATA DATA ANSWER

	Drugs: None.
	Exercise: None currently. Ran 3 times a week until ankle sprain in 1989.
Family history	Father: died 62 of GI bleed, alcoholism.
	Mother: age 68, arthritis, H/A.
	Brother: 46, HTN.
	Sister: 38, healthy.
	Children: 1 son, 22; daughter 18; son, 13; all healthy.
Social organizations	Veterans group (no history of combat during service).
	AA for 6 months in 1994.
	Church activities until 1 year ago.
	Coached son's baseball team until 3 years ago.
Relationship with wife	Expresses resentment about being "kicked out" of the house because of anger outbursts, spending habits, and withdrawal from family.
Relationship with children	Believes younger son and daughter miss him. Older son resents him for not taking better care of himself and family, as well as for being intoxicated in front of his friends.
Relationship with mother/siblings	Visits mother 2 times each month, sister weekly. Both are supportive. Last saw brother during holidays.
Employment/insurance	$35,000/year earned in factory. 3rd job in past 5 years. Wife works in retail. Family coverage medical/dental through his work.
Length of symptoms	Pain for 3 years since MVA. Increased pain for 8 months.
How has pain affected your ADLs?	Misses work at least 2 times a month. Does not participate in family activities. "Always" going to health care providers. "They can't find a cause for my pain."
Losses in your life?	Separation from family. Father's death. Refinanced home due to spending problems.
Legal charges	DUI after MVA 1994. No ongoing litigation.
What do you do for the pain?	Take more medication and drink alcohol.
Do you ever think about hurting yourself?	No.
Do you ever think about hurting others?	No.

What additional information do you need in terms of pain assessment?

PAIN ASSESSMENT*	ANSWER
On a scale of 1–10 with 0 being no pain and 10 being the worst pain you can imagine, rate your pain at its worst in the past 24 hours.	8.
What number best describes the least pain you've felt in the past 24 hours?	5.
Rate the amount of pain you have now	7.
In the past 24 hrs, how much relief has medication given you? (0–100%)	50%.
Describe how your pain interferes with the following activities in the past 24 hours: (0: does not interfere; 10: completely interferes)	General ability, 7. Walking ability, 6. Relation with other people, 5. Enjoyment of life, 8. Mood, 6. Normal work, 8. Sleep, 9.
What is the quality of the pain?	Sharp, constant.
Onset of pain?	Always present.
What makes it better?	Tylenol with codeine.
What makes it worse?	Walking, physical labor.
What is an acceptable level of pain for you?	3.
What was the pain like that made the MD put you on Tylenol with codeine?	Constant severe pain.

*Pain Assessment, U.S. Department of Health and Human Services (1994).

● PHYSICAL ASSESSMENT

What are the significant portions of the physical examination that should be completed for Bill?

SYSTEM	RATIONALE	FINDINGS
Vital signs	Baseline data	BP, 142/88 mm Hg left arm sitting and, 146/90 mm Hg right arm sitting; P, 92; RR, 20; T, 98.0 °F; Ht, 5'10"; Wt, 190 lbs.

(continued)

SYSTEM	RATIONALE	FINDINGS
General appearance/Skin	Mental status and mood help assess psychological status and stability. Status of skin helps assess presence/absence of drug withdrawal, IV drug abuse, liver disease, and bleeding disorder.	Appears anxious with labile affect. Cooperative. Skin cool; mild diaphoresis on trunk; no needle marks (tracks); no jaundice or petechiae.
HEENT	Could defer VA and exam of ears. Condition of nasal mucosa helps assess drug use. Fundoscopy, thyroid, venous distention, and carotid exams are indicated when patient has HTN.	Eye: VA OD 20/40; OS 20/30; O/U 20/30 uncorrected. Fundoscopy: red reflex intact bilaterally. No AV nicking. No lesions. Ear: Left cerumen occluding canal. Right canal clear. TM pearly gray, + cone of light. Nose: thin clear discharge bilaterally. Mucosa pink. Septum deviated right. No perforation. Mouth: poor dentition; receding gums; no lesions. No erythema, lesions, or exudate. Neck: no carotid bruits; no JVD; thyroid nonpalpable; no masses; no enlarged lymph nodes.
Lungs	Bill smokes, so respiratory status should be evaluated.	CTA.
Heart	Assess CV status in middle-aged smoker with HTN.	S1, S2 WNL; no MRG.
Back	C/o severe back pain; assess for objective evidence.	Mild tenderness of paravertebral muscles to palpation. Negative SLR and crossover SLR.
Abdomen	Bill c/o of constipation. In addition, because Bill is hypertensive, the abdomen should be checked for bruits. Because he has a history of ETOH dependence, it is important to evaluate liver size.	Hyperactive BS, no bruit. Soft, with mild tenderness throughout. No rebound. No masses or HSM.
Rectal	C/o constipation. 44-year-old man at lower age range for BPH.	Anus without lesions and with intact tone. Rectum without masses. Prostate firm, symmetric, not enlarged; no masses or tenderness.

(continued)

SYSTEM	RATIONALE	FINDINGS
Genital	May defer if Bill has no symptoms.	Penis circumcised, no lesions or urethral discharge. Testes descended, nontender, no masses or lesions bilaterally. No inguinal hernia palpated.
Neurological assessment	Especially important to assess neurological status of lower extremities in patient with low back pain to establish baseline and determine objective evidence of deficits.	CN II–XII intact. Strength/sensation WNL. Steady gait, negative Romberg. Intact tandem walk, heel/toe walk. DTRs 2+; alert, oriented ×3.
Extremities	Evaluate for edema because he has history of HTN. Important to assess musculoskeletal status of arms and legs, given history of MVA, shoulder injury, and low back pain.	Pulses 2+ bilaterally. No edema or lesions. ROM: decreased neck extension, left shoulder abduction and external rotation. Otherwise full ROM neck, shoulders, elbows, wrist, trunk, hips, knees, and ankles. No deformity.

● DIFFERENTIAL DIAGNOSIS

What are the significant positive and negative findings that support or refute your diagnoses for Bill? (In order to assist with the development of differential diagnoses in this case, it will be helpful to become familiar with definitions of terms found in substance abuse and pain literature.)

DIAGNOSIS	POSITIVE DATA	NEGATIVE DATA
Chronic pain disorder associated with psychological factors	Pain is the predominant focus of the clinical presentation, severe enough to warrant clinical attention. Pain causes significant distress or impairment in work and social relationships. Psychological factors present. Pain does not	Pain may have a physiological basis not yet revealed on history and physical. History of MVA in 1994 with significant trauma.

(continued)

DIAGNOSIS	POSITIVE DATA	NEGATIVE DATA
	appear to be intentionally produced. Medical condition appears to play no role or minimal role in onset or maintenance of pain. For chronic pain, symptoms are present more than 6 months (American Psychiatric Association [APA], 1994).	
Chronic pain disorder with both psychological factors and a general medical condition	Pain is the predominant focus of the clinical presentation, severe enough to warrant clinical attention. Pain causes significant distress or impairment in work and social relationships. Psychological factors present. Pain does not appear to be intentionally produced. Medical condition appears to play no role or minimal role in onset or maintenance of pain. For chronic pain, symptoms are present more than 6 months (APA, 1994).	Physical exam did not reveal objective source of pain.
Chronic pain disorder associated with a general medical condition	History of MVA.	Physical exam did not reveal source of pain.
Opiate withdrawal	Decrease in use after prolonged (over several weeks) period of use. Symptoms of dysphoric mood, nausea, muscle aches, lacrimation, rhinorrhea, pupillary dilatation, diarrhea, insomnia (APA, 1994).	None.
Opiate abuse	Recurrent use leads to failure to fulfill major role obligation, recurrent use in situations where it is	Evidence of tolerance and withdrawal. Great deal of time involved in obtaining substance. Family, social, and occupational

(continued)

DIAGNOSIS	POSITIVE DATA	NEGATIVE DATA
	physically hazardous, continued use despite having persistent social or interpersonal problems (APA, 1994).	activities given up. (Meeting criteria for dependence overrides diagnosis of abuse [APA, 1994].)
Opiate dependence	Evidence of tolerance and withdrawal. Substance taken in larger amounts over longer period of time than intended. Great deal of time spent in activities necessary to obtain substance (ED visits). Work, social activities reduced (APA, 1994). History of problems with alcohol in past (Vallerand, 1991).	None.
Malingering	Bill states he wants Tylenol with codeine for pain. Discrepancy between claimed degree of pain and lack of physical findings.	He cooperated during the history and exam. No ongoing litigation.
Back pain	MVA 3 years ago. Mild paravertebral tenderness to palpation.	Discrepancy between claimed degree of pain and lack of physical findings; -SLR, crossed SLR; DTRs 2+; able to heel-and-toe walk. ROM WNL. No bowel/bladder dysfunction. Strength/sensation intact.
Constipation secondary to drug use and poor dietary habits	Takes laxative every week. Poor dietary habits. No or little exercise.	None.
Alcohol abuse	History of alcohol abuse; received treatment for abuse in 1994; DUI; family history of alcohol abuse. Admits he drinks alcohol to combat pain when out of medications.	None.

● DIAGNOSTIC TESTS

Based on the history and physical examination, what, if any, diagnostic testing or additional data would you obtain?

DIAGNOSTIC TEST	RATIONALE	RESULTS	INTERPRETATION
Stool for guaiac	Test for GI bleeding.	Negative.	No GI bleeding.
Urine toxicology screening test	Identify the presence of current opioids. Identify other drugs Bill may be using to cope with withdrawal or pain. In addition, he may be abusing (opioids may be present from 12 hours to several days in urine) (APA, 1994).	Positive for opioids	Currently taking opioids.
CBC, liver function, electrolytes, renal	History of alcohol use puts Bill at increased risk for GI bleeding and liver dysfunction. Also, baseline liver and renal status helps determine safety/risks for alternative and possibly long-term medication regimens that may be indicated for pain management.	H/H, 15.1 g/dL/45.2%. RBC, 5.2 million/mm³. WBC, 7,100/mm³. Platelets, 250,000. AST, 35 IU/L. ALT, 27 IU/L. GGT, 45 U/L. Alkaline phosphatase, 70 ImU/mL. BUN, 10 mg/dL. Creatinine, 1.0 mg/dL. Na, 142 mEq/L. Cl, 110 mEq/L. K, 4.2 mEq/L. CO_2, 26.0 mEq/L.	GGT elevated. AST/ALT ratio, > 1. Both are sensitive indicators of chronic excessive alcohol intake.
Serum alcohol	Identify if Bill has been drinking before appointment. Level > 250 mg/dl indicates someone who will need hospitalization for detoxification.	50 mg/dL.	Indicates Bill has been drinking but does not show legal intoxication.

(continued)

DIAGNOSTIC TEST	RATIONALE	RESULTS	INTERPRETATION
Electromyograph, computed tomography, magnetic resonance imaging	Other tests to evaluate physiological source of pain as indicated by exam.	Not done. Exam revealed no signs and symptoms that required further testing. All these tests were completed within 2 months of initial injury.	
Clinical interview DSM-IV or CAGE to assess alcohol dependence	Assess current severity of alcohol use. History is suggestive of alcohol abuse/ dependence, with a period of remission. Alcoholics are at increased risk for use/dependence upon other substances, and individuals dependent on other substances are at increased risk for alcohol dependence (Savage, 1993).	Bill is struggling to **cut down** amount of alcohol; **annoyed** when wife asked him to decrease alcohol. Has felt **guilty** about drinking. Bill states he does not drink in morning.	Yes to 3 of 4 questions. More than one yes is a strong indication that alcohol abuse exists.
Assess social supports	Family, 12-step recovery network, or church group may be available to help Bill. A recovery setting increases Bill's chances of success and is critical to pain management (Savage, 93).	Bill identifies sister and mother as supportive. He is willing to call them today to discuss today's visit.	N/A.

(continued)

DIAGNOSTIC TEST	RATIONALE	RESULTS	INTERPRETATION
Seek information from family or friends	Confirm Bill's history of drug, medication, and alcohol use (Wesson, Ling, & Smith, 1993).	Bill gives written permission for NP to speak with sister.	
Self report and if indicated clinician-completed depression scale	Persons with chronic pain are at increased risk for suicide, especially if associated with severe depression or terminal illness, such as cancer (APA, 1994).	Bill says he has no thoughts or plans of harming himself and agrees to call sister if mood worsens.	N/A.

● DIAGNOSES

What diagnoses do you determine as being appropriate after a review of the subjective and objective data?

Opiate Dependence
Alcohol Abuse
Tobacco Dependence
Constipation secondary to opiate use
Chronic pain disorder

Data Supporting the Diagnosis of Opiate Dependence

- Evidence of tolerance and withdrawal
- Substance taken in larger amounts over longer period of time than intended.
- Great deal of time spent in activities necessary to obtain substance (ED visits).
- Work, social activities reduced

Pathophysiology

Addictive substances stimulate the neural reward pathway in the limbocortical region of the brain, which regulates basic emotions and behaviors. The substances stimulate the reward pathway and entice people to sacrifice other pleasures or to endure pain to get the substance.

● THERAPEUTIC PLAN

1. *What are the issues to consider for Bill when deciding on treatment?*
   - Need to treat withdrawal symptoms without simply giving another prescription of same drug and telling client to "cut down."
   - Explain that pain may very well improve, or at least not become worse, if opiate use is discontinued.
   - A trial off opiates and all other substances of abuse or dependence, such as alcohol, is key to assessing pain and planning long-term treatment (Savage, 1993).
   - Identify appropriate setting for withdrawal; Bill needs adequate support and monitoring, such as a supervised detoxification program on an inpatient or outpatient basis.
   - Explain rationale for diagnosis of opiate dependence, while acknowledging the significance of pain and the need for pain treatment.

2. *List short-term and long-term goals appropriate to include in a health care contract with Bill. Set short-term and long-term goals with Bill for health care contract. Discuss realistic expectations for course of treatment and outcomes. Negotiate NP/client responsibilities in the treatment plan. There are no "quick fixes." Different therapies will be tried. Improvement of pain is expected, but there are no guarantees of complete resolution of pain. Refer to pain rating scales for perspective.*

   Examples of goals:
   Short term goals: detoxify from opiates; remain substance free; resume job responsibilities; identify any life-threatening diseases.
   Long-term goals: improve pain; resolve family conflict; identify physiologic contributors to pain; maintain active support group; be substance free until alternatives have been systematically tried; continue care with one provider/team

3. *What is the necessary first step in treatment for Bill?*
   The first step is a supervised detoxification program in an inpatient or outpatient setting.

   You should consider an inpatient setting for detoxification because he is male, over 40, has been drinking more than 10 years, drinks round the clock to maintain a steady blood level, has an unstable home environment, has prior treatment for alcohol dependence, and has polydrug abuse.

   The appropriate next step?

   Refer Bill to a substance abuse treatment/rehabilitation program, either an inpatient or intensive outpatient setting.

4. *What other health care providers could be included on the interdisciplinary team to assess Bill and help manage the therapeutic plan?*
   An addiction specialist could help assess the severity of the substance dependence and monitor the response to treatment. A physician is needed for consultation and referral and to aid in interpreting test results and

ordering procedures to determine any physiological source of pain. A physician also may collaborate in supervising the outpatient detoxification plan. A psychiatrist/psychologist could determine if Bill meets the criteria for other mental disorders that may take precedence over the determination of chronic pain disorder. A licensed clinical social worker, psychiatric nurse specialist could provide referral/consultation regarding addiction assessment, mental disorder determination, family counseling, relaxation training, and biofeedback. Physical therapists could support alternative pain management modalities, such as transcutaneous electrical nerve stimulation (TENS), hot packs, and muscle strengthening. A pain specialty consultant/team, which can consist of physicians, physical medicine and rehabilitation specialists, advanced practice nurses, psychologists, social workers, and others.

5. *If Bill did not have a substance dependence problem, how might management of his pain differ?*
   Although physiological dependence on narcotics for pain is common if such agents are used regularly, most people stop taking narcotics when the pain stops (McCaffery & Parero, 2001). Unless a client has a prior substance dependence problem, chances are low for development of psychological dependence on narcotic analgesics (Vallerand, 1991). Opiates may be appropriate for a client with chronic pain without a history of substance dependence. Remember that the pain-relieving effects of nonnarcotic analgesics are underestimated and under used (McCaffery & Parero, 2001). In addition, consider alternative and adjuvant therapies.

6. *Based on the information given so far about Bill, what impact do you think this situation has had on his family?*
   Bill was organizing his life around opiates (and probably alcohol), while his family was organizing itself around responses to his substance dependence (Janosik & Green, 1992), reacting to the moods and money problems he created. They, especially his wife, may have had difficulty developing individual identities separate from the troubled family (codependence). The unpredictable nature of life with a person dependent on substances, creates fear of losing control of what normality exists in the family (Janosik & Green). The children often experience neglect, if not abuse, and can be confused by the adults' denial of the severity of the family's problems (Janosik & Green).
   What would be appropriate interventions for Bill's family?
   Family counseling and involvement of the family in the client's treatment enhance the chances for successful recovery from substance dependence (Martin, 1982; Janosik & Green, 1992) and management of chronic pain (Vallerand, 1991).

7. *Bill returns in 6 weeks with reports of successful withdrawal from opiates and participation in a recovery program. Bill says he is feeling better in general but still needs help with pain relief. Lab work reveals no anemia, and normal*

liver and renal function. What adjustments could you make to the therapeutic plan?

- Review client/NP contract.
- Revise goals as appropriate. Total relief of pain may not be a realistic goal (Vallerand, 1991).
- Strive for a level of pain the client can live with.

8. *What are the principles of pain management?*

Principles

- Cultivate a sense of control in the client.
- Encourage client activities that keep him active and productive.
- Involve the client's family and friends in the plan.

Pharmacology

- Use the least potent analgesic with the fewest side effects.
- Give each medication an adequate time trial.
- Use a regular dosing schedule, not PRN.
- Recognize side effects and avoid oversedation.

Medications

- Acetaminophen
- Acetylsalicylic acid (ASA)
- Nonsteroidal anti-inflammatory drugs (NSAIDs)

Adjuvant analgesics

- Tricyclic antidepressants
- Caffeine
- Phenothiazines
- Anticonvulsants

Controlled Drugs

- In the case of a client with a history of substance dependence, alternative modalities must be exhaustively tried before a return to controlled drugs is indicated. In additions to opiates, benzodiazepines have the potential for abuse and dependence and can trigger cross addiction (Savage, 1993).

Nonpharmacologic Treatments

- Nerve block
- Transcutaneous electrical nerve stimulation (TENS)
- Biofeedback
- Massage
- Local heat and/or cold application
- Activity scheduling
- Relaxation training (Savage, 1993; Sees & Clark, 1993; Vallerand, 1991).

9. *Where can a nurse practitioner obtain more information concerning substance dependence and pain management and/or additional resources for assisting affected clients?*

- See local Yellow Pages for Alcoholics Anonymous (AA), Narcotics Anonymous (NA), and Adult Children of Alcoholics (ACOA). These organizations provide meetings lists, literature, and support groups.
- Identify local referral sources for detoxification and chemical dependence treatment programs and mental health counseling.
- Write or call for information:

> Alcoholics Anonymous, General Service Office
> A.A. World Services, Inc.
> PO Box 459, Grand Central Station
> New York, NY 10163
> 212/870-3400

> National Clearinghouse for Alcohol and Drug Information
> 800/729-6686
> *www.health.org*
> Action on Smoking and Health
> *http://ash.org*

Action on Smoking and Health (ASH) is a national nonprofit legal action and educational organization fighting for the rights of nonsmokers against the many problems of smoking.

Addiction Technology Transfer Center locations can be found on the web site http://www.nattc.org. The web site furnishes information and training resources that translate into better care for people with substance use disorders.

AlcoholMD: *http://www.alcoholmd.com.* This web site is designed to provide clinicians, patients, recovering alcoholics, families, children, and the general public broad access to information and services in the field of alcohol and care.

Centre for Addiction and Mental Health: *http://www.camh.net.* The Centre for Addiction and Mental Health is a clinical and multidisciplinary research center offering a unique model for understanding people with addiction and mental illness, preventing substance abuse and promoting mental health. Formed in 1998 in Toronto, Canada, with the former Addiction Research Foundation being one of its founding partners, it is both a teaching hospital of the University of Toronto and a World Health Organization Centre of Excellence.

Moderation Management: *http://www.moderation.org.* MM is a behavioral change program and national support group network for people who have made the decision to reduce their drinking and make other lifestyle changes. MM empowers individuals to accept personal responsibility for choosing and maintaining their own path, whether moderation or abstinence. MM promotes early self-recognition of risky drinking behavior, when moderation is an achievable goal. Individuals who are not able to successfully reduce their drinking either find a local abstinence-only program to attend or remain in MM and choose abstinence as their goal.

National Institute on Drug Abuse: *http://www.nida.nih.gov*. The mission of NIDA is to lead the Nation in bringing the power of science to bear on drug abuse and addiction.

Narcotics Anonymous
World Service Office, Inc.
P.O. Box 9999
Van Nuys, CA 91409
(818)780-3951

To order clinical practice guidelines for pain management, contact:

AHCPR Publications Clearinghouse
P.O. Box 8547
Silver Spring, MD 20907
(800)358-9295
FAX: (301) 594-2800

Information and educational materials on chemical dependence and related topics are available from

Hazelden Education Materials
PO Box 176
Center City, MN 55012-0176
800/328-9000 (U.S., Canada, and the Virgin Islands)
612/257-4010 (Outside the U.S. and Canada)
612-257-1331 (24-hour FAX)
http://www.hazelden.org/library

REFERENCES

American Psychiatric Association. (1994). *Diagnostic and statistical manual of mental disorders* (4th ed.). Washington, DC: Author.

Caulker-Burnett, I. (1994). Primary care screening for substance abuse. *Nurse Practitioner: American Journal of Primary Health Care, 19*(6), 42, 44–48.

Compton, P., Monahan, G., & Simmons-Cody, H. (1999). Motivational interviewing: An effective brief intervention for alcohol and drug abuse patients. *Nurse Practitioner: American Journal of Primary Health Care, 24*(11), 27–28, 31–32, 34.

Cukr, P. L., Jones, S. L., Wilberger, M. E., Smith, R., & Stopper, C. (1998). The psychiatric clinical nurse specialist/nurse practitioner: An example of a combined role. *Archives of Psychiatric Nursing, 12,* 311–318.

Dyer, J. G., Hammill, K., Regan-Kubinski, M. J., Yurick, A., & Kobert, S. (1997). The psychiatric primary care nurse practitioner: A futuristic model for advanced practice psychiatric mental health nursing. *Archives of Psychiatric Nursing 11,* 2–11.

Edmands, M. S., Hoff, L. A., Kaylor, L., Mower, L., & Sorrell, S. (1999). Bridging gaps between mind, body, & spirit: Healing the whole person. *Journal of Psychosocial Nursing and Mental Health Services, 37*(10), 35–42, 44–45.

Fleming, M., & Barry, K. (1992). *Addictive disorders.* St. Louis: Mosby.

Janosik, E., & Green, E. (1992). *Family life: Process and practice.* Boston: Jones and Bartlett.

McCaffery, M. & Parero, C. (2001). Pain control. *American Journal of Nursing, 101*(5), 778–781.

Miller, N. S., Gold, M. S., & Smith, D. E. (1997). *Manual of therapeutics for addictions.* New York: John Wiley & Sons.

Savage, S. R. (1993). Addiction in the treatment of pain: Significance, recognition, and management. *Journal of Pain and Symptom Management, 8*(5), 265–278.

Sees, K. L., & Clark, W. (1993). Opioid use in the treatment of chronic pain: Assessment of addiction. *Journal of Pain and Symptom Management, 8*(5), 257–264.

U.S. Department of Health and Human Services. (1994). *Management of cancer pain: Clinical practice guideline number 9* (AHCPR Publication No. 94–0592). Rockville, MD: Government Printing Office.

Vallerand, A. H. (1991). The use of narcotic analgesics in chronic nonmalignant pain. *Holistic Nursing Practice, 6*(1), 17–23.

Wenrich, M. D., Paauw, D. S., & Carline, J. D. (1995). Do primary care physicians screen patients about alcohol intake using CAGE questions. *Journal of General Internal Medicine, 10,* 631–634.

Westreich, L., & Rosenthal, R. (1995). Physical examination in substance abusers: How to gather evidence of concealed problems. *Postgraduate Medicine, 97,* 111–123.

Wesson, D. R., Ling, W., & Smith, D. E. (1993). Prescription of opioids for treatment of pain in patients with addictive disease. *Journal of Pain and Symptom Management, 8*(5), 289–296.

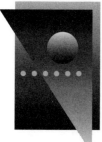

Appendix

COMMONLY USED CLINICAL ABBREVIATIONS

Abbreviation	Definition	Abbreviation	Definition
AARP	American Association of Retired Persons	CA	cancer
		CABG	coronary arterial bypass graft
ABGs	arterial blood gases	CAD	coronary artery disease
AC	acromioclavicular	CBE	clinical breast exam
AC>BC	air conduction greater than bone conduction	CDC	Centers for Disease Control
		CHF	congestive heart failure
ADHD	attention deficit hyperactivity disorder	CMT	cervical motion tenderness
		CN	cranial nerve
ADL	activities of daily living	COPD	chronic obstructive pulmonary disease
AFP	alpha-fetoprotein		
ALT	alanine transaminase	CPR	cardiopulmonary resuscitation
AP	anteroposterior	CSF	cerebrospinal fluid
AROM	active range of motion	CTA	clear to auscultation
ASA	aspirin	CV	cardiovascular
ASAP	as soon as possible	CVA	cerebrovascular accident
AST	aspartate transaminase	CVAT	costovertebral angle tenderness
AUA	American Urology Association		
AV	anteverted	CXR	chest x-ray film
AV nicking	arteriovenous nicking	D & C	dilation and curettage
Bands	banded neutrophils	d/c	discharge
BASO	basophil	DDST	Denver Developmental Screening Test
BCP	birth control pill		
BID	two times a day	D & E	dilation and evacuation
BM	bowel movement	DIP	distal interphalangeal
BP	blood pressure	DM	diabetes mellitus
BPH	benign prostatic hypertrophy	DMPA	Depo-Provera
BPPV	benign paroxysmal positional vertigo	DOE	dyspnea on exertion
		DTAP	diptheria, tetanus, acellular pertussis
BS	bowel sounds, breath sounds		
BSE	breast self exam	DTR	deep tendon reflexes
BUN	blood urea nitrogen	DUI	driving under the influence
BUS	Bartholin's, urethral, and Skene's glands	DVT	deep venous thrombosis
		ELISA	enzyme-linked immunosorbent assay
CBC	complete blood count		
C & S	culture and sensitivity	ED	emergency department
c/o	complains of	EDC	estimated date of confinement

(continued)

COMMONLY USED CLINICAL ABBREVIATIONS *(Continued)*

Abbreviation	Definition	Abbreviation	Definition
EMG	electromyogram	L & D	labor and delivery
ENT	ear, nose, throat	LA	lymphadenopathy
EOMI	extraocular movements intact	LCTA	lungs clear to auscultation
ESR	erythrocyte sedimentation rate	LD	learning disabled
		LDL	low density lipid
ETOH	ethyl alcohol	LH	luteinizing hormone
FB	foreign body	LLQ	left lower quadrant
FBS	fasting blood sugar	LNMP	last normal menstrual period
FEV1	forced expiratory volume in 1 second	LOC	loss of consciousness
		LUQ	left upper quadrant
FH	family history	LVH	left ventricular hypertrophy
FROM	full range of motion	Lymph	lymphocytes
FSH	follicle-stimulating hormone	mammo	mammogram
FTT	failure to thrive	MCH	mean corpuscular hemoglobin
FVC	forced vital capacity	MCHC	mean corpuscular hemoglobin concentration
FX	fracture		
GAS	general anxiety syndrome	MCL	midclavicular line
GBS	group B streptococcus	MCP	metacarpal phalanx
GC	gonococcus	MCV	mean corpuscular volume
GERD	gastroesophageal reflux disease	MDI	multi-dose inhaler
		MGF	maternal grandfather
GGT	gamma-glutamyl transpeptidase	MGM	maternal grandmother
GI	gastrointestinal	MI	myocardial infarction
GPA	gravida para abortions	ML	midline
Gtt	drop	MMR	measles, mumps, rubella
GU	genitourinary	Monos	monocytes
Gyn	gynecological	MRG	murmur, rub, gallop
H/A	headache	MS	multiple sclerosis
HCG	human chorionic gonadotropin	MSG	monosodium glutamate
HCT	hematocrit	MTP	metatarsal phalanx
HCTZ	hydrochlorothiazide	MVA	motor vehicle accident
HDL	high density lipid	MVI	multi-vitamin
HEENT	head, ears, eyes, nose, throat	N/V	nausea and vomiting
Hep B	hepatitis B vaccine	NAD	no acute distress
Hgb	hemoglobin	neuro	neurologic
Hib	hemophilus B influenza	NIDDM	non–insulin dependent diabetes mellitus
HIV	human immunodeficiency virus		
HJR	hepatojugular reflex	NKA	no known allergies
HPV	human papilloma virus	NKDA	no known drug allergies
HR	heart rate	NSAIDs	nonsteroidal anti-inflammatory drugs
HRT	hormone replacement therapy		
HS	hour of sleep	NSR	normal sinus rhythm
HSM	hepatosplenomegaly	NVD	nausea/vomiting/diarrhea
Ht	height	NVD	neck vein distention
HTN	hypertension	OA	osteoarthritis
HZ	herpes zoster	OBG	obstetrical/gynecological
IADL	independent ADL	OC	oral contraceptives
IBD	irritable bowel disease	OCP	oral contraceptive pills
IBS	irritable bowel syndrome	OD	right eye
IPV	intermuscular polio vaccine	ODD	oppositional defiant disorder
IVDA	IV drug abuser	OM	otitis media
JVD	jugular vein distention	OPV	oral polio vaccine

(continued)

COMMONLY USED CLINICAL ABBREVIATIONS *(Continued)*

Abbreviation	Definition	Abbreviation	Definition
OS	left eye	RDW	red (cell) distribution width
OTC	over the counter	RLQ	right lower quadrant
OU	both eyes	ROM	range of motion
PCN	penicillin	ROS	review of systems
PE	physical examination	RR	respiration rate
PEFR	peak expiratory flow rate	RRR	regular rhythm, rate
PERRL	pupils equal round reactive to light	RTC	return to clinic
		RUQ	right upper quadrant
PERRLA	pupils equal round reactive light and accommodation	S/P	status post
		SEG	segmented neutrophils
PFT	pulmonary function test	SEM	systolic ejection murmur
PGF	paternal grandfather	SLR	straight leg raise
PGM	paternal grandmother	SOB	shortness of breath
PID	pelvic inflammatory disease	SPF	sun protection factor
PIP	proximal interphalangeal	STD	sexually transmitted disease
PMI	point of maximal impulse	T	temperature
PND	paroxysmal nocturnal dyspnea	T&A	tonsillectomy and adenoidectomy
PPD	purified protein derivative		
PRN	as needed	TID	three times a day
PSA	prostate specific antigen	TM	tympanic membrane
PTT	partial thromboplastin time	trich	trichomoniasis
PUD	peptic ulcer disease	TSH	thryroid-stimulating hormone
QD	every day	U/A	urinalysis
QID	four times a day	UGI	upper gastrointestinal
QOD	every other day	URI	upper respiratory infection
QS	quantity sufficient	UTI	urinary tract infection
R	respirations	VA	visual acuity
RA	right arm	VS	vital signs
RAM	rapid alternating movements	WBC	white blood cell (count)
RBC	red blood cell (count)	w/o	without
RCM	right costal margin	WNL	within normal limits
RDA	recommended daily allowance	Wt	weight
		y/o	years old

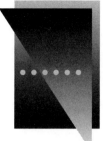

Index